Psychology, Pain and Anaesthesia

Edited by

H. B. Gibson

*Honorary Research Fellow,
formerly Head of Psychology,
University of Hertfordshire,
Hatfield
UK*

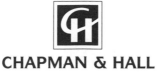

CHAPMAN & HALL

London · Glasgow · New York · Tokyo · Melbourne · Madras

Published by Chapman & Hall, 2–6 Boundary Row, London SE1 8HN

Chapman & Hall, 2–6 Boundary Row, London SE1 8HN, UK

Blackie Academic & Professional, Wester Cleddens Road, Bishopbriggs, Glasgow G64 2NZ, UK

Chapman & Hall Inc., One Penn Plaza, 41st Floor, New York 10119, USA

Chapman & Hall Japan, Thomson Publishing Japan, Hirakawacho Nemoto Building, 6F, 1–7–11 Hirakawa-cho, Chiyoda-ku, Tokyo 102, Japan

Chapman & Hall Australia, Thomas Nelson Australia, 102 Dodds Street, South Melbourne, Victoria 3205, Australia

Chapman & Hall India, R. Seshadri, 32 Second Main Road, CIT East, Madras 600 035, India

Distributed in the USA and Canada by Singular Publishing Group Inc., 4284 41st Street, San Diego, California 92105

First edition 1994

© 1994 Chapman & Hall

Typeset in Palatino 10/12pt by Intype, London

Printed in Great Britain by the Alden Press, Oxford

ISBN 0 412 33650 2   1 56593 129 7 (USA)

A catalogue record for this book is available from the British Library

Library of Congress Cataloging-in-Publication data available

∞ Printed on permanent acid-free text paper, manufactured in accordance with ANSI/NISO Z 39.48–1992 and ANSI Z 39.48–1984

Contents

Contributors

P. A. Alden BA (Hons) Psychology Consultancy, Grimsby General Hospital, South Humberside, UK

John I. Alexander FRCA Consultant in Anaesthesia and Pain Management to the United Bristol Hospitals and Clinical Lecturer in the University of Bristol, Sir Humphry Davy Department of Anaesthesia, Bristol Royal Infirmary, Bristol, UK

Robert I. Block PhD Department of Anaesthesia, College of Medicine, University of Iowa, Iowa City, Iowa, USA

C. Kerry Booker BA, MSC MPhil Principal Clinical Psychologist, Department of Behavioural Medicine, Hope Hospital, Salford and Psychological Specialist in Pain Management, The Manchester and Salford Back Pain Centre, Ladywell Hospital, Salford, UK

Keith Budd FRCA Consultant in Anaesthesia and Pain Management, The Royal Infirmary, Bradford, UK

Laurel Archer Copp PhD Doctor of Humane Letters, Fellow of the Institute of Arts and Humanities, Fellow of the American Academy of Nursing, University of North Carolina, Chapel Hill, North Carolina, USA

Freda V. Gardner PhD Clinical Psychologist, Pain Relief Clinic, Bristol Royal Infirmary and University Department of Cardiac Surgery, Bristol, UK

M. M. Ghoneim MD Department of Anaesthesia, College of Medicine, University of Iowa, Iowa City, Iowa, USA

Hamilton B. Gibson PhD Department of Psychology, University of Hertfordshire, UK

Anne K. Goddard MSC District Clinical Psychologist, Psychology Department, Swindon Health Authority, Swindon, UK

Barry B. Hart PhD Department of Clinical Psychology, Community Health Unit, Scunthorpe General Hospital, South Humberside, UK

Steven P. Mewaldt PhD Departments of Psychology and Pharmacology, Marshall University, Huntington, West Virginia, USA

Michael O'Connor FRCA Consultant Anaesthetist, The Pain Clinic, Princess Margaret Hospital, Swindon, UK.

A. G. Oswald BSC, MB, ChB, MRCPsych Consultant Psychiatrist, Royal Cornhill Hospital, Aberdeen, UK

Pam Price SRN Clinical Nurse Specialist in Pain Management, The Royal Infirmary, Bradford, UK

Peter Salmon DPhil Department of Clinical Psychology, University of Liverpool, Liverpool, UK.

Karen H. Simpson MB, FRCA Consultant Anaesthetist and Senior Clinical Lecturer, St James's University Hospital, Leeds, UK

Frank J. Vingoe PhD Consultant Clinical Psychologist, Department of Clinical Psychology, University Hospital of Wales, Cardiff, UK

CHAPTER 1

Prevention and management of postoperative pain

John I. Alexander and Freda V. Gardner

1.1 INTRODUCTION

The prevention and management of postoperative pain are undergoing rapid and radical change. The working parties of the Australian Health Service (Atkinson *et al.*, 1988), of the Royal Colleges of Surgeons of England and Anaesthetists (1990) and of the Agency for Health Care Policy and Research of the United States of America (Jacox and Carr, 1991) have reported that the monitoring and treatment of pain after surgery are inadequate. They made recommendations to correct this inadequacy, improve training, increase resources for postoperative pain control and establish 'acute pain teams' in all major hospitals.

Stimulated both by these reports and by previous example, the challenge of acute pain has been taken up in many hospitals. Worldwide, since 1987, 'the growth of acute pain services, acute pain research, and the education in this field has been extraordinary' (Cousins, 1992). The improvements already made in regional and systemic analgesia have engendered enthusiastic co-operation in those involved in postoperative care. Actions are taken before and during the operation to reduce the incidence of persistent pain. There is also a change in medical and surgical practice and some major surgical procedures are being replaced by pharmacotherapy or by minimally invasive techniques.

Better managed analgesia usually requires less nursing time and reduces the time spent by the patient in hospital after operation. This can release resources to continue and improve the provision of analgesia. The tolerant acceptance of unrelieved pain by the patient (Owen, McMillan and Rogowski, 1990) and by the staff is disappearing (Semple and Jackson, 1991).

1.2 NATURE OF POSTOPERATIVE PAIN

Postoperative pain may be the result of the operative trauma and of the changed condition of the patient as a result of the procedure. Pain may arise from distension, spasm or traction, from infection, inflammation and ischaemia of tissues. Pain caused by provocation or exacerbation of other conditions can present in the postoperative period. Prolonged immobilization and relaxation of joints can cause persistent pain. Pain and nerve damage may be caused by supporting harness, by unguarded movement and by any compressive dressing.

Pain may arise from continuing noxious stimulation or from non-noxious stimuli in the presence of hyperalgesia. In the hyperalgesic state, pain is perceived with greater severity, for longer and over a wider area than normal. It may result from local factors such as inflammatory swelling, release of algogenic substances, of neural processing, changes in second messengers and induction of proto-oncogenes (Bond, Charlton and Woolf, 1991). This state is opposed by the inhibition of nociceptive activity at the spinal level by descending controls from the brain stem (Le Bars *et al.*, 1986), which may be the result of the acute noxious stimulus itself or during periods of extreme excitement or repetitive stress (Willer, Dehen and Cambier, 1981). Increased thresholds to electrically induced sensation (increased inhibition) (Lund, Hansen and Kehlet, 1990) and decreased thresholds to pain (Dahl *et al.*, 1992b) coexist in the postsurgical state.

1.3 PSYCHOLOGICAL ASPECTS OF ACUTE PAIN

Both the physiological and the psychological components of postoperative pain determine the magnitude of the experience. Similar trauma can engender very different responses in patients and pain relief may be unnecessary for some patients and impossible to achieve in others. The central processing of acute pain is influenced by the psychological state. Hospitalization and surgery frequently engender anxiety and distress which alter the patients' expression of pain, their demand for analgesia and their postoperative complications.

The interpretation of a sensation of pain depends on context as well as intensity. A patient observing a scalpel enter locally anaesthetized skin may interpret the sensation incorrectly, based on expectation. When a patient is anxious or psychologically distressed, the pain threshold and tolerance are decreased and the threshold approaches the level of tolerance.

The psychological factors associated with the experience of acute pain are now widely recognized and psychological interventions that reduce pain in surgical and dental contexts are becoming used increasingly for both adult and paediatric patients (Wilson *et al.*, 1982).

1.3.1 Acute pain in paediatrics

The normal response of a healthy infant to a painful stimulus involves a non-purposive movement of all limbs often accompanied by grimacing or crying. Crying is a process that involves higher level nervous system function. More painful stimuli generate louder and more distressed cries from an infant with non-vocal signs of agitation and distress. These responses may be due to a lack of differentiation of the mechanisms for expression or to the locus of the stimulus not being identified (Booker and Nightingale, 1985). Grunau, Johnston and Craig (1990) found that invasive procedures were associated with cry responses which were distinctive in pitch and intensity, a stress-specific facial expression in combination with a short latency of onset of cry and a long duration of the first cry cycle.

Rudimentary forms of affective development exist very early in infancy (Stern, 1985) and infants are less sensitive to painful stimuli when they are being cuddled. In neonatal intensive care units, parents are being encouraged to touch and hold their pre-term infants in an attempt to reduce the infants' distress and anxiety and to facilitate the development of the association between human contact and non-painful stimuli.

With older children invasive procedures frequently cause fear and anxiety which may compound the child's perception of pain and many children who have repeated painful procedures develop conditioned generalized anxiety in situations that become associated with acute pain. As with adults, intervention takes account of the interaction of behavioural, cognitive–affective and physiological responses. Overt behavioural pain responses refer to observable behaviours such as crying, screaming and physical resistance. Cognitive–affective, or covert, responses refer to the child's perceptions, imagery and thoughts during invasive procedures.

Varni (1983) described two forms of psychological interventions for the management of paediatric pain:

- Pain behaviour regulation methods, such as contingency management, which identify and modify socio-environmental factors which may influence the expression of pain;
- Pain perception regulation methods which alter the child's perception of pain through self-regulatory processes such as hypnosis, guided imagery, meditation, relaxation and biofeedback.

Pain perception regulation, or cognitive intervention, is more commonly used for the management of acute pain in children whereas the behavioural form of intervention is more frequently used in the treatment of chronic pain. Psychological interventions aim to reduce or minimize anxiety, thereby also reducing the experience of pain.

Most interventions designed for children have used a combination of techniques which use the child's capacity for fantasy and imagery following progressive relaxation or hypnotic induction (Fielding, 1985). These commonly include preparation, hypnosis, behavioural and cognitive therapy.

Preparation of a child for hospitalization or for surgery has been shown to be effective in reducing pre- and postoperative distress and postoperative pain (Melamed and Siegel, 1975). 'Preparation' is a generic term which includes such interventions as hospital tours, modelling in play or video films. It provides children with information about the operation, encourages emotional expression and attempts to establish a trusting relationship with hospital staff. The child is also able to see that there are positive aspects to a children's ward such as a wide range of toys and other children with whom to play.

Pre-operative instruction is the most frequently used method of preparation for children. It helps the child to understand the reason for procedures and corrects misconceptions. Preparatory information is either sensory or procedural. Sensory information provides details of sensations the child will experience during the procedure, such as being aware of smells and movement. Procedural information describes each of the steps of the procedure so that the child will be aware of what will happen. A combination of procedural and sensory preparation has been found to be the most effective (Anderson and Masur, 1983).

Puppet therapy (Cassell, 1965) and play therapy (Dimock, 1960) have been used to enable younger children to act out or to express their fears vicariously while providing information about medical procedures. Filmed modelling is effective (Peterson and Mori, 1988). Children who were shown a peer model film relating to hospitalization showed less anxiety-related behaviour and had fewer medical concerns before and after surgery (Melamed and Siegel, 1975). A combination of coping techniques (deep muscle relaxation, imagery distraction and self instruction) and filmed modelling is more effective than coping techniques or modelling alone (Peterson and Shigetomi, 1981).

Modelling may be contraindicated in some of the more experienced children such as those who require frequent invasive procedures (Melamed and Siegel, 1980; Melamed, Dearborn and Hermecz, 1983). Faust and Melamed (1984) found that these children may be sensitized by viewing modelling preparation and that their levels of distress may increase. A relationship exists between optimal timing of preparation and age (Dimock, 1960). Older children benefit from a longer time interval between preparation and surgery, while younger children benefit from preparation closer to surgery.

Much of the research in preparing children for surgery has been focused on minor surgery such as tonsillectomy and there is a need to develop this research in paediatric areas where children are undergoing more complex and life-threatening surgery such as open-heart surgery and renal transplanation. In these circumstances, the complications of chronic ill health, severe parental and child anxiety, and higher expected and actual levels of post-operative pain create greater difficulty for the patients and their parents. They are also a greater challenge for the various forms of psychological intervention.

1.3.2 Acute pain in adults

Adult surgical patients are often anxious about the diagnosis, the findings and outcome of the operation, the possibility of death and disability, about awareness during paralysis and about postoperative pain and distress (Norris and Baird, 1967). Patients may also be anxious about hospitalization, the stress of the unfamiliar environment, and about those left at home. Separation from partners is stressful as is isolation and inadequate information. These all have an effect on a patient's experience of pain. It has been found that there is a linear relationship between anticipatory anxiety and anxiety related specifically to the event (Scott, Clum and Peoples, 1983). Patients who are more anxious before surgery are more distressed postoperatively and the intensity of reporting of postoperative pain is related to state (context-based) rather than to trait (personality-based) anxiety (Johnson, 1980). Some patients are able to control the debilitating effects of anxiety by, for example, refusing to think of the potential dangers of the operative experience. When confronted with pain, however, some patients may have difficulty in maintaining denial and Janis (1958) found that patients with extremely low levels of pre-operative anxiety had high levels of emotional distress postoperatively.

Patients who have had surgery may feel vulnerable, helpless and out of control. An aversive experience may cause distress as a result of several different forms of loss of control, including behavioural and cognitive control (Thompson, 1981). Many forms of psychological intervention for postoperative patients attempt to return behavioural and cognitive control to the patient and to augment their own resources. Simple and practical interventions are used widely. Patients are given information and reassurance about the surgical procedure and consequences. They are shown around the ward by nursing staff, introduced to other patients and given information about visiting arrangements and ward routine. Information and reassurance has been shown to reduce the patient's anxiety and make it more manageable (Egbert *et al.*, 1964). Distraction and imagery also help (Reading, 1979).

The manipulation of attention is very useful. Levine and Gordon

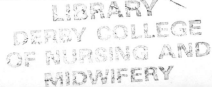

(1982) found that the degree of postoperative pain varied with the amount of attention paid to the injury. Pickett and Clum (1982) used altered attention in the form of imagery of pleasant situations to distract patients from general concerns about surgery. This was effective in reducing postoperative anxiety, but not postoperative pain.

Behavioural techniques such as relaxation, slow controlled breathing and self-hypnosis also have a significant effect on postoperative pain (Wells, 1982). The separation of cognitive and behavioural methods of psychological management, however, is often arbitrary and most frequently, in practice, a combination of both methods would be used.

1.4 MONITORING OF PAIN

Pain should be monitored to prevent moderate and severe pain, to audit the prevalence and severity of pain, and to improve techniques of surgery and of pain relief.

The severity of pain can be assessed by the patient and expressed in words, pictures, numbers or distance along a line. Subjective reporting is not always reliable. The ability to interpret, assess and to co-ordinate movements necessary in recording visual analogue scores may be impaired in the early postoperative period. Subjective reporting by patients under-reports the presence of considerable pain (Wilder-Smith and Schuler, 1992) and the assessment of pain by an observer is usually less than that of the subject. Pain may be present at more than one site. The sensory, emotional and temporal character, and reactivity, of the pain may be as important as the severity in determining the cause and treatment of the pain, This can be recorded on the full or short form of the McGill Pain Questionaire (Melzack, 1987).

The presence and severity of pain may be inferred by clinical signs and changes in behaviour but, although rises in pulse rate and blood pressure, pallor, rigidity, groaning, crying, may indicate pain, they may occur for other reasons. After thoracic and abdominal operations, the pain is associated with muscle spasm. Oesophageal and transpulmonary pressure rise, functional residual capacities fall and airway closure increases. All these variables can be measured and may be assumed to be related to the severity of the pain or stimulus.

Pain relief (rather than pain) can be assessed after analgesic measures: the relief being expressed as a proportion of the pre-existing pain. Pain and pain relief can also be inferred by the quantity of standard analgesic drug required to alleviate the pain. Patient controlled intravenous analgesia fulfils the two demands of pain monitoring: a numerical measurement of the pain perceived and immediate pain relief.

In most cases, the severity and, if relevant, the site and character of pain should be recorded on the chart which records other vital signs –

so that adjustments of analgesia or re-assessments of pain can be made frequently. Other details may be necessary if the pain is of unusual character or resistant to treatment.

1.5   CONSEQUENCES OF POSTOPERATIVE PAIN

Pain is associated with a stress response by the patient and with an attempt to avoid further pain. These may be a mechanism for survival but are themselves causes of morbidity. Relative immobility avoids distraction of the wound and diversion of a large part of the cardiac output to active muscles; the inability to gain access to food and water is offset by the responses of catabolism of body tissues and salt and water retention (Bond, Charlton and Woolf, 1991).

The breakdown of proteins to simpler peptides provides a source of energy and flexible constructional material. Glucose availability is increased by the changes in insulin, glucagon, cortisol and adrenaline. The uptake of insulin by the cell and the plasma insulin response to a glucose load are reduced. The secretion of insulin is inhibited by raised levels of adrenaline. The levels of adrenaline are raised by pre- and postoperative anxiety, by nociception and other stressors even during anaesthesia. Adrenaline increases glucose production transiently, but also decreases glucose utilization. The plasma cortisol concentrations are raised following the start of surgery and the rise in concentration is related to the severity or extent of the trauma. The plasma levels remain raised during the first postoperative week following major trauma. The level of glucagon is raised postoperatively, at least in part because of a raised level of cortisol. Glucagon increases glucose production and increases peripheral utilization. The combined effect is protein breakdown and hyperglycaemia. This increases endogenous substrates for energy requirements but leads to muscle wasting, weakness and net loss of nitrogen and glucose.

Fluid balance is controlled by renal blood flow, fluid intake, the antidiuretic hormone and aldosterone. Reduction of renal blood flow is inhibited by the secretion of prostaglandin. Renin secretion, which increases aldosterone levels, may rise during surgery and anaesthesia. Antidiuretic hormone (ADH) acts on the distal tubule of the nephron and the collecting ducts to increase their premeability to water, with a resultant decrease in the volume of the urine. The level of ADH rapidly rises in response to haemorrhage, pyrexia, emotional distress or pain and to changes in levels of adrenergic amines, probably through the baroreceptor mechanism.

The sympathetic response to pain causes a rise in blood pressure and pulse rate, renal and peripheral vasoconstriction and hyperglycaemia. The cardiac contractility, irritability, output and work are increased

(Reiz *et al.*, 1982) and cardiac reserves of output and oxygenation may be exceeded.

However, not all the stress responses are related to pain. The rise in acute phase proteins and changes in white blood cells are related to the severity of surgery and tissue damage and to the rise in cytokines which promote the development of a prolonged stress response (Hall and Desborough, 1992).

Pain avoidance behaviour may lead to postoperative morbidity. Prolonged immobility can lead to pressure sores and ulceration, renal stasis and stone formation, deep vein thrombosis and pulmonary embolus, muscle weakness and loss of postural stability. Pain of the thorax and abdomen can lead to the avoidance of truncal movement, deep breathing and coughing. This in turn leads to a fall in the resting lung volume, increased airway closure and hypoxaemia, a tendency to pulmonary collapse, retention of secretions and pulmonary infection.

1.6   CHANGES IN MEDICAL AND SURGICAL PRACTICE

Histamine–2 antagonists and proton pump inhibitors have replaced vagotomy and gastric drainage as the management of choice for peptic ulceration. The long-term costs and relapse rates are similar and the mortality is less (Sontag, 1988). Many traumatic operations have been replaced by endoscopy, ultrasound, radio-imaging and minimally-invasive surgery. Stones of the biliary or renal tract may be redissolved by pharmacotherapy or be broken into excretable pieces by percussive ultrasonic lithotripsy. Some surgical procedures such as drainage of cysts and abscesses can be performed radiologically. Endoscopy is being found increasingly useful in many forms of thoracic, abdominal, pelvic, vascular and joint surgery (Zucker, Bailey and Reddick, 1991). Some hysterectomies are being superseded by transcervical resection of endometrium. The advantages are many. The reduction in tissue damage, pain and in the use of analgesic drugs and techniques results in shorter hospital stay, reduced convalescence and an earlier return to normal activity (Mealy *et al.*, 1992).

1.7   THE RISK: BENEFIT BALANCE OF ANALGESIA

In any system of analgesia, the benefit to the patient in improved pain relief, greater freedom of movement, decreased morbidity and more rapid recovery must outweigh the dangers of the technique and the risks of unwanted side-effects. The balance can be shifted towards analgesia and safety by increases in monitoring and intervention.

After almost any operation, there is a proportion of patients whose

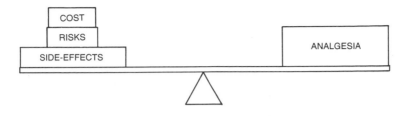

Fig. 1.1 The analgesic balance.

pain is tolerable and who are content without any form of pain relief. Others require analgesics for a short time, on predictable occasions (physiotherapy etc.) or on few, if unpredictable, occasions. For these, there is no justification for the risks and side-effects of uninterrupted analgesic medication. Conversely, others have severe pain which requires sequential medication. This may have to be applied regionally, be adjusted frequently by patient controlled analgesia devices or, when given continuously, be associated with support of vital functions. The more aggressive is the attempt to relieve pain, the greater must be the monitoring to prevent and control life-threatening events. The use of apnoea alarms, pulse oximeters and the placement of patients at risk within sight of the nursing station reduce the incidence of uncorrected complications.

1.8 METHODS AVAILABLE FOR THE RELIEF OF PAIN

In general, postoperative pain is usually relieved by:

- treatment of a reversible cause of the pain. Treatment can limit or reverse damage from pressure or ischaemia, infection, tumour, etc.;
- increasing the ability of the patient to suppress or inhibit the perception of pain: the ability to 'cope' with pain, as described above;
- systematic analgesia;
- regional anaesthesia
  - to the wound
  - to nerve trunks serving the operated area
  - intrapleurally
  - spinally;
- Regionally applied analgesics: These are usually applied as a single dose to the subarachnoid space or as repeated doses or as a constant or variable infusion, to the epidural space. Opioids are most commonly used, but local anaesthetics or alpha–2 adrenergic agonists may be added to the opioid solution;
- stimulation analgesia.

1.8.1 Pre-emptive analgesia

Experimental evidence suggests that if the pain of injury is prevented by opioids or local anaesthetics, less processing occurs within the spinal cord, impulse generation is less and the total pain experience is reduced (Wall, 1988). However, while one group of researchers (Katz *et al.*, 1992) have found that the totality of postoperative pain is less if local anaesthetics and opioids are given before the pain is experienced rather than to treat established pain, other workers (Dierking, Dahl and Kanstrup, 1992; Dahl *et al.*, 1992a) have found no such benefit.

1.8.2 Systemic analgesia

The most convenient method of analgesia is to apply to the whole body a drug which has a relatively large effect on the perception of pain and a relatively small effect on other systems. With few exceptions, the drugs used to provide analgesia postoperatively are either an opioid or a prostaglandin synthase inhibitor.

(a) Opioids

Opioids are powerful analgesics, acting on the spinal cord and brain and, probably, in higher concentration, at peripheral receptors (Stein *et al.*, 1991). They can be administered by almost any route. Some are rapid in onset when given intravenously, such that the dose of analgesic can be titrated against the severity of pain. Most are strong mu opioid agonists and are capable of relieving all acute pain. All these can cause depression of ventilation, nausea and vomiting, delay in gastric emptying and micturition, and tolerance. Some cause euphoria. The partial mu agonists in clinical use also cause ventilatory depression equivalent to their analgetic effect, but, with use and tolerance, this effect and that of psychic dependence become less. They are therefore less liable to abuse. Some are antagonists at the mu opioid receptor and agonists at the kappa receptor (e.g. pentazocine, nalbuphine). Kappa receptor activation is not capable of achieving the same degree of analgesia for all kinds of pain (e.g. thermal) at any dosage and are less widely applicable. Opioids, given pre-, intra- or postoperatively remain the mainstay of analgesia for moderate or severe postoperative pain, although the requirements may be reduced by other analgesic methods.

(b) Prostaglandin synthase inhibitors

These are also known as the cyclo-oxygenase inhibitors, the endoperoxidase inhibitors, or the non-steroidal anti-flammatory drugs (NSAID). Prostaglandins increase the algogenic effect of bradykinin and histamine and increase leucocyte motility. Paracetamol inhibits brain cyclo-oxy-genase, but has little, if any, anti-inflammatory activity. The peri-operative use of non-steroidal anti-inflammatory drugs has been reviewed recently by Dahl and Kehlet (1991). There is still concern that the side-effects may increase morbidity and affect surgical outcome, yet NSAID, alone or in combination with opioids, can improve pain relief without disadvantage in most cases. For dental and minor orthopaedic pain, the NSAID are at least as effective as low doses of opioids. For moderate and more severe pain, NSAID reduce the need for opioids in most patients and the combination of NSAID and opioid may be more effective than similar doses of either, used alone. In renal colic, NSAID may be more effective than pethidine.

The analgesic properties of NSAID can be partially dissociated from their anti-flammatory effects (McCormack and Brune 1991). Ketorolac, a potent prostaglandin synthase inhibitor, is 500–800 times more potent than aspirin in relieving the pain of pressure or flexion of an inflamed limb, but only 2–3 times more potent than naproxen in prevention of inflammation (Rooks, 1990).

The limiting side-effects are those related to the bronchial and intesti-nal tract, the process of haemostasis, and the kidney. Some NSAID may cause leukotriene-induced bronchoconstriction. The erosive effects on the stomach are less common in the limited duration of therapy of the perioperative period. Increased bowel permeability and diaphrag-matic disease of the bowel are uncommon side-effects of NSAID, usually after prolonged therapy. Bleeding time is prolonged after all NSAID, even after low doses, but a clinically significant increase in operative blood loss has not been shown to occur. NSAID may cause sodium and potassium retention and a significant fall in renal plasma flow especially when renal function is already deficient or when renal blood flow is protected by prostaglandin release as in the presence of cardiac failure, shock or during rapidly developing hypovolaemia (Harris, 1992). Monitoring of postoperative micturition is always advis-able.

NSAID are especially useful for day-case surgery, because they have minimal effects on the sensorium, bladder or vomiting centre.

(c) Administration of systemic analgesia

In the early postoperative period, orally administered drugs may be unreliably absorbed and analgesics are commonly given by another route. Opioids and NSAID can be given intravenously, intramuscularly or rectally. Some opioids can be given by any route. Intravenous anal-gesics are fastest in onset, have the greatest peak effects and the shortest duration. (NSAID, however, are delayed in onset because of their mech-anism of action and the intravenous route probably has little advantage in this respect.) Drugs by other routes are, in general, slower in onset, less in maximal effect but longer in duration. Transdermal fentanyl, for example, has a latency of onset of peak action of 15 hours and an apparent half-life of 21 hours, even after removal of the transdermal patch (Holley and Van Steenis, 1988). It is therefore more suitable for prevention of pain or the maintenance of basal analgesic levels than for treatment of established pain.

The analgetic level of a drug can be found by titration before the patient is returned to the ward and half that required dose, given every half-life of that drug, will re-establish analgesia. This prescription reflects the inter-patient variability of plasma analgesic concentration but not the variability with time, activity, nor metabolic/excretion rates. The tendency to administer more than the optimal requirement for analgesia and to prolong the interval between doses leads to periods of both overdosage and pain. The optimal level can also be maintained by a continuous infusion. However, the requirements for analgesia vary from time to time depending upon activity and usually decline with healing.

Unless the pain is continuous, pain is most often treated as it occurs and as the pain tolerance of the patient is exceeded. The administration can be requested by the patient and administered by the nurse, usually by the oral or intramuscular route. This entails delay in making contact, in dispensing and in absorption. The patient can be offered pain relief at regular intervals to reduce the pain before the pain tolerance is exceeded and this is rarely more expensive of nursing time. In High Dependency Units, severe pain can be pre-empted more frequently and opioids can be administered intravenously, thereby reducing the delay during absorption.

Analgesia can be administered by the patient. At home, those in pain administer their own analgesics and rarely exceed the recommended dose or frequency. In hospital, the ability to self-administer is usually removed. Patient analgesic administration is effective, is responsive to the needs of the patient and restores to the patient the sense of control which may reduce the need for analgesia.

(d) *Patient-controlled analgesia*

The most successful, but not the only, method is by patient-controlled intravenous opioids. Bioavailability is maximal and latency of onset is short. The patient should be rendered pain-free before patient control is instituted. The dose of drug delivered at each demand is pre-set. Each delivery is followed by a pre-set lock-out interval during which further demands are unrewarded. This allows the analgesic to have an effect before another dose delivery is made. In some devices, the total amount delivered over a period, say, of four hours can be predetermined. If the drug is delivered through a dedicated intravenous cannula and used only occasionally, free flow should be maintained by flushing with saline. The drug can be delivered into an existent intravenous infusion line. In such, the 'dead space' between the entry of the drug delivery line and the vein must be small and a valve must be inserted to ensure that the drug is not introduced, retrogradely, up the infusion line. The reservoir should be placed at or below the level of the patient to prevent siphoning of the drug solution into the patient.

The size of the bolus dose and lock-out interval affect the patient's perception of efficacy. Too small a bolus dose results in a lack of perceived effect and loss of confidence. If the bolus dose is too large, side-effects such as nausea occur and lead to a failure of acceptance by patients and staff. If the lock-out interval is too long, the patient has little sense of control over the pain; if too short, repeated drug delivery is made while the plasma and brain levels are rising and lead to cumulation beyond the optimal effect. The feed-back to the patient of the knowledge of which demands are successful and which are within the lock-out period increases the acceptance of the method (Owen *et al.*, 1986) but does not decrease the frequency of demand (Johnson and Luscombe, 1992).

A background infusion is sometimes used to prevent the brain concentration of the drug falling below analgetic levels during periods of reduced demand. However, even when a significant proportion of the expected demanded dose is infused constantly, the number of demands is not reduced and the total amount administered is increased (Owen, Kluger and Plummer, 1990). The chosen analgesic drug should be capable of achieving noticeably greater effect with increasing dose. It should have a relatively rapid response and sufficient duration of effect to allow titration of drug against severe pain. Many drugs have been used by this method, but the most satisfactory have been the full opioid agonists. Alfentanil has the fastest onset of action of the opioids in clinical practice but the short duration of action necessitates frequent drug demands to prevent pain. Morphine, with a 1 mg bolus and a lock-out interval of 5 minutes, appears now to be the most usual regimen.

The principal disadvantage of this technique is the associated high incidence of nausea and vomiting (Semple *et al.*, 1992) and the dangers are those of the occasional incidences of programming errors and equipment malfunction. The danger of ventilatory depression and arterial desaturation is probably no greater than that of intermittent intramuscular opioids (Wheatley *et al.*, 1990).

1.8.3 Local anaesthesia

Local anaesthetic blockade can prevent pain both at rest and on movement. Large and bilateral wounds may require application in multiple sites, in large volume or to be centrally placed. Visceral anaesthesia generally requires blockade of the visceral afferent plexuses or of the spinal cord. Used alone, prolonged local anaesthesia must be maintained by repeated injection percutaneously or by repeated bolus or infusion through indwelling cannulae.

Local anaesthesia also reduces function and protective mechanisms. Sympathetic blockade leads to vasodilatation, sometimes to hypotension and cooling. Systemic toxicity is related to the identity, amount and rate of absorption of the local anaesthetic agent. Local or regional neurotoxicity is seen as a result of intraneural or intra-arterial injection, or of continuous infusion of local anaesthetic in high concentration. Other complications arise from the introduction of infection or damage to adjacent structures.

The site of local anaesthetic blockade is also a balance of benefit and risk. Application of local anaesthetic to the operative wound before closure is simple to perform and causes little local damage or loss of function. Cannulae can be laid in the wound to allow maintenance of the local anaesthetic block for long periods. It is sufficient after operations on the skin and cutaneously innervated structures such as the breast and helps in the pain management of other deeper operations. Local anaesthesia by rectus sheath cannulation has been shown to be effective for upper midline abdominal surgery (Watson *et al.*, 1991) and by intercostal or paravertebral cannulation for both upper abdominal and thoracic surgery (Hashimi, Stewart and Ah-fat, 1991; Sabanathan *et al.*, 1988; Sabanathan *et al.*, 1990). Cannulation of the perivascular sheath surrounding the brachial plexus can achieve intermittent or continuous analgesia of the arm and relieve vascular insufficiency (Audenaert, Vickers and Burgess, 1991). Topical anaesthesia can produce long-lasting postoperative pain relief after operations on the skin and mucous membranes. Parietal and visceral pain relief can be achieved by local anaesthesia applied in the subarachnoid, epidural and interpleural spaces.

(a) Interpleural anaesthesia

Local anasethetic injected into the interpleural space spreads throughout the space and diffuses easily through the pleura to the intercostal nerves and to the visceral afferents. It can also block the lower part of the brachial plexus, the vagus or the phrenic nerves. Bilateral interpleural block risks bilateral pneumothoraces and paralysis of the muscles of ventilation. Unilateral block is rarely sufficient for operative procedures but may relieve postoperative pain without the lability of heart rate and blood pressure associated with subarachnoid or epidural anaesthesia.

Relatively large amounts of local anaesthetic are required (Strømskag *et al.*, 1988). Higher concentrations give a longer duration of block and higher volumes give a wider spread of analgesia. The addition of adrenaline reduces the relatively high peak plasma concentration (Kambam *et al.*, 1989) which is maximal after 15 to 20 minutes, and is not as toxic as the same level achieved in a shorter time (Wood, 1986). For unilateral incisional pain after cholecystectomy and renal operations, it has been found to be more effective than intercostal blocks (Blake, Donnan and Novella, 1989) and similar both in efficacy and in reducing ventilatory function to epidural local anaesthesia (Scott *et al.*, 1989). The analgesia may be relatively short after thoracotomy (Scheinin Lindgren and Rosenberg, 1989), and, in general, the use of this technique is not increasing at the rate expected of a significantly superior method of analgesia.

(b) Spinal anaesthesia

Spinal – subarachnoid or epidural – local anaesthesia blocks both somatic and sympathetic, afferent and efferent nerves. While unilateral block can sometimes be achieved, it cannot be achieved reliably, and some loss of proprioceptive and motor function is inevitable. Spinal anaesthesia can achieve total anaesthesia of a segment of the body and be sufficient for operation and postoperative pain relief, but with associated loss of sensory, motor and reflex activity which may be unacceptable. Vasodilatation resulting from sympathetic blockade may cause heat loss and hypotension, especially in response to volume depletion or venous pooling. Nevertheless, anaesthesia of even large incisions of the body wall can usually be achieved without respiratory embarrassment or uncorrected hypotension.

Profound regional anaesthesia is more readily achievable with subarachnoid block. The risk of low pressure headaches has been reduced by the introduction of smaller, Whitacre or Sprotte needles. Cannulation through atraumatic fine spinal needles is also possible, but associated with (small) spinal fluid leakage and with a toxic cauda equina syndrome when 5% lignocaine with adrenaline is used (Rigler *et al.*, 1991). Local anaesthesia in the postoperative period is thus usually still maintained by cannulation of the epidural space. The site of placement of the epidural cannula is critical in reducing the required volumes of local anaesthetic and systemic toxicity.

(c) Spinal analgesia

In many patients with major thoracic or abdominal postoperative pain, regional anaesthesia and systemic analgesia are either insufficient for postoperative comfort or associated with unacceptable hypotension or loss of function. The spinal application of opioids has been reviewed many times during its development (e.g. Cousins and Mather 1984,

Morgan, 1989). It can achieve powerful regional analgesia without these side-effects, but it may be associated with sudden and severe respiratory depression even after an interval of several hours from administration. Epidurally-applied opioids are absorbed mainly into the bloodstream from the spinal canal, but that part which diffuses into the spinal cord causes profound regional analgesia. Distribution of a drug is determined by lipid solubility. The rate of distribution is determined by lipid solubility and dissociation constants. Intradurally, morphine, which is relatively hydrophilic, is distributed predominantly in the cerebrospinal fluid (csf). Here, it can act as depot of analgesic to prolong the duration of action of epidural or subarachnoid morphine. The drug in the csf may reach the brain slowly by diffusion, or suddenly by mass movement, and cause itching, somnolence, and depression of breathing. Opioids depress ventilation by reduction of sensitivity to carbon dioxide, reduction of the hypoxic drive and by causing disorder in the rhythmicity of the ventilatory pattern. Hypercarbia can cause somnolence, airway occlusion and sudden ventilatory arrest. Morphine within the spinal cord is distributed preferentially to the non-lipid parts of the cord such as the synapses which are the site of action. Highly lipid soluble opioids such as fentanyl, given systemically, are distributed preferentially to the richly-perfused lipid tissues of the body such as the brain and spinal cord and the advantage of injection directly into the spinal canal is less than for morphine. From the epidural space, they diffuse more easily into the epidural veins, but that part which diffuses into the csf is distributed predominantly to the spinal cord. Less drug is in the mobile phase of the csf, able to move suddenly rostrally. Rostral spread is still possible within the substance of the cord. Lipid-soluble undissociated drugs also pass more easily from the cord substance into the veins of the cord. However, even fentanyl has been shown to be more potent and more long-lasting when given by the spinal route rather than systemically.

Diamorphine may have the advantages of both lipophilicity and hydrophilicity. It is two hundred times more lipid soluble than morphine and it is less dissociated at body temperature so that it is absorbed more completely and more rapidly into the spinal cord than morphine (Stevens and Wooton, 1988). The intermediate analgesic metabolite of diamorphine – 6-acetyl morphine – also crosses membranes more readily than would be expected from its polar properties (Shelly and Park, 1991). Morphine and its metabolites are metabolized to morphine within the spinal cord (Way, Young and Kemp, 1965), distributed to the non-lipid sites and is subject to the same delay in release from neural tissue as is morphine. By infusion, it may be the most ideal opioid for intraspinal use.

Delayed, sudden cessation of ventilation is also more probable if the opioid is given as a bolus rather than as a slow infusion (Chrubasik *et al.*, 1984), if it is dissolved in a large volume of solvent, if it is administered into the cervical or thoracic spine or if it is given intrathecally rather than epidurally (Rawal *et al.*, 1987). The ventilatory rate, rhythm and the level of consciousness should be monitored (see above). The risks of the procedure have to be measured against the risk of ventilatory arrest from an intravenous or intramuscular bolus of opioid and against the benefit of effective analgesia (Yeager *et al.*, 1987). Other side-effects which occur more commonly than after systemic administration are urinary retention and pruritus (Rawal *et al.*, 1987). Pruritus can be severe, especially after intrathecal morphine, relieved by naloxone and partly relieved by antihistamines in high dose.

Opioids applied intrathecally are more potent, last longer, have fewer systemic effects but, because they are more potent and are given as a bolus, the incidence of respiratory arrest and other side-effects is greater. Monitoring the ventilation by apnoea detectors and pulse oximetry, and the use of high dependency areas, reduce this risk.

Opioids have been combined with other drugs in the spinal space. The combination of local anaesthetic with opioid appears to enhance the analgesic effect and duration of both agents. (Hjortsø *et al.*, 1986; Jones *et al.*, 1989), but it introduces the additional risk of gradual or sudden hypotension. Similarly, epidural clonidine has been shown to enhance the analgesia of epidural opioids, allowing the reduction of the dose of opioid and the incidence of ventilatory depression, but again at the increased risk of hypotension (Vercauteren *et al.*, 1990).

(d) Postoperative stimulation analgesia

Acupuncture and electroacupuncture can produce effective postoperative analgesia but the response may be inconsistent (Leong and Chernow, 1988) and, in variance to the response in chronic pain, short-lived (Christiansen *et al.*, 1989). Similarly, postoperative transcutaneous nerve stimulation (TENS) has a very variable analgesic response. Some investigators (e.g. Rooney, Jain and Goldiner, 1983) showed a significant reduction in opioid requirement during TENS, whereas others (e.g. McCallum *et al.*, 1988) found any benefit to be minimal and insignificant.

The benefits are uncertain and less than can be achieved by other methods. Where resources are limited, acupuncture and TENS may be best reserved for those unsuitable or unresponsive to more conventional treatment.

1.8.4   Acute pain teams

The acute pain team (Ready *et al.*, 1988) can bring expertise to interventionist pain management, supervise and change management, change cannula sites or drugs depending upon individual response, explain and reassure, and diagnose incision-unrelated pain. It provides a source of reference and help for continuous management and consultation for postoperative pain management problems (e.g. in cases of myasthenia, narcotic abuse, etc.) before they occur. The team will educate other staff involved in pain management and provide decision trees or algorithms for treatment of inadequate pain relief or side-effects.

1.8.5 Specific problems

(a) Postoperative pain in very young children

The widespread belief, until recently, that the infant's nervous system was insufficiently developed to feel pain in the same way as older children and adults led to signs of distress being overlooked. The problem of assessment of pain in children has been reviewed (McGrath, 1987; 1990) and pain management has become more interventional and more carefully monitored (Lloyd-Thomas, 1990). Opioids tend to cause more ventilatory depression in the neonate and the premature. The metabolism and excretion of drugs are more variable but usually more prolonged. In the ventilated patient, intravenous infusions of opioids are effective and relatively safe. In the spontaneously breathing neonate, opioids, when indicated, should be used in conjunction with monitoring such as apnoea alarms or pulse oximetry. The need for opioids in neonates and older children can be diminished by the use of local anaesthesia applied regionally or spinally. The development of the 24 G epidural catheter and small Tuohy needles has helped the wider adoption of continuous epidural anaesthesia for paediatric pain. Hypotension appears to be less prevalent than in adult practice. The caudal epidural block is easiest to perform and is effective for most sacral and lower abdominal surgery. The catheter can even be threaded from the caudal to the thoracic epidural space in small children for use after thoracic and upper abdominal surgery. Paracetamol and, in most cases, NSAID such as ibuprofen can be used as a sole analgesic or to reduce the need for opioids. Patient-controlled intravenous or subcutaneous analgesia has been used successfully in children as young as four years old. Injections, themselves, can be regarded as aversive by children and analgesia in this form may be refused. If intermittent parenteral analgesia is required in children, a cannula should be inserted in the appropriate site before recovery of consciousness.

(b) Pain after laparoscopy

Despite the small incisions and lesser damage to the parietes and viscera, the anaesthetic required for laparoscopy may be as great as for laparotomy (Joris *et al.*, 1992) and the amount of postoperative pain varies widely. This pain does not decline with time in a simple manner but may increase several hours after surgery, often in association with mobilization (Dobbs *et al.*, 1987). It has at least three probable causes: the skin and muscle incisions, visceral damage and traction of the supporting mesentery. The pain of visceral damage is shown by the large difference in pain between laparoscopic sterilization by Falope rings and sterilization with Hulka clips (Dobbs *et al.*, 1987). Falope rings cause ischaemia and death of a large section of the fallopian tube whereas the Hulka clip compresses only the width of the clip. Application of local anaesthetic to the mesosalpinx (Alexander, Wetchler and Thompson, 1987) or to the mesosalpinx and rectus sheath (Smith *et al.*, 1991) can modify the pain following Falope (Yoon) ring sterilization but not that of the lesser pain of Hulka clip sterilization (Cook and Lambert, 1986).

The pain which arises or persists after several hours, and which is often referred to the costal margin or shoulder tip, is unaffected by this local anaesthetic application. Its incidence and severity can be reduced by the insertion of a tube to allow egress of gas during closure of the laparoscopy ports (Alexander and Hull, 1987). The cause of this pain is not certain but the nerve supply of the shoulder tip is shared by part of the diaphragm and by the falciform and coronary ligaments of the liver. When gas is introduced into the peritoneum and cohesion of the two layers of peritoneum surrounding the liver is lost, these ligaments of peritoneum are subject to greater traction.

1.9 CONCLUSION

Although the search continues for drugs and techniques which can produce analgesia without the side-effects which presently limit effective analgesia, much can be achieved with that which is available. Postoperative pain should be a consideration throughout the operative process – in the decision to operate, in the choice of procedure and incision, in the use of pre-emptive and local anaesthetic techniques and in evaluating the effect of pain and pain relief on the medical condition of the patient. Greater use should be made of the psychological techniques available and control of pain relief should be returned to the patient where possible. Pain severity and relief should be monitored and recorded. Aggressive techniques should be considered for severe pain and accompanied by reliable monitoring. Analgesia should be individualized for the patient, the cause of pain and the level of optimal activity. Postoperative pain relief should be made the responsibility of one or more designated clinicians who will educate and lead other members of the staff caring for the patient.

REFERENCES

Alexander, J. I. and Hull, M. G. R. (1987) Abdominal pain after laparoscopy: the value of a gas drain. *British Journal of Obstetrics and Gynaecology*, **94**, 267–9.

Alexander, C. D., Wetchler, B. V. and Thompson, R. E. (1987) Bupivacaine infiltration of the mesosalpinx in ambulatory surgical laparoscopic tubal sterilisation. *Canadian Anaesthetists' Society Journal*, **34** 362–5.

Anderson, K. O. and Masur, F. T. (1983) Psychological preparation for invasive medical and dental procedures. *Journal of Behavioural Medicine*, **6** (1), 1–37.

Atkinson, L., Bogduk, N., Cousins, M. J. *et al.* (1988) *Management of Severe Pain*, Australian Government Publishing Service, Canberra, Australia.

Audenaert, S. M., Vickers, H. and Burgess, R. C. (1991) Axillary block for vascular insufficiency after repair of radial club hands in an infant. *Anesthesiology*, **74**, 368–70.

Blake, D. W., Donnan, G. and Novella, J. (1989) Interpleural administration of bupivacaine after cholecystectomy: a comparison with intercostal nerve block. *Anaesthesia and Intensive Care*, **17**, 269–74.

Bond, M. R., Charlton, J. E. and Woolf, C. J. (eds) (1991) Proceedings of the VIth World Congress on Pain, Elsevier Science Publishers, Amsterdam.

Booker, P. D. and Nightingale, D. A. (1985) Postoperative analgesia for children. In *The Management of Post-operative Pain in Children*. (ed. M. E. Dodson) Edward Arnold, London, pp. 141–56.

Cassell, S. (1965) Effects of brief puppet therapy upon the emotional responses of children undergoing cardiac catheterization. *Journal of Consulting and Clinical Psychology*, **29**, 1–8.

Christiansen, P. A., Noreng, A., Andersen, P. E. *et al.* (1989) Electroacupuncture and postoperative pain. *British Journal of Anaesthesia*, **62**, 258–62.

Chrubasik, J., Scholler, K. L., Wiemers, K., *et al.* (1984) Low dose infusion of morphine prevents respiratory depression. *Lancet*, **i**, 793.

Cook, P. T. and Lambert, T. F. (1986): An investigation of the effectiveness of bupivacaine applied to the abdominal wall and fallopian tubes in reducing pain after laparoscopic tubal ligation. *Anaesthesia and Intensive Care*, **14**, 148–51.

Cousins, M. J. and Mather, L. E. (1984) Intrathecal and epidural administration of opioids. *Anesthesiology*, **61**, 276–310.

Cousins, M. J. (1992) Foreword in *The Management of Acute Pain: a Practical Guide* (eds L. B. Ready and W. T. Edwards,) IASP Publications, Seattle, p.v.

Dahl, J. B. and Kehlet, H. (1991) Non-steroidal anti-inflammatory drugs: rationale for use in postoperative pain. *British Journal of Anaesthesia*, **66**, 703–12.

Dahl, J. B., Hansen, B. L., Hjortsø, N. C. *et al.* (1992a) Influence of timing on the effect of continuous extradural analgesia with bupivacaine and morphine after major abdominal surgery. *British Journal of Anaesthesia*, **69**, 4–8.

Dahl, J. B., Erichsen, C. J., Fuglsang-Frederiksen, A. *et al.*, (1992b) Pain sensation and nociceptive reflex excitability in surgical patients and human volunteers. *British Journal of Anaesthesia*, **69**, 117–21.

Dierking, G. W., Dahl, J. B. and Kanstrup, J. (1992) Effect of pre- vs postoperative inguinal field block on postoperative pain after herniorrhaphy. *British Journal of Anaesthesia*, **68**, 344–8.

Dimock, H. G. (1960) *The Child in the Hospital: A Study of his Emotional and Social Well-being*, Davis, Philadelphia.

Dobbs, F. F., Kumar, V., Alexander, J. I. *et al.* (1987) Pain after laparoscopy related to posture and ring-versus-clip sterilization. *British Journal of Obstetrics and Gynaecology*, **94**, 262–6.

Egbert, L. D., Battit, G. E., Welch, C. E. and Bartlet, M. K. (1964) Reduction of postoperative pain by encouragement and instruction of patients. *New England Journal of Medicine*, **270**, 825–7.

Faust, J. and Melamed, G. (1984) Influence of arousal, previous experience and age on surgery preparation of same day of surgery and in-hospital pediatric patients. *Journal of Consulting and Clinical Psychology*, **52**, 359–65.

Fielding, D. (1985) Chronic illness in children. In *New Developments in Clinical Psychology*. (ed. F Watts), British Psychological Society, Wiley, Leicester.

Grunau, R. V. E., Johnston, C. C. and Craig, K. D. (1990) Neonatal facial and cry responses to invasive and non-invasive procedures. *Pain*, **42**, 295–305.

Hall, G. M. and Desborough, J. P. (1992) Interleukin-6 and the metabolic response to surgery. *British Journal of Anaesthesia*, **69**, 337–8.

Harris, K. (1992) The role of prostaglandis in the control of renal function. *British Journal of Anaesthesia*, **69**, 233–5.

Hashimi, H., Stewart, A. L. and Ah-fat, G. (1991) Continuous intercostal nerve block for postoperative analgesia after surgical treatment of the upper part of the abdomen. *Surgery, Gynecology and Obstetrics*, **173**, 116–18.

Hjortsø, N. C., Lund, C., Morgensen, T. *et al.* (1986) Epidural morphine improves pain relief and maintains sensory analgesia during continuous epidural bupivacaine after abdominal surgery. *Anaesthesia and Analgesia*, **65**, 1033–6.

Holley, F. O. and Van Steenis, C. (1988) Postoperative analgesia with fentanyl: Pharmacokinetics and pharmacodynamics of constant rate IV and transdermal delivery. *British Journal of Anaesthesia*, **60**, 608–13.

Jacox, A. and Carr, D. B. (1991) *Clinical Practice Guideline for Acute Pain Management: Operative or Medical Procedures and Trauma* (DHHS publication Number (AHCPR) 91–0046), Agency for Health Care Policy and Research, Rockville, Maryland.

Janis, I. L. (1958) *Psychological Stress*, Wiley, New York.

Johnson, D. W. (1980) Attitude modification methods. In *Helping People Change*. (2nd ed) (eds F. H. Kanfer and A. P. Goldstein), Pergamon, Oxford.

Johnson, T. W. and Luscombe, F. E. (1992) Patient-controlled analgesia – assessment of machine feedback to patients. *Anaesthesia*, **47**, 899–901.

Jones, G., Paul, D. L., Elton, R. A. *et al.* (1989) Comparison of bupivacaine and bupivacaine with fentanyl in continuous extradural analgesia during labour. *British Journal of Anaesthesia*, **63**, 254–9.

Joris, J., Cigarini, I., Legrand, M. *et al* (1992) Metabolic and respiratory changes after cholecystectomy performed via laparotomy or laparoscopy. *British Journal of Anaesthesia*, **69**, 341–5.

Kambam, J. R., Hammon, J. Parris, W. C. *et al.* (1989) Intrapleural analgesia for post-thoracotomy pain and blood levels of bupivacaine following intrapleural injection. *Canadian Anaesthestists' Society Journal*, **36**, 106–9.

Katz, J., Kavanagh, B. P., Sandler, A. N. *et al.* (1992) Preemptive analgesia. Clinical evidence of neuroplasticity contributing to postoperative pain. *Anesthesiology*, **77**, (3) 439–46.

Le Bars, D., Dickenson, A. H., Besson, J. M. *et al.* (1986) Aspects of sensory processing through convergent neurons. In *Spinal Afferent Processing*, (ed T. L. Yaksh), Plenum Press, New York, pp. 467–504.

Leong, R. J. and Chernow, B. (1988) The effects of acupuncture on operative pain and the hormonal response to stress. *International Anesthesiology Clinics*, **26** (3), 213–17.

Levine, J. D. and Gordon, N. C. (1982) Pain in prelingual children and its evaluation by pain induced vocalization *Pain*, **14**, 85–93.

Lloyd-Thomas, A. R. (1990) Pain management in paediatric patients. *British Journal of Anaesthesia*, **64**, 85–104.

Lund, C., Hansen, O. B. and Kehlet, H. (1990) Effect of surgery on sensory threshold and somatosensory evoked potentials after skin stimulation. *British Journal of Anaesthesia*, **65**, 173–6.

McCallum, M. I. D., Glynn, C. J., Moore, R. A. *et al.* (1988) Transcutaneous electrical nerve stimulation in the management of acute postoperative pain. *British Journal of Anaesthesia*, **61**, 308–12.

McCormack, K. and Brune, K. (1991) Dissociation between the antinociceptive and anti-inflammatory effects of the non-steroidal anti-inflammatory drugs: a survey of their analgesic efficacy. *Drugs*, **41**, 533–47.

McGrath, P. A. (1987) An assessment of children's pain: a review of behavioral, physiological and direct scaling techniques. *Pain*, **31**, 147–76.

McGrath, P. J. (1990) Paediatric pain: a good start. *Pain*, **41**, 253–4.

Mealy, K., Gallagher, H., Barry, M. *et al.* (1992) Physiological and metabolic responses to open and laparoscopic cholecystectomy. *British Journal of Surgery*, **79**, 1061–4.

Melamed, B. G. and Siegel, L. G. (1975) Reduction of anxiety in children facing hospitalization and surgery by use of filmed modeling. *Journal of Consulting and Clinical Psychology*, **43**, 511–21.

Melamed, B. G. and Siegel, L. G. (1980) *Behavioural Medicine: Practical Applications in Health Care*, Springer, New York.

Melamed, B. G., Dearborn, M., and Hermecz, D. A. (1983) Necessary considerations for surgery preparation: Age and previous experience. *Psychosomatic Medicine*, **45**, 517–25.

Melzack, R. (1987) The short-form McGill Pain Questionnaire. *Pain*, **30**, 191–7.

Morgan, M. (1989) The rational use of intrathecal and extradural opioids. *British Journal of Anaesthesia*, **63**, 165–88.

Norris, W. and Baird, W. L. M., (1967) Pre-operative anxiety: a study of its incidence and aetiology. *British Journal of Anaesthesia*, **39**, 503–9.

Owen, H., Glavin, R. J., Reekie, R. M. *et al.* (1986) Patient-controlled analgesia. Experience of two new machines. *Anaesthesia*, **41**, 1230–5.

Owen, H., Kluger M. T. and Plummer, J. L. (1990) Variables of patient-controlled analgesia. 4: the relevance of bolus size to supplement a background infusion. *Anaesthesia*, **45**, 619–22.

Owen, H., McMillan, V. and Rogowski, D. (1990) Postoperative pain therapy: a survey of patients' expectations and their experiences. *Pain*, **41**, 303–7.

Peterson, L. J. and Mori, L. (1988) Preparation for hospitalization. In *Handbook of Pediatric Psychology*, (ed D. K. Routh), Guilford Press. New York, pp. 460–91.

Peterson, L. and Shigetomi, C. (1981) The use of coping techniques to minimize anxiety in hospitalized children. *Behaviour Therapy*, **12**, 1–14.

Pickett, C. and Clum, G. A. (1982) Comparative treatment strategies and their interaction with locus of control in the reduction of post-surgical pain and anxiety. *Journal of Consulting and Clinical Psychology*, **50**, 439–41.

Rawal, N., Arner, S., Gustafsson, L. L. *et al.* (1987) Present state of extradural and intrathecal opioid analgesia in Sweden. A nationwide follow-up survey. *British Journal of Anaesthesia*, **59**, 791–9.

Ready, B. L., Oden, R., Chadwick, H. S. *et al.* (1988) Development of an anesthesiology-based postoperative pain management service. *Anesthesiology*, **68**, 100–6.

Reading, A. E. (1979) The short-term effects of psychological preparations for surgery. *Social Science and Medicine,* **ISA,** 641–54.

Reiz, S., Balfors, E., Sorensen, M. *et al.* (1982) Coronary hemodynamic effects of general anesthesia and surgery. Modification by epidural analgesia in patients with ischemic heart disease. *Regional Anesthesia,* **7,** S8–18.

Rigler, M. L., Drasner, K., Krejce, T. C. *et al.* (1991) Cauda equina syndrome after continuous spinal anesthesia. *Anesthesia and Analgesia,* **72,** 275–81.

Rooks, W. H. (1990) The pharmacologic activity of ketorolac tromethamine. *Pharmacotherapy,* **10,** 30S–32S.

Rooney, S. M., Jain, S. and Goldiner, P. L. (1983) Effect of transcutaneous nerve stimulation on postoperative pain after thoracotomy. *Anesthesia and Analgesia,* **62,** 1010–12.

Royal College of Surgeons (1990) Pain after Surgery. *Report of the Working Party of the Commission on the Provision of Surgical Services of The Royal College of Surgeons of England and The College of Anaesthetists.*

Sabanathan, S. Hashimi, H., Bickford-Smith, P. *et al.* (1988) Continuous intercostal nerve block for pain relief after thoracotomy. *Annals of Thoracic Surgery,* **46,** 425–6.

Sabanathan, S., Mearns, A. J., Bickford-Smith, P. J. *et al.* (1990) Efficacy of continuous extrapleural intercostal nerve block in post-thoracotomy pain and pulmonary mechanics. *British Journal of Surgery,* **77,** 221–5.

Scheinin, B., Lindgren, L. and Rosenberg, P. H. (1989) Treatment of post-thoracotomy pain with intermittent instillation of intrapleural bupivacaine. *Acta Anaesthesiologica Scandinavica,* **33,** 156–9.

Scott, L. E., Clum, G. A., Peoples, J. B. (1983) Preoperative predictors of postoperative pain. *Pain,* **15,** 283–93.

Scott, N. B., Mogensen, T., Bigler, D. *et al.* (1989) Comparison of the effects of continuous intrapleural vs epidural administration of 0.5% bupivacaine on pain, metabolic response and pulmonary function following cholecystectomy. *Acta Anaesthesiologica Scandinavica,* **33,** 535–9.

Semple, P. and Jackson, I. J. (1991) Postoperative pain control. A survey of current practice. *Anaesthesia,* **46,** 1074–6.

Semple, P., Madej, T. H., Wheatley, R. G. *et al.* (1992) Transdermal hyoscine with patient-controlled analgesia. *Anaesthesia,* **47,** 399–401.

Shelly, M. P. and Park, G. R. (1991) Speed of onset of analgesia of diamorphine or morphine. *British Journal of Anaesthesia,* **67,** 666–7.

Smith, B. E., MacPherson, G. H., de Jonge, M. *et al.* (1991) Rectus sheath and mesosalpinx block for laparoscopic sterilization. *Anaesthesia,* **46,** 875–7.

Sontag, S. J. (1988) Current status of maintenance therapy in peptic ulcer disease. *American Journal of Gastroenterology,* **83,** 607–17.

Stein, C., Comisei, K., Haimeri, E. *et al.* (1991) Analgesic effect of intra articular morphine after arthroscopic knee surgery. *New England Journal of Medicine,* **325,** 1123–6.

Stern, D. N. (1985) *The Interpersonal World of the Infant.* Basic Books, New York.

Stevens, L. A. and Wooton, C. M. (1988) The pharmacokinetic properties of diamorphine, in *Diamorphine: Its Chemistry, Pharmacology and Clinical Use,* (ed D. B. Scott.) Woodhead Faulkner, Cambridge.

Strømskag, K. E., Reiestad, F., Holmqvist, E. L. O. *et al.* (1988) Intraplural administration of 0.25%, 0.375% and 0.5% bupivacaine with epinephrine after cholecystectomy. *Anesthesia and Analgesia,* **67,** 430–4.

Thompson, S. C., (1981) Will it hurt less if I can control it? A complex answer to a simple question. *Psychological Bulletin,* **90,** 89–101.

Varni, J. W. (1983) *Clinical Behavioural Paediatrics,* Pergamon, New York.

Vercauteren, M., Lauwers, E., Meert, T. *et al.* (1990): Comparison of epidural sufentanil plus clonidine with sufentanil alone for postoperative pain relief. *Anaesthesia*, **45**, 531–4.

Wall, P. D. (1988) The prevention of postoperative pain. *Pain*, **33**, 289–90

Watson, D., Farquhar, I. K., Dennison, A. R. *et al*. (1991) Postoperative analgesia by infusion of local anaesthetic into the rectus sheath. *British Journal of Anaesthesia*, **67**, 656P.

Way, E. L., Young, J. M. and Kemp, J. W. (1965) Metabolism of heroin and its pharmacological inplications. *Bulletin of Narcotics*, **17**, 25–33.

Wells, N. (1982) The effect of relaxation on post-operative muscle tension and pain. *Nursing Research*, **31**, 236–8.

Wheatley, R. G., Somerville, I. D., Sapsford, D. J. *et al*. (1990): Postoperative hypoxaemia: comparison of extradural, i.m. and patient-controlled opioid analgesia. *British Journal of Anaesthesia*, **64**, 267–75.

Wilder-Smith, C. H. and Schuler, L. (1992) Postoperative analgesia: pain by choice? The influence of patient attitudes and patient education. *Pain*, **50**, 257–62.

Willer, J. C., Dehen, H., and Cambier, J. (1981) Stress-induced analgesia in humans; endogenous opioids and naloxone – reversible depression of pain reflexes. *Science*, **212**, 689–91.

Wilson, J. F., Moore, R. W., Randolph, S. and Hanson, B. J. (1982) Behavioural preparation of patients for gastrointestinal endoscopy: information, relaxation and coping style. *Journal of Human Stress*, **8**, 13–23.

Wood, N. (1986) Plasma drug binding: implications for anesthesiologists. *Anesthesia and Analgesia*, **65**, 786–804.

Yeager, M. P., Glass, D. D., Neff, R. K. *et al*. (1987) Epidural anesthesia and analgesia in high-risk surgical patients. *Anesthesiology*, **66**, 729–36.

Zucker, K. A., Bailey, R. W., Reddick, E. J. (eds) (1991) *Surgical Laparoscopy*, Quality Medical Publishing inc., St. Louis, Missouri.

CHAPTER 2

Rehabilitation of the chronic pain patient

C. Kerry Booker

2.1 INTRODUCTION

The development of chronic pain and incapacity in the absence of progressive disease or neuropathy, is a complex and poorly understood process. Nevertheless, it has important implications for the decision to treat, and the timing and efficacy of intensive (and expensive) rehabilitation. The aim of the present chapter is to explore the issues pertinent to the selection, assessment and treatment of patients with Chronic Intractable Benign Pain (CIBP), in intensive interdisciplinary rehabilitation and Pain Management Programmes (PMPs). The issues raised and techniques discussed can, however, with little modification be employed with other chronic pain conditions, in group or individual therapy.

2.2 THE DEVELOPMENT OF CIBP

Nachemson (1982) estimated that 90% of cases of acute back pain injuries will remit naturally within an average of four weeks, or 12 weeks at the latest. The remaining 10% of cases consume 80% of the costs of chronic care. Given that soft and bony tissue healing is adjudged to be complete within three months post-injury, the International Association for Pain (Classification of Chronic Pain, 1986) have used this period to mark the transition to chronicity.

Chronic Intractible Benign Pain (CIBP) is one symptom amongst a constellation of other symptoms. Essentially therefore, it is but one component of a syndrome and not a disease. The primary distinguishing feature of the CIPB syndrome (Pinsky and Crue, 1984) is that of an on-going pain problem that cannot at the time of presentation be causally connected with any active patho-physiological or patho-anatomic

process. A history of generally ineffective medical and surgical interventions unfolds as the pain generalizes from the original site, and this
takes place against a background of disturbed psychosocial functioning.
The patient's dissatisfaction with health-care professionals and the
health-care system can culminate in conflict and hostility with each
failed treatment, and each failed communication. Burdened by the con-
viction and fear that increasing pain signifies bodily harm and tissue
damage, the individual becomes increasingly inactive in an attempt to
avoid activities which are thought of as 'dangerous'. Further passive
attempts to control pain by escalating the amount of drugs consumed, is
not only ineffective but counterproductive, as the pain relief habituates
leaving CNS disturbance, lability of mood and feelings of worthlessness
and helplessness. Eventually as illness behaviour fails to elicit a benevol-
ent response, the scene is set for interpersonal conflict with family and
friends, psychosocial withdrawal from sources of interpersonal and
environmental gratification, and the prospect of profound demoralization, or sometimes clinical depression. By this stage individuals have
become divested of most of their social and occupational responsibilities, and have developed a demeanour of dependency and hostility.
In effect, they have become prisoners of pain.

In terms of physical status the inactive patient presents with a disuse
or deconditioning syndrome (Waddell, 1992). This is characterized by
a loss of muscle bulk, loss of muscle strength and endurance, loss of
cardiovascular fitness, demineralization of bone, inhibition of tissue
healing (musculo-ligamentous structures are large and have poor blood
supply), adhesions and deficits in joint lubrication, and a general feeling
of debility and malaise. Such organic sequelae can further aggravate
existing disturbances of biomechanical function in the lumbar spine
articulations produced by asymmetrical scar formation.

2.3   THE AETIOLOGICAL DEBATE

Recently, Philips and Grant (1991) having followed 117 patients with
acute back pain injury from onset to six months post-injury, have challenged the IASP designation of chronicity (more than three months).
Finding that 40% of their cohort fell within this category, they concluded:

*Of particular importance for the understanding of the evolution of chronic
pain is the evidence that, far from chronic pain evolving and growing, it
may be better perceived as a persistence of the acute presentation. By this
is meant the continuing presentation of pain as if it were an acute injury,
rather than the development of new types of behaviour or increases in
reaction. If this interpretation is correct, studies of the prevention of chronic*

pain problems would be wise to consider factors that retard the extinction of pain experience and emotions provoked by acute pain, rather than concentrate an exclusive interest on reinforcers that promote increases in reactivity and pain behaviour. (p. 441)

If these results are representative of the general population of acutely injured persons, then it would help to explain why many medical practitioners continue to treat chronic pain as if it were an acute condition. Alternatively, the physician may hold the view that medically unexplained pain is of psychological origin, and therefore requires psychological treatment, or simply that in any event there is no alternative treatment approach. Chronic patients also tend to attribute their pain to some unresolved or unidentified organic cause, or occasionally to recurrent injury. Such reductionist views ignore the complex genesis and maintenance processes involved, and lead patients and practitioners into a collusive relationship which reinforces the acute pain model of treatment.

Endeavours to explore the aetiology of chronic pain pose substantial methodological problems. Unfortunately, theories attempting to explain it are not well defined. One of the more plausible theories has been proposed by Turk and Flor (1984). Their 'diathesis/stress' model proposes that organismic predisposition (the diathesis) is a necessary, but not sufficient condition, for the development of a disorder which is likely to occur when there is a coexistent stress component. Another interesting biopsychosocial perspective is provided by Feuerstein *et al.* (1987). They propose a schema to highlight the major psychosocial and behavioural factors presumed to be associated with the development, exacerbation, and/or maintenance of CIBP. The major factors (and their components) are:

- predictors of accident/symptom onset (individual, system, pathophysiological);
- accidents or symptoms;
- reactions to accidents or symptoms at individual (behavioural, psychological, psychophysiological) and broader system (family, work environment) levels;
- psychobiological mechanisms (environmental/behavioural, cognitive/perceptual, and psychophysiological); and
- subsequent outcomes related to adjustment at work and/or recreation, family and social activities.

In their Fear-Avoidance Model of Exaggerated Pain Perception, Lethem *et al.* (1983) postulated a process by which the motivational-affective (pain perception) component of pain, and the consequent pain behaviour, can become out of synchrony with the sensory-discriminative (pain sensation) component of pain and its associated organic pathology. Two extremes of coping, **confrontation** or **avoidance** were viewed as being adaptive or maladaptive, respectively. Thus they hypo-thesized that an individual who confronts acute pain would tend to view it as a temporary nuisance, be strongly motivated to resume normal work and social responsibilities, and be prepared to challenge his or her personal pain tolerance during this recuperative phase. Con-fronters would continually recalibrate the synchrony between moti-vation-affective and sensory-discriminative information processing. The non-adaptive pain avoider, on the other hand, motivated by fear, avoids anticipated pain (cognitive avoidance) and painful activities (behavioural avoidance). Deconditioning is the physical consequence of this strategy. Exaggerated pain perception (desynchrony), resulting from a lack of exposure to disconfirming experiences, reduced behavioural repertoires and increased responsiveness to reinforcement of invalid status, constitutes the psychological consequences. The psychosocial context within which the original injury and its therapeutic management occurred is thought to be influenced by four major factors:

- stressful life events;
- personal pain history/memory;
- personal coping strategies;
- personality characteristics.

Taking a cognitive-behavioural perspective of avoidance behaviours and the maintenance of chronic pain behaviour, Philips (1987) attributes a more central role to individuals' beliefs about their ability to control pain, and expectations of pain increase prior to activation.

Unfortunately, discussion of the relative merits of the various theories pertinent to pain management is beyond the scope of this chapter. However, chronic pain patients demand and deserve a clear explanation of the mechanisms likely to govern their distress. It is incumbent upon the clinical psychologist to provide an honest appraisal of the basic mechanisms which integrate, within a systems or process model, the biological, psychological and social parameters of the chronic pain experience. A good working knowledge of pain neurophysiology and the Gate Control Model (Melzack and Wall, 1988; LaRocca, 1992) is also invaluable.

In addition to the chapters by O'Connor, and Budd (this volume), a useful insight into the role of the anaesthetist (Spanswick and Main, 1989), physiotherapist and occupational therapist (Mayer and Gatchel, 1988), has been carefully explained elsewhere. A succinct distillation of the multi-disciplinary management of chronic low back pain can be found in Nordin and Vischer (1992). Issues relating to the reliability of medical assessment of the chronic back pain patient have also been extensively explored (Waddell *et al.*, 1984; Waddell *et al.*, 1992). Finally, patients may find Parker and Main's (1990) self-help book friendly and very informative.

2.4 SELECTION AND ASSESSMENT

Central to the success of intensive inter-disciplinary PMPs is the disciplined approach to the selection of patients whose medical status and degree of disability leaves considerable scope for functional improvement. Perusal of the medical case notes is often the first filter in the selection process. A systematic and thorough evaluation of cognitive and behavioural response to chronic pain and the degree to which these are associated with distress and disability is also fundamental. Assessment techniques include standardized questionnaires, structured interviews with the patient and significant other, and direct observations by staff. Frequently, self-monitoring devices such as diaries are also useful to enable the gathering of subjective estimates of pain intensity, activity, mood and cognitions.

2.4.1 Selection criteria

In order to assist referral agents a set of inclusionary and exclusionary criteria must be decided upon. The provision of criteria such as those listed below may help to promote appropriate referral practices.

Objectives are to promote a greater understanding of chronic back pain, to increase fitness and mobility, and to teach stress management techniques with the aim of producing changes in lifestyle through rehabilitation.

(a) Inclusionary criteria

Behavioural – at least two of the following:

- magnified illness presentation;
- major interference, due to pain, of activities of daily living; (e.g. work, home duties, social life, hobbies and leisure pursuits);
- long periods resting or lying down during the day;
- over-activity/under-activity cycles;
- inappropriate consumption of analgesics or other medication.

Emotional – at least two of the following:

- major interference, due to pain, of personal relationships;
- maladaptive pain-related feelings of anger, hostility, or anxiety;
- negative outlook with low mood;
- disturbed sleep due to pain;

- other signs of maladaptive coping (e.g. dishevelled appearance).

(b)   Exclusionary criteria

- Patient has come to end of sensible medical intervention and PMP is seen as last resort.
- Further physical investigation/intervention is planned.
- Patient has major structural abnormalities.
- Patient has progressive rheumatological or neoplastic disease.
- Primary drug abuse.
- Patient requires immediate psychiatric intervention.
- Patient aged less than 18 or more than 65 years of age.
- Patient is not willing to accept rehabilitation approach.

Of course, one should not assume that all persons who meet the inclusionary criteria would benefit from an intensive pain management approach. Ultimately, in order to promote group cohesion and optimize successful outcome it is necessary to conduct an in-depth and structured psychological interview.

2.4.2   Structured psychological interview

The clinical interview is often viewed as the first stage of therapeutic intervention, providing the patients with the opportunity to articulate verbally the transition from acute onset to their present state of chronicity. By conducting a structured and systematic exploration of their medical and psychosocial history, the clinician helps patients to conceptualize the multidimensional nature of their pain and distress. The first difficulty however, is to engage patients in the assessment process. Not infrequently, patients will arrive with the expectation that the psychologist will try to persuade them that their pain is 'imaginary', or will attempt to determine whether or not they are malingering. It is important at the outset to dispel these misconceptions by reassuring them that their pain is 'real'. It is indicated that by its very nature chronic pain frequently leads to unwanted changes in lifestyle and interpersonal tensions. Moreover, it places strenuous demands on coping resources and abilities to tolerate pain. Once 'defused', an interview such as that outlined below can proceed.

(a)   History of pain and illness

- Onset of present episode (be rigorous about dates).
- Was onset sudden, traumatic or insidious?
- Previous episodes of pain and illness.

(b)   History of treatment and treatment outcome

- List all previous interventions.
- Perceived long/short-term efficacy.
- Change over time (i.e. static vs gradual improvement or decline).
- Evidence of previous commitments to rehabilitation.

(c)   Present pain experience

- Frequency, intensity, duration, location and quality of pain and other sensations.
- Alleviating and exacerbating factors.
- Impact of pain on mood and disability.

*(d)   History and current use of drugs and alcohol**

- Type and amount (good day vs. bad day).
- Drug-taking contingencies (i.e. pain, activity, superstition, time).
- Drug-effects (positive vs. negative, physical vs. cognitive).
- Beliefs about addiction and tolerance.

*(e)   Analysis of pain behaviour and lifestyle**

- Patient's routine domestic/work activities (cf. with premorbid activity).
- Co-habitant's routine domestic/work activities (cf. with premorbid activity).
- Views about any changes in role.
- Up-time vs. down-time.
- Verbal and non-verbal pain communications; co-habitant's response.
- Engagement in mastery/pleasure activities; co-habitant's response.
- Development of avoidance behaviours over time.
- Sleep habits: delayed onset, (no. of) early awakenings, pain or toilet reason, hypersomnia, day-time napping, effect on spouse, restorative vs. non-restorative.
- Social skills (e.g. assertive vs. non-assertive, submissive vs. manipulative).
- Impact of pain/mood on co-habitants.

(f)   Coping skills

- Describe behavioural coping response to pain increase.
- Reactive thoughts and feelings.
- Future expectations.

* Categories of information to address when interviewing co-habitants or significant others.

(g)   Causal attributions*

- Perceived cause of present pain and disability.
- Evidence of morbid health fears/preoccupations.
- Interpretation of previously conveyed medical information.

(h)   Current life stress*

- Conflicts with co-habitants, work associates, welfare-system.
- Impact of above on pain, disability, mood.
- Other psychological dysfunction – phobias, obsessions, pathological anger, suicidal ideation/intention.

(i)   Psychosocial history (establish accurate dates)

- Previous psychological dysfunction and treatment.
- As above for co-habitants and family of origin.
- Response to loss experiences – bereavement, divorce, desertion.
- Physical/sexual abuse or neglect.
- Incidents leading to post-traumatic distress.
- History of pain and illness in spouse and family of origin.

(j)   Occupational assessment and employment prospects

- Satisfaction with present/former job.
- Education and work experience.
- Transferrable skills.
- Motivation to return to work vs. disincentives.

(k)   Medico-legal issues

- Is claim contemplated or in progress (? settlement date).
- Perceived implications of functional improvements on litigation or welfare claims.
- Query response to (expected) settlement (e.g. sense of hostility).

(l)   Efficacy appraisal and commitment to engage in intensive rehabilitation programme

- Is the patient holding out for some other type of treatment or investigation?
- If no to the above, does he/she think programme would have beneficial or adverse effects on the condition?

*Categories of information to address when interviewing co-habitants or significant others.

- Is there willingness to comply with treatment regimen despite initially increased discomfort, medico-legal/welfare rights implications?
- Has he/she the ability to make all necessary logistical arrangements to enable full-time attendance?

2.4.3 Psychometric assessment

Comprehensive though the clinical interview may be, time constraints limit the amount of information which can be obtained. Therefore the use of standardized questionnaires covering topics such as pain beliefs and attitudes, personal control beliefs, coping strategies, cognitive distortion, psychological adjustment, lifestyle impact, disability and pain intensity and quality, is recommended. Several excellent books and research papers are available (Jensen *et al.*, 1991; Karoly and Jensen, 1987; Main and Waddell, 1991; Main *et al.*, 1992).

2.4.4 Introduction to cognitive-behavioural interventions

Cognitive-behaviour therapy is primarily a collaborative problem-solving approach. It seeks to teach the patient to recognize the association between sensation, thoughts, feelings, behaviours, environmental and social stimuli, and subsequently to alter maladaptive emotional and behavioural responses contingent upon the occurrence of such events. Although reconceptualization is the general goal of treatment, therapeutic gain would be limited were the approach merely didactic in nature. Involvement in the setting and completion of behavioural goals (e.g. visiting the library for 30 minutes) provides the opportunity for the monitoring of thoughts, feelings and physical reactions to activities and experiences from which the individual has gradually and progressively withdrawn. Participation in the pain management programme provides the opportunity to practise a great variety of functionally important tasks in an environment that allows accurate feedback on performance, and reinforcement contingent upon the completion of tasks. Engagement in this process fosters acceptance of personal responsibility for one's actions and reactions and fosters a sense of personal competence or self-efficacy (Bandura, 1977). A typical ninety minute session (Philips, 1988) involves a discussion of previous homework assignments, a short didactic presentation, demonstration and practice, and the setting of new homework tasks. The approach comprises both cognitive and behavioural techniques which are applied in parallel, each interfacing with the other. For the purpose of simplicity, however, the main components will be described separately.

2.4.5　Behavioural analysis

The use of behavioural modification techniques in chronic pain management stems from the need to increase the frequency of functional
behaviours, and decrease the frequency of dysfunctional behaviours.
The principles governing behavioural modification are as follows. When
a behaviour is closely followed in time by a positive consequence or
reinforcer (e.g. attention from a solicitous spouse) the behaviour which
elicits this **positive reinforcement** will increase in rate of future occurrence and acquire greater reinforcement-strength or value. Conversely,
when a behaviour is closely followed in time by a negative consequence,
the future occurrence of that behaviour will be less frequent, and in all
likelihood, will be replaced by behaviours designed to avoid the negative consequence. Successful escape is **negatively reinforcing**. The concept of **punishment** in behavioural terms, relates to the application of
an aversive consequence or the removal of a positive consequence; the
aim being to reduce the likelihood of the targeted behaviours being
emitted. In the latter case it is not uncommon however, to find that
the rate and intensity of the maladaptive behaviour increases initially.
Withdrawal of the punishing consequence at this juncture serves to
further strengthen the maladaptive behaviour. Behaviour which fails to
elicit either a positive or negative consequence, will reduce in frequency
or be eliminated altogether, a process known as **extinction**.

　　Fordyce (1976) has the distinction of demonstrating the systematic
application of these principles in chronic pain management. He posited
that individuals whose behaviour is inconsistent with the presumed
pathological status or is excessive, may function in an environment in
which (1) positive reinforcement of such pain behaviour operates; or,
(2) well behaviour is punished or not rewarded. Such behaviours are
called **operants** because they operate on the environment. Behavioural
responses which are presumed to be consistent with known pathology
and occur in a reflexive manner following noxious stimulation, are
called **respondents**.

　　The first distinction between respondent and operant learning, therefore, is that the former learned response occurs because of an ante-
cedent stimulus, whereas the latter occurs because of the expected
consequences. The second difference concerns the concept of **resistance
to extinction**. Respondent behaviours are unlikely to persist when the
noxious stimulus remits. Operant behaviours, on the other hand,
require only intermittent reinforcement in order to be maintained and
are thus more resistant to extinction. Lest we view the manifestation of
these processes in simple dichotomous terms, Fordyce (1990) cautions:

> It is important to recognize that these distinctions between 'respon-
> dent' and 'operant' pain are not mutually exclusive. In actuality,
> most chronic pain patients show a mixture of the two. It is almost

impossible for pain behaviours occurring mainly under operant control to be totally free of nociception and respondent pain behaviour, nor can it be assumed that chronic pain problems under essential control of continuing nociception are entirely free of operant pain behaviours. (p. 293)

In line with the principles outlined above a detailed and specific assessment of behaviours which occur too infrequently (e.g. walking, bending forward), too frequently (e.g. medication-taking, reclining), or that are absent should be undertaken. Maladaptive or undesirable behaviours which occur most frequently should be targets for change as these are the ones for which most reinforcement is obtained. Getting patients to complete a daily pain diary on a hourly basis for two weeks aids clinical decision-making. Relevant activities for monitoring are: sitting, standing, walking, reclining, pain intensity, and medication intake.

Clinicians may find that it is difficult to structure the information gathered during a brief interview and behavioural observation. The profiles set out in Table 2.1 may help to enhance the probability of correctly attributing responses to either operant or respondent processes. The profiles are based on the author's clinical experience and the insights of Fordyce (1976, 1990) but have yet to be empirically substantiated. Chris Main, in a personal communication discussing work in progress, urges caution when interpreting interview data.

2.4.6 Contingency management

The most appropriate and expedient way to modify behaviour is to employ **incompatible responses**. That is, it is easier to accomplish an increase in a target behaviour than it is to decrease it. For example, because the body strives biomechanically for economy of motion, such behaviours as gait distortions, limping, and a giving-way of the leg can be remedied by speed-walking quotas. Fordyce (1990) recommended gradual approximations from baseline to an optimal 20–26 seconds per 50 metres for females, and 20–24 seconds per 50 metres for males. Consistent failure to meet quotas results in a review assessment, or goal setting, with continued treatment contingent upon successful completion of quotas. Getting patients to set realistic quota levels and chart their own progress, increases compliance. Such work-to-quota schedules, based on rest and social reinforcement contingencies, stand in contrast to pain contingent or work-to-tolerance models operated by non-behavioural professionals.

Where excessive behaviours are involved, the goal of treatment is extinction. The clinician endeavours to provide social encouragement for well behaviours, but should the patient begin to engage in pain behaviours, eye contact should not be averted lest an impression of

Table 2.1 Guidelines for the behavioural analysis of pain

Pain severity profile				Effect of activity	Behavioural discrep.	Episodic vs. contin.	Evidence vs. disuse	Freq. sex	Delayed sleep onset	Times awake	Reasons for awakenings	Daytime nap	Change over 6/12	Probable operant (O), respondent (R)
AM	PM	EVE	REST											
+	++	+++	↓	↑	yes	C	yes	↓	no	1	Change position Go to toilet	no	=/↑	O
+	++	+++	↓	↑	yes	C	yes	=	no	≥2	Medication Pace around TV/book	yes	=/↑	O
+	++	+++	=	↑	no	E	no	↓	yes	>2	Medication TV/book	no	=	R
+++	++	+	↑	↓	no	E	no	=	no	>2	Medication TV/book	no	=	R
+++	++	+	→	↑	yes	C	yes	↓	yes	≥2	Change position Go to toilet	yes	=/↑	O
+++	+++	+++	=	↑	yes	C	yes	=	yes	≥2	Change position Go to toilet	yes	=/↑	O

Notes:
Degrees of pain intensity: +, ++, +++
Decreased pain intensity: ↓
Increased pain intensity: ↑
No change: =

disregard or escape-avoidance is conveyed. Likewise, if the patient wants to discuss pain during activities, do not change the subject, rather ask for a restatement of the programme's criteria for activity cessation (i.e. sharp, unaccustomed pain). Getting the patient to graphically illustrate performance on each task provides a sound basis for self-reinforcement, which also enables significant others to respond accordingly. Graphs should show tolerance baseline levels and quotas.

2.4.7 Detoxification

Drug rationalization is a major goal of rehabilitation and a major anxiety for patients. Drugs should be scheduled for administration in 4–6 hourly intervals, and not on a pain contingent basis. It is advisable therefore, that the schedule should be fully explained and informed consent secured before commencement. Drug reduction is accompanied by increased mobilization, and the acquisition of coping and relaxation skills. *Detoxification* (i.e. the reduction of narcotic intake), can be achieved by the conversion to equivalent amounts of methadone at a withdrawal rate of 10–20% per day. Conversion of sedative-hypnotics to phenobarbital with a reduction of 10% per day, and the discontinuation of tranquilizers is also recommended (Fordyce, 1990). Drugs are usually suspended in taste and colour masked syrup in 10cc doses. Increased reports of pain or exaggeration of pain behaviour should be monitored for one or two days and analgesia subsequently raised if complaints persist. After stabilization, fading should resume.

The operant approach has been the subject of constructive criticism over the last decade, and the primary issue relates to the use or abuse of such powerful techniques. This matter should be the concern of every clinician.

2.4.8 The pain-behaviour controversy

Fordyce (1976) sets out the first detailed descriptions of pain behaviour, which briefly include: (a) verbal complaints of pain and suffering; (b) para-verbal sounds (e.g. groans, sighs); (c) body posturing and gesturing (e.g. bracing, guarding, rubbing, grimacing); and (d) display of functional impairments (e.g. excessive time spent in a reclined position – i.e. downtime).

Over the last two decades, usage of the term pain behaviour has been absorbed into the vocabulary of the majority of professionals working with chronic pain patients. Letters from referral agents frequently mention the display of such behaviours. But can it be assumed that they are of equal importance, that they serve only a communicative function, that this communication is unambiguous, and that they are in some way more objective than other self-report measures? The major issues relating to the reliability and utility of pain behaviour constructs, and the reliability and validity of behaviour observation methods, have been the subject of several excellent reviews (Fordyce *et al.*, 1985; Keefe and Dunsmore, 1992; Turk and Flor, 1987; Turk and Matyas, 1992).

One of the earliest criticisms of the operant approach, is that in failing to address pain directly as a subjective experience, the behaviourist denies the existence of pain. This is easily refuted. To monitor the posture, verbal and para-verbal sounds, facial expressions, or peripheral autonomic responses of an individual, is the nearest one can get to acknowledging pain itself. Since one cannot directly measure pain, one must measure the related phenomena. The retort that in reinforcing the suppression of pain behaviour, we cruelly punish suffering in the pursuit of stoicism is only a little problematic. To answer this complaint one must return to the goal of rehabilitation, that is to help restore function for those individuals who are more functionally disabled than is necessary. Fordyce *et al.* (1985) explain this more fully:

> The problem arises from confusing the hypothesis that pain *behaviours* can be learned and unlearned. Behavioural treatments for chronic pain are intended to reduce the *disability* associated with chronic pain problems. That large numbers of patients report decreasing pain following the application of these methods is not surprising, but decreased pain per se has never been a primary goal of these rehabilitation methods. (pp. 120–1)

However pain behaviour can serve multiple functions. It can be a means of social communication, avoidance response, a strategy to reduce pain (e.g. rubbing as a means of counterstimulation). Moreover, there is a need to consider medical status variables when attempting to attach meaning to behaviour. For example, McDaniel *et al.* (1986) reported that in rheumatoid arthritis patients, there was a high positive correlation between overt pain behaviours and functional disability. Anderson *et al.* (1988) and Keefe, Wilkins and Cooke (1984) found similar associations in arthritis and low back pain patients, respectively. Merskey (1992) also provides sobering food for thought, thus:

> Problems that have been called hysterical have often been found to be based on physical illness. In a notable follow-up study Slater and Glithero (1965) showed that some 60% of patients diagnosed by distinguished neurologists as having hysteria did suffer from, or develop, relevant physical disease that might account for their symptoms. There is increasing evidence that signs and symptoms that were taken as proof of hysteria – or of behavioural disorder – such as failures of complaints to observe anatomical boundaries, may have a physical basis (Mersky, 1986). Regional pain syndromes and regional loss of sensitivity can have a pathophysiological origin

related to an expansion of receptor fields through the responses of peripheral injury of spinal cord neurons (Mersky, 1986; Wall and Melzack, 1989). If we decide that a set of complaints is due to fibromyalgia, or to myofascial pain dysfunction á la Travell and Simons (1986), or to involvement of zygapophyseal joints á la Bogduk and Marsland (1986; 1988), we may feel that there is a physical mechanism for pain behaviour that has not been recognized, in addition to any physical mechanisms that was observed. Thus the hazards of pain behaviour as a sign of psychological illness, and as an object for psychological/behavioural treatment are even greater. (p. 103)

The foregoing should not avert our efforts to measure or modify pain behaviours. We do need to be particular about how we target behaviours so that adaptive strategies are not included in a blanket approach to behaviour modification – for ultimately such efforts to change will fail. While insightful and ingenious measures of pain behaviour have recently been developed (Keefe and Block, 1982; Craig *et al.*, 1991), a more sophisticated analysis of behavioural principles is required. Keefe and Dunsmore (1992) suggest that future research directions should include:

- a means of classifying maladaptive pain behaviours according to the contingencies that control them;
- the sequential analysis of antecedents and consequences;
- behavioural sampling in naturalistic settings;
- observation of behaviours seen by the patient as problematic;
- the inclusion of both pain behaviours and well behaviours in any functional analysis.

Of course, these objectives, based on the tenets of behavioural analysis accord with the advice given to clinicians by Fordyce (1976). Unfortunately, if researchers are analysing such criteria, they are not reporting them in the scientific literature (Hardardottir, James and Owen, 1988).

2.5 THE COGNITIVE–BEHAVIOURAL PERSPECTIVE

According to the lay conception of illness cognition (Leventhal, Meyer and Nerenz, 1980) physical symptoms such as pain are attributed to discrete pathophysiological or pathoanatomical insults, the intensity of which varies in direct proportion to the size or extent of the pathology. This mechanistic view eases the process of socialization into the acute disease model whereby patients come to expect the medical profession to be able to cure all ills. It is not surprising therefore, that some chronic sufferers view their plight as being the result of medical mismanagement, to their being regarded as 'head cases' or more generally due to a lack of empathy on the physician's behalf. The goal of cognitive-behavioural interventions is to guide the patients to a reconceptualization of their status, in line with the four central assumptions of the cognitive-behavioural perspective (Turk and Rudy, 1987). These are:

- individuals are active processors of information and not passive recipients, or reactors, to or of environmental stimuli;
- thoughts can mediate sensation and response to sensation. That is, they can modulate mood, influence physiological processes, and motivate behaviours, which in turn, can change environmental contingencies. Thoughts can also be reactive to mood, physiology or environmental factors;
- behaviour is reciprocally determined by individual or environmental factors;
- individuals can learn more adaptive ways of thinking, feeling and behaving;
- patients should be encouraged to be actively involved in the transformation to more adaptive cognitive styles.

Cognitive-behavioural strategies and techniques can be characterized under three broad headings: (1) cognitive restructuring; (2) coping skills training; and (3) problem-solving (Mahoney and Arnkoff, 1978).

2.5.1   Cognitive restructuring

Generally speaking, every component of a pain management programme is intended to help patients to revise maladaptive beliefs and attitudes about their status. There are however, specific components which warrant examination.

2.5.2   Education

This phase provides the first opportunity for the clinical psychologist to build upon the rapport established during the initial interview. It is crucial that a therapeutic allegiance be forged at this juncture as it is then that potentially challenging issues relating to pain perceptions and experience are introduced. It is helpful prior to the first didactic session to use group introductory techniques to forge group cohesion, and by getting individuals to relate their pain history. The resulting use of pain descriptors can be picked up by the clinician to acknowledge pain as a legitimate experience of group members, which can be thought of in sensory – discriminative, motivational–affective, and cognitive–evaluative terms. This provides an intriguing introduction to a simple mini-lecture about pain perception based on the Gate-Control Model. The concepts of ascending and descending influences on a pain gate mech-

Table 2.2 Factors which influence the pain gate

Mode of influence	Open gate	Close gate
Physical	Degree and location of tissue damage, over-exertion, contracture, muscular tension, residual scarring	Optimal dosage of medication, paced activity, counter-stimulation, muscular relaxation
Emotional	Negative emotions, e.g. anxiety, depression, anger	Positive emotions, e.g. happiness, optimism, mental relaxation
Thinking style	Pain pre-occupation, boredom, catastrophizing	Distraction techniques and activities, coping self-statements

anism can be made more personally relevant to patients by helping them to identify factors which increase or decrease pain. That is, factors which open or close the pain gate. Socratic dialogue is the preferred form of communication at this point. These observations are reinforced by the discussion of issues in Table 2.2.

Core issues that follow naturally from a discussion of the physical mode of influence relate to the patient mis-attributions that: (1) hurt is synonymous to harm; and (2) pain limited functioning is synonymous to anatomically limited functioning. Patients having defended these beliefs on numerous occasions, both to themselves and others, are very sensitive to, and indeed anticipate messages which smack of patronizing pontification by the non-afflicted. A brief didactic presentation explaining the deconditioning syndrome, is the preferred vehicle by which to address these issues. Particular emphasis should be placed on inactivity as the sensible and natural response during the first few days of injury, and the recognition that until very recently it appeared to be the sensible and natural approach to the management of chronic back pain (i.e. do not apportion blame to either patients or practitioners).

The third core issue to be addressed during the educational module is that of drug tolerance and the benefits of rationalization. Patients who have been taking pain killers, or indeed any medication, may acknowledge that they provide little positive effect and perhaps some negative effects. Nevertheless, the continued *abuse* is maintained as a form of superstitious behaviour. Any suggestion that their pain killers will be withdrawn leaves anticipatory anxiety etched on many faces. Emphasis therefore, must be placed on the optimal or sensible use of drugs.

The educational modules may be co-chaired by a consultant anaesthetist whose expertise and experience lends credibility to what remain in patients' eyes medical matters. Such expert status is valuable both in ratifying the role of the clinical psychologist and in explaining why other members of the medical profession may have offered seemingly contradictory advice.

2.5.3 Attributional retraining

Basically, the educational phase is intended to convey knowledge and correct misattributions (i.e. causal cognitions) about the perceived source or locus of internal states (e.g. pain experience and other symptoms). That is, whether control of symptoms lies within the individual (i.e. internal) or under the influence of forces outside the individual's control (i.e. external). Attributional retraining (Försterling, 1985; Weiner, 1988), in addition, attempts to determine and modify the extent to which: (1) people believe that they can do something to control the cause through intentional actions; and (2) the presumed *stability* of the cause can be affirmed or disconfirmed. The central assumption of attributional retraining is that many behaviours, affects, and cognitions (e.g. phobic avoidance, anger, low expectations of success) are the consequences of causal attributions one makes about events or behavioural outcomes, such as successful or unsuccessful completion of certain tasks.

Application of re-attribution theory to therapeutic intervention in PMPs begins with the identification of adaptive or maladaptive attributions for success or failure. For example, a maladaptive ascription of successful task completion to chance factors (e.g. it was a good day for some reason) would be expected to lead to little enhancement of positive affect, minimally increased expectations of future success, and consequently, a consistently low probability of future adaptive efforts. This attribution probably represents an external, unstable and uncontrollable cause for success. Likewise, following a failed task attempt, the maladaptive assumption 'the pain won't let me continue' (in my view, an internal, stable and uncontrollable assumption) might be expected to lead to feelings of helplessness, decreased expectancies of success and a lack of persistence on task. In contrast, a more adaptive interpretation for successful task completion might identify enhanced pain tolerance (an internal, unstable but controllable cause) presumably would lead to increased confidence, enhanced self-esteem, and a greater likelihood of future task approach. Note that unstable attributions can be adaptive insofar as failure can be attributed to reduced tolerance (for example) which should precipitate re-appraisal, problem-solving and instigation of effective coping strategies. Consquently, the probability of future task approach should be undiminished as individuals reaffirm their resourcefulness.

To date, the efficacy of this approach in a sample of chronic pain patients has yet to be empirically tested. However, findings of other achievement motivation studies indicate that (1) attribution of failure to lack of effort maximizes subsequent persistence; and, (2) compared to persistent triers, subjects who are less persistent are less likely to use lack of effort ascriptions. Re-attribution training also has much in common with other models of action such as self-efficacy theory (Bandura, 1977) which has proved useful in predicting outcome (O'Leary *et al.*, 1988, Council *et al.*, 1988). Self-efficacy theory holds that task-approach is dependent upon the perceived probability that one can perform a particular behaviour which is necessary to produce a desired outcome (e.g. concentrate on a pleasant image when experiencing a moderate level of pain), and the expectancy that successful completion of that task will lead to the desired outcome (i.e. pain relief).

2.5.4 Rational Emotive Therapy (RET) techniques

In common with re-attribution training and other cognitive-behavioural therapies, Rational Emotive Therapy (Ellis, 1962) is a Stimulus–Cognition–Response model. Because RET lends itself to a phased approach to implementation it can be worked into homework assignments in meaningful modules. Thus the identification of Activating event → Beliefs → emotional/behavioural Consequence (ABC) format (Phase I) can be extended in Phase II to include the patient's definition of rational/irrational, adaptive/maladaptive thoughts, beliefs and evaluations. The third phase involves systematic Socratic disputation of beliefs before going on to the creation of rational/adaptive alternatives (Phase IV).

Wessler and Wessler (1980) described and expanded a model of the ABCs known as the Emotional Episode. The model has eight stages which relate to events in Schachter's (1964) Theory of Emotions (the latter posits that heightened autonomic arousal engenders anxiety and provokes avoidant thoughts and images).

Dawson (1991) has suggested a six-stage model for the modification of the basic irrational beliefs (i.e. Demandingness, Catastrophizing, Low Frustration Tolerance, and Condemnation) which emphasizes the affective, cognitive and action dimensions of behaviour. Outlined under the acronym REGIME, the model emphasizes the therapeutic Relationship, Emotional responsibility, Goal setting, Interventions (that are specific goal-directed), Monitoring of homework, and Evaluation/Exit. Exit or discharge is indicated when changes in problem-focused emotionality are consistent with changes in cognition and overt behaviour.

2.5.5 Anger management

Chronic pain sufferers are frequently noted to exhibit thinly disguised anger, pent-up hostility and an aggravated sense of entitlement. Anger is directed towards employers and agents of the medico-legal and welfare systems with whom an adversarial relationship may have developed. Ultimately these grievances leave the individual in a no-win situation, being unable to attain sufficient satisfaction even when emotions are expressed openly. Typically, however, interactions with authority figures are dealt with in an unassertive fashion; only the family takes the brunt of angry outbursts. While assertiveness training is a useful component in pain management, when there are several angry people in the group anger control takes priority.

A cognitive–behavioural approach to anger control (Deffenbacher, 1991) is suitable for groups. Treatment involves the integration of several strategies. One such strategy aimed at **increasing personal awareness** uses self-monitoring of environmental, cognitive, emotional, physiological, and behavioural cues for anger. Monitoring is practised during visualization and simulation exercises. **Time-out** or **Leave-taking** entails removing oneself, physically or mentally, from the provocative situation. In order to facilitate leave-taking attention should be paid to challenging self-denigrating cognitions (e.g. 'I chickened-out again').

It is necessary to rehearse specific exit lines in order to avoid creating further acrimony and ease re-entry. Strategies which shift attention from angry ruminations should also be taught. In common with most stress management programmes, **Applied Relaxation** and systematic desensitization techniques are employed. The penultimate component addresses the modification of the following anger-engendering cognitive distortions: (1) catastrophic interpretations; (2) demanding/coercing rules (e.g. use of shoulds, oughts and musts); (3) over-generalizations; (4) use of inflammatory labels; (5) egocentric misattributions; and, (6) dichotomous thinking. Finally the use of coping self-statements, problem-solving and assertiveness skills are intended to encourage active, problem-focused coping skills and a sense of self-efficacy.

Many patients find a mnemonic device aids implementation. In this instance the acronym ANGER can be helpful. ANGER stands for: Anticipate provocative situations; Notice the physical and mental cues; Get out of the situation (physically or mentally); Engage in coping and problem-solving skills; and Return to the situation and address the issue assertively.

2.5.6   Stress inoculation training and systematic desensitization

Meichenbaum and Turk (1976) have explained the application of Stress-inoculation Training (SIT), to problems of anxiety, anger and pain. In order to effect cognitive manipulation, particular emphasis is placed on imaginal rehearsal, self-instructional training and muscular relaxation techniques, which are introduced in three phases (i.e. educational, rehearsal, application training).

The educational phase seeks to provide the individual with an explanatory scheme for understanding cognition and behavioural responses to stressful events. Schachter's Theory of Emotion provides the conceptualization for multiphobic and angry patients, while the Gate Control Theory is offered to provide an understanding of the pain experience. This phase concludes with a discussion of four stages of coping: (1) preparing for a stressor; (2) confronting or handling a stressor; (3) possibly being overwhelmed by a stressor; and (4) reinforcing oneself for having coped. Meichenbaum and Turk give examples of self-statements for each stage.

During the rehearsal phase, coping techniques are practised. This entails the collection of stimulus-specific information and the learning of the relaxation response (Direct action model) and translation and transformation of appraisals, attributions and self-perceptions into self-statements (Cognitive coping mode). Once proficient in the use of these behaviours and cognitive coping skills, they are tested either *in vivo* or *in situ*. When working with chronic pain patients, it is useful to indicate that the use of relaxation and breathing exercises may help to control sensory and discriminative aspects of pain experience, while the use of imagery-based techniques may help counteract feelings of helplessness, in line with the motivational-affective component of pain control. Application of the four phases of coping (i.e. preparatory, confronting, coping with being overwhelmed and self-reinforcement) can be presented as one way of dealing with the cognitive-evaluation component of pain experience. Moreover, the clinician may consider applying SIT within a Systematic Desensitization (Wolpe, 1969) framework, which involves three sets of operations: (1) training in deep muscle relaxation; (2) the construction of symptom-specific hierarchies; (3) the counterposing of relaxation and arousal-evoking stimuli from the hierarchies.

2.6 COPING SKILLS

2.6.1 Breathing control and relaxation

Deep diaphragmatic breathing control is usually the first treatment component in relaxation training. Patients are instructed that the introduction of slow, paced breathing and relaxation leads to a generalized decrease in sympathetic nervous activity. Generally speaking therefore, proficient use of relaxation can help by: (1) reducing pain caused by muscle tension; (2) reducing pain by capturing attention; (3) ameliorating anxiety-related pain; (4) helping to facilitate sleep onset; and, (5) providing an adaptive strategy for use before, during and after a painful experience (Turk, Meichenbaum and Genest, 1983).

Hyperventilation is a major problem with chronic pain patients (Glynn, Lloyd and Folkhard, 1981) and the typical shallow, fast, upper thoracic breathing pattern results in the chronic anxiety response. The likelihood of lapsing into a hyperventilation episode is decreased by bracing the lower back, thus elevating the rib-cage and diaphragm and partly compressing the lungs. The procedure, which is explained more fully elsewhere (Davis, Eshelman and McKay, 1982; Syrjala, 1990), involves nasal inhalation over a four second period, beginning with abdominal expansion and a raising of the chest and shoulders towards the end of the inhalation. The breath is held for a further four seconds, followed by oral exhalation of the same duration. Practice should be a minimum of five minutes, three times daily. This skill is sometimes difficult for patients to grasp, and progress which may take up to a fortnight can be aided by practising in the supine position, finger tips touching each other at the midriff during exhalation and partly during inhalation as a means of monitoring diaphragmatic expansion and con-traction respiration.

Progressive Muscular Relaxation (Jacobson, 1974), the most common form of relaxation in contemporary usage, is fully explained in a manual by Bernstein and Borkovec (1973). This involves the systematic tensing and relaxation of 16 muscle groups. Though it has good face validity, and is a simple technique to learn, continued practice must be moni-tored in order to correct problems of rhythm and to reinforce its value as a fundamental coping skill. Once accomplished in the basic skills, patients can practise a shortened regime involving nine muscle groups (i.e. legs, arms, stomach and midriff, buttocks, thighs and pelvic floor, chest, neck, jaw and facial muscles).

Having mastered diaphragmatic breathing and the shortened muscu-lar relaxation exercises, the patient can be introduced to *cue-controlled* relaxation. This merely requires the patient to repeat a word or visualize a pleasant image associated with the relaxed state during exhalation. With massed practice the cue can powerfully evoke the relaxation response and be easily adopted as a crisis intervention skill. Novice trainees may be over-zealous in tensing certain muscles which are already close to their threshold for spasm and should be cautioned to monitor this closely. However, such fundamental skills can only be fully effective if applied during activities of daily living, paying due attention to kinaesthetics and proprioception.

2.6.2 Activity pacing

Were patients not to have developed dysfunctional activity patterns they probably would never have been referred to a PMP. Pacing activi-ties, therefore, may be the single most important but difficult skill for the chronic musculo-skeletal pain sufferers to learn. By asking patients to review graphs of their activity in the fortnight prior to intervention, they can be asked to classify themselves as one of two types: (1) the camels, whose frenetic cycles of activity are constrained only by severe exacerbation of pain leaving them with the hump; or (2) those whose activity has remained at immediate post-injury levels, and who, like a greyhound's tail are stuck to the bottom and declining rapidly! If presented adeptly, it can be one of many humorous tactics which may help them to re-learn how to laugh at themselves and fix in their mind a critical point.

Pacing entails doing less than the maximum on good days and more than the minimum on bad days. Both camels and greyhounds should adopt the following guidelines:

- begin by following the fitness programme to build up abdominal and leg muscles;
- plan rest periods after a period of activity which had been adjudged to be comfortably within their limits;
- if the targets were set too high, make a note on an activity schedule for future reference, then increase the frequency of rest breaks, and employ relaxation and cognitive coping skills – they should not give up altogether;
- base non-programme activity on knowledge of experience quota achievements;
- prior to beginning a challenging task, do stretching and other warm-up exercises;
- should the patient feel inclined to avoid a planned task, either (a) the task is too physically demanding, or (b) motivation is lacking. If the former is the case, consider a task analysis, while an analysis of reinforcing contingencies is required where the latter case transpires;
- finally, patients should be encouraged not to persist stoically but rather it is advisable to remember PAMPERS (i.e. Plan Activities which Motivate Pleasure-seeking, Efficacy experiences and Responsibility for Self-care).

2.6.3 Controlling attention

Clinical psychologists have drawn upon limited-capacity models of information-processing to design strategies aimed at displacing the processing of nociceptive stimuli, thereby attenuating perceived pain. Turk, Meichenbaum and Genest, (1983) provided the description of six strategies:

(1) Imaginative inattention, involves ignoring pain sensations by focusing on mental images or memories, which are personally meaningful and pleasant, thus incompatible with the pain experience.
(2) Imaginative transformation of pain, requires the patient to view the

sensations as harmless, unreal, impersonal (e.g. electro-mechanical dysfunction such as that which might affect fictional characters like the Six Million Dollar Man):

(3)   Imaginative transformation of context, entails one in mentally transposing oneself from the actual situation to (fictional) scenarios which demand total concentration, in order to ensure successful task completion. Where sensations impinge upon concentration those stimuli can be interpreted as constituent of the scenario, but non-threatening (e.g. muscle strain while traversing an Alpine track):

(4)   Attention-diversion (external), requires the patient to focus on physical characteristics of the environment (e.g. the number of leaves on a living-room plant).

(5)   Attention-diversion (internal), involves the use of self-generated thoughts (e.g. write a story or poem).

(6)   Somatization, entails scrutinizing the painful area in a detached or analytic fashion.

Fernandez and Turk (1989), conducted a meta-analysis of empirically derived multi-dimensional categories of cognitive coping strategies (i.e. pleasant imagining, neutral imagining, dramatized coping, external focus of attention, rhythmic cognitive activity, and pain acknowledging) and found that such strategies were effective in alleviating pain. Bandura *et al.* (1987) demonstrated their efficacy even when endogenous endorphin release had been blocked by naloxone.

Unfortunately, the strategies have limited face validity, and extreme care must be taken when introducing them, in order to ensure that the credibility of cognitive-behaviour techniques in general are not undermined. Prior to advocating their use, it may help to ask patients to engage in one of the strategies, pre-empting failure by stressing that, as yet they are probably unpractised in this respect; indeed that 20% of the population cannot generate clear visualizations. Following completion of this task, introduce the concept of limited-capacity attention and its possible role in the secretion of endogenous pain substances (e.g. endorphin, substance P, bradykinin), before returning to practise each strategy in turn.

McCaffery (1979) provided guidelines which have much in common with those used when introducing hypnosis. Patients should be assured that during tuition successful induction of imagery, requires alertness and concentration, accompanied by a willingness to respond to instructions. This does not however entail any sacrifice of control on their part as they can terminate the procedure at any time, and techniques for termination will be taught. Nor is the protective function of pain depleted with prolonged use of imagery. Initial learning and practice will be facilitated by preceding practice by relaxation, preferably during periods of low pain intensity. The use of images chosen by patients from their personal experience is an appropriate starting exercise. Patients should be encouraged to employ all five senses. Finally, presentation using soothing and positive descriptions, peppered with permissive directions (e.g. perhaps you would like to imagine . . .) rather than authoritarian commands, helps to expedite acceptance. Difficulties encountered or concerns arising from practice, should be addressed following each session.

2.7 PROBLEM-SOLVING

When faced with new treatment regimes or other changes in lifestyle, chronic sufferers frequently encounter difficulties in problem-solving and decision-making. This is probably associated with their gradual accommodation to the dependent role, whereby the responsibility for decision-making is handed over to others. In the event of social withdrawal, a poverty of life experience leads to a poverty of choice experience. Ultimately, they get out of the habit of analytical thinking, and their difficulties are compounded during periods of low mood. Paradoxically they may feel angered by being left out of things yet feel unable to provide solutions which are not constrained by their functional limitations. In order to enhance their feelings of self-efficacy, therefore, patients should be set tasks and be encouraged to participate in decisions concerning programme logistics.

It is likely that a host of problems relating to physical, emotional, social and vocational domains have accrued over time. Use of an algorithm from Turk and Fernandez (1991), can assist in systematizing the problem-solving task. Guidelines are:

- Construe the source of distress or stress reaction as the problem to be solved.
- Give priority to problems in terms of ease of manageability and time-frame.
- Consider the consequences of successful/unsuccessful strategy. Is the proposed strategy a precursor to further adaptive change?
- Define the problem in behavioural terms, specifying discrete tasks.
- Use a brain-storming technique to generate alternative options.
- Order the solutions according to desireability, identifying reinforcers.
- Consider what options (significant) others might suggest – are there hidden agendas?
- Target the most acceptable and feasible solution.
- Employ imaginal and behavioural rehearsal and graduated practice techniques prior to implementation.

- Congratulate positive efforts, even if unsuccessful.
- Use knowledge gained from previous experience to revise under-standing of other problems and proposed solutions.
- When satisfactory outcome is achieved consider the next problem.

2.7.1 Management of sleep disturbance

Disturbed sleep pattern is one of the most disabling sequelae of chronic pain. Typically patients present with a mixture of sleep onset disturb-ance, sleep maintenance disturbance, and early morning awakening. Sleep loss can exacerbate pre-existing deficits in physical and psycho-logical functioning. Fortunately, most patients do not have a sleep disorder, rather they are disordered sleepers. The process of imposing order is the task of the patient but is often adversely hampered by medication effects.

In addition to problems of tolerance and dependency, the use of alcohol, sedatives and hypnotics in the longer term can disturb the normal four-stage pattern of sleep. The deeper stages of sleep (Slow Wave Sleep) are disrupted, as is dream-sleep (Rapid Eye Movement sleep). This eventually leads to a dream-sleep hang-over (REM rebound) which can disturb the patient prior to awakening. Ironically, the pre-scription of amitriptyline to increase the deep restorative type of sleep (Stage 4) can also cause REM rebound.

Below are outlined the self-control strategies employed in combating disturbances in circadian rhythm, sleep-avoidance behaviour, and heightened cognitive arousal. These techniques can be facilitated by the use of sleep diaries (Haythornthwaite, Hegel and Kerns, 1991; Lacks and Morin, 1992).

Guidelines for sleep control:

(a)   Sleep hygiene

- Optimize medication-intake under medical supervision.
- Exclude stimulants (e.g. tea, coffee, cola, chocolate, smoking) within 4–6 hours of retiring.
- Do not eat vegetables within 4 hours of bed-time so as to reduce gastrointestinal motility and gaseous production.
- Retire after regular, disturbing environmental noises have ceased.

(b)   Stimulus control

- Go to bed only when sleepy.
- Use the bed only for sleep and sex (i.e. no reading or TV watching).
- When unable to fall asleep or return to sleep within 20 minutes,

leave the bedroom, relax or do mundane task (no TV). Return only when sleepy.

- Get up at a regular time each morning irrespective of hours slept.
- Avoid day-time napping.

(c) *Cognitive control*

- Wind-down one hour before bed-time; schedule relaxation exercise.
- Write down worries and possible solutions before retiring; resolve to address these issues in the morning.
- Challenge catastrophic thoughts and use calming self-statements.

(d) *Sleep restriction*

- Restrict occupation of bed to the average hours slept in the previous week (to a minimum of 5). Increase this period by 15 minutes nightly, only if a sleep efficiency of 80% is achieved (i.e. (time asleep)/(time in bed) × 100).

2.7.2 Treatment efficacy and adherence

Extensive reviews of treatment outcome following cognitive-behavioural intervention (Turner and Chapman, 1982; Flor, Fydrich and Turk, 1992) conclude that multi-disciplinary pain management programmes are efficacious. For example, compared to untreated patients or those treated with a single mode of treatment, these patients showed improvements in medication use, health-care use, exercise, and reductions in pain behaviour (63% vs 21%; 35% vs 4%; 53% vs 13%; 62% vs 0%; respectively). They were almost twice as likely (68% vs 36%) to return to work (Flor *et al.*).

Unfortunately, long-term adherence to treatment recommendations has been inconsistent. Between 30% and 70% of patients failed to maintain all or some of their acquired skills (Keefe, Gil and Rose, 1986). The need to build treatment adherence strategies into every sphere of the protocol has been stressed by a number of authors (Dunbar, 1980; Meichenbaum and Turk, 1987; Turk and Rudy, 1991) from whom the recommendations below have been drawn.

Guidelines for treatment adherence

(a) *Reconceptualization phase*

- Establish patient's causal attributions about pain onset, maintenance and expected treatment effects.
- Attempt to resolve misattributions.

- Use plain language when explaining diagnosis and treatment rationale.
- Present information in logical categories (e.g. diagnosis, pain experience, treatment, and outcome expectancy).
- Present information gradually so as not to overwhelm.
- Summarize all salient information in take-home folder.
- Place more emphasis on the how rather than the why of therapy.
- Work to enhance the patient-practitioner relationship.

(b) Skill-acquisition phase

- Make patient a partner in treatment-planning.
- Tailor instructions for each patient.
- Ensure short and long term goals are realistic.
- Incorporate mastery and pleasure activities in goal-planning.
- Set homework assignments for core components.
- Obtain patient's commitment to adhere to negotiated plans.
- Work with patient to overcome obstacles to adherence.
- Choose activities which do not require special equipment.
- Deliver social reinforcement on intermittent and delayed schedule.
- Include significant other (SO) in treatment programme.
- Obtain commitment from SO to reinforce activity.
- Have patient and SO teach the how and why to each other as an aid to assimilation.

(c) Preparation for discharge

- Provide rules for managing flare-ups and set-backs.
- Get patient and SO to discuss changes in rewards and expectancies.
- If forgetful, work to identify stimulus cues and memory aids.
- Provide supply of self-monitoring material.
- Be persistent in following-up patients during first year.
- Provide family doctor with guidelines for future maintenance.

2.8 FUTURE DIRECTIONS

Leading centres of pain management are placing renewed effort in the assessment and application of strategies relating to self-efficacy, coping skills, cognitive restructuring and memory for pain. Attempts to identify the most efficacious aspects of multi-disciplinary pain management is also ongoing. In the UK, the Manchester and Salford Back Pain Centre and Department of Behavioural Medicine are taking advantage of technological advances to explore psychophysiological indicators (paraspinal EMG and autonomic reactivity) of both acute and chronic incapacity and distress. Paradoxically, however, some of the major barriers to recovery arise not from inadequate rehabilitation techniques, but as a result of financial disincentives imposed by welfare benefit schemes and medico-legal compensation schemes. The future aspirations of national Governments therefore, should favour phased integration schemes for return to work and no-loss compensation.

REFERENCES

Anderson, K. O., Keefe, F. J., Bradley, L. A. *et al* (1988) Prediction of pain behaviour and functional status of rheumatoid arthritis patients using medical status and psychological variables. *Pain*, **33**, 25–32.

Bandura, A. (1977) Self-efficacy: toward a unified theory of behavioral change. *Psychology Review*, **84**, 191–215.

Bandura, A., O'Leary, A., Taylor, C. B. *et al*. (1987) Perceived self-efficacy and pain control: opioid and nonopioid mechanisms. *Journal of Personality and Social Psychology*, **53**, 563–71.

Bernstein, D. A. and Berkovec, T. D. (1973) *Progressive Relaxation Training: A Manual for the Helping Professionals*, Research Press, Champaign, Illinois.

Bogduk, N. and Marsland, A. (1986) On the concept of third occipital headache. *Journal of Neurology Neurosurgery and Psychiatry*, **49**, 775–80.

Bogduk, N. and Marsland, A. (1988) The cervical zygapophyseal joints as a source of back pain. *Spine*, **13**, 610–17.

The Classification of Chronic Pain (1986) *Pain*, suppl. 3.

Council, J. R., Ahern, D. K., Follick, K. J., *et al*. (1988) Expectancies and functional impairment in chronic low back pain. *Pain*, **33**, 323–31.

Craig, K. D., Hyde, S., and Patrick, C. J. (1991) Genuine, suppressed, and faked facial behavior during exacerbation of chronic low back pain. *Pain*, **46**, 161–72.

Davis, M., Eshelman, E. F., and McKay, M. (1982) *The Relaxation and Stress Reduction Workbook*. New Harbinger Publications, Oakland.

Dawson, R. W. (1991) Regime: A counselling and educational model for using RET effectively, in *Using Rational Emotive Therapy Effectively: A Practitioner's Guide*, (ed M. E. Bernard), Plenum Press, London, pp. 111–32.

Deffenbacher, J. L. (1991) Cognitive-behavioural approaches to general anger reduction. Paper presented at the first International Congress of Stress, Anxiety and Emotional Disorders, University of Minho, Braga, Portugal, (July, 1991).

Dunbar, J. (1980) Adhering to medical advice: a review. *International Journal of Mental Health*, **9**, 70–87.

Ellis, A. (1962) *Reason and Emotion in Psychotherapy*, Lyle Stuart, New Jersey.

Fernandez, E. and Turk, D. C. (1989) The utility of cognitive coping strategies for altering pain perception: a meta-analysis. *Pain*, **38**, 123–35.

Feuerstein, M., Papciak, A. S. and Hoon, P. E. (1987) Biobehavioral mechanisms of chronic low back pain. *Clinical Psychology Review*, **7**, 243–73.

Flor, H, Fydrich, T. and Turk, D. C. (1992) Efficacy of multidisciplinary pain treatment centers: a meta-analytic review. *Pain*, **49**, 221–30.

Fordyce, W. E. (1976) Behavioral concepts in chronic pain and illness, in *The Behavioral Management of Anxiety, Depression and Pain*, 2nd edn, (ed P.O. Davidson), Brunner/Mazel, Inc., New York, pp. 147–88.

Fordyce, W. E. (1990) Learned pain: pain as behavior, in *The Management of Pain*, 2nd edn. (ed J. Bonica), Lea & Febiger, Philadelphia, pp. 291–9.

Fordyce, W. E., Roberts, A. H. and Sternbach, R. A. (1985) The behavioral management of chronic pain: a response to critics. *Pain*, **22**, 113–25.

Försterling, F. (1985) Attributional retraining: a review. *Psychological Bulletin*, **98**, 495–512.

Glynn, C. J., Lloyd, J. W. and Folkhard, S. (1981) Ventilatory responses to chronic pain. *Pain*, **11**, 201–12.

Hardardottir, D., James, J. E. and Owen, N. (1988) Do operant treatments of chronic pain adhere to precepts of behavioural analysis? *Behavioural Psychotherapy*, **16**, 153–64.

Haythornthwaite, J. A., Hegel, M. T. and Kerns, R. D. (1991) Development of a sleep diary for chronic pain patients. *Journal of Pain and Symptom Management*, **6**, 65–72.

Jacobson, E. (1974) *Progressive Relaxation*. University of Chicago Press, Midway Reprint, Chicago.

Jenson, M. P., Turner, J. A., Romano, J. M., *et al.* (1991) Coping with chronic pain: a critical review of the literature. *Pain*, **47**, 249–83.

Karoly, P. and Jensen, M. P. (1987) *Multimethod Assessment of Chronic Pain*, Psychology Practitioner Guidebooks, Pergamon Press, Oxford.

Keefe, F. L. and Block, A. R. (1982) Development of an observation method for assessing pain behavior in chronic low back pain patients. *Behavior Therapy*, **13**, 363–75.

Keefe, F. J. and Dunsmore, J. (1992) Pain Behavior: concepts and controversies. *American Pain Society Journal*, **1**, 92–100, 112–14.

Keefe, F. J. Gil, K. M. and Rose, S. C. (1986) Behavioral approaches in the multidisciplinary management of chronic pain: programs and issues. *Clinical Psychological Review*, **6**, 87–113.

Keefe, F. J., Wilkins, R. H. and Cook, W. A. (1984) Direct observation of pain behavior in low back patients during physical examination. *Pain*, **20**, 59–68.

Lacks, P. and Morin, C. M. (1992) Recent advances in the assessment and treatment of insomnia, *Journal of Consulting and Clinical Psychology*, **60**, 586–94.

LaRocca, H. (1992) A taxonomy of chronic pain syndromes. *Spine*, **17**, S344–55.

Lethem, J., Slade, P. D., Troup, J. D. G. *et al.* (1983) Outline of a fear-avoidance model of exaggerated pain perception–1. *Behavioural Research Therapy*, **21**, 401–8.

Leventhal, H., Meyer, D. and Nerenz, D. (1980) The common sense representation of illness danger, in *Contributions to Medical Psychology* (Vol. 2), 2nd edn. (ed S. Rachman), Pergamon, Oxford, pp. 7–30.

Mahoney, M. J. and Arnkoff, D. (1978) Cognitive and self-control therapies, in *Handbook of Psychotherapy and Behavior Change: An Empirical Analysis*, (eds S. L. Garfield and A. N. Bergin), John Wiley & Sons, New York, pp. 689–722.

Main, C. J. and Waddell, G. (1991) A comparison of cognitive measures in low back pain: statistical structure and clinical validity at initial assessment. *Pain*, **46**, 287–98.

Main, C. J., Wood, P. L. R., Hollis, S. *et al.* (1992) The distress and risk assessment method: a simple patient classification to identify distress and evaluate the risk of poor outcome. *Spine*, **17**, 42–52.

Mayer, T. G. and Gatchel, R. J. (1988) *Functional Restoration for Spinal Disorders: The Sports Medicine Approach*, Lea & Febiger, Philadelphia.

McCaffery, M. (1979) *Nursing Management of the Patient with Pain*, (2nd edn), J. B. Lippincott, Philadelphia.

McDaniel, L. K., Anderson, K. O., Bradley, L. A. *et al.* (1986) Development of an observation method for assessing pain behavior in rheumatoid arthritis patients, *Pain*, **24**, 165–84.

Meichenbaum, D. and Turk, D. (1976) The Cognitive-behavioral management of anxiety, anger and pain, in *The Behavioral Management of Anxiety, Depression and Pain*, 2nd edn, (ed. P. O. Davidson), Brunner/Mazel Inc., New York, pp. 1–34.

Meichenbaum, D. and Turk, D. C. (1987) *Facilitating Treatment Adherence: A Practitioner's Guidebook*, Plenum, New York.

Melzack, R. and Wall, P. D. (1988) *The Challenge of Pain*, 3rd edn, Penguin Books, London.

Merskey, H. (1986) The importance of hysteria. *British Journal of Psychiatry*, 149, 23–8.

Merskey, H. (1992) Limitations of pain *American Pain Society Journal*, **1**, 101–4.

Nachemson, A. (1982) The natural course of low back pain, in *Symposium on Idiopathic Low Back Pain*, (eds A. A. White and S. L. Gordon), Mosby, St Louis, Mo., pp. 46–51.

Nordin, M. and Vischer, T. L. (1992) *Common Low Back Pain: Prevention of Chronicity*, Clinical Rheumatology Series, Bailliére Tindall, London.

O'Leary, A. Shoor, S., Lorig, K. *et al.* (1988) A cognitive-behavioral treatment for rheumatoid arthritis. *Health Psychology*, **7**, 527–44.

Parker, H. and Main, C. J. (1990) *Living with Back Pain*, Manchester University Press, Manchester and New York.

Philips, H. C. (1987) Avoidance behaviour and its role in sustaining chronic pain. *Behaviour Research and Therapy*, **25**, 273–9.

Philips, H. C. (1988) *The Psychological Management of Chronic Pain: A Treatment Manual*, Springer Publishing Company, Inc., New York.

Philips, H. C. and Grant, L. (1991) The evolution of chronic pain problems: a longitudinal study. *Behaviour Research and Therapy*, **29**, 435–41.

Pinsky, J. J. and Crue, B. L. (1984) Intensive group therapy, in *Textbook of Pain*, (eds P. D. Wall and R. Melzack), Churchill Livingstone, Edinburgh.

Schachter, S. (1964) The interaction of cognitive and physiological determinants of emotional state, in *Advances in Experimental Social Psychology*, (ed L. Berkowitz), Academic Press, New York.

Spanswick, C. C. and Main, C. J. (1989) The role of the anaesthetist in the management of chronic low back pain, in *Back Pain: New Approaches to Rehabilitation and Education*, (eds M. O. Roland and J. R. Jenner), Manchester University Press, Manchester, pp. 108–28.

Syrjala, K. L. (1990) Relaxation techniques, in *The Management of Pain*, 2nd edn, (ed J. Bonica), Lea & Febiger, Philadelphia, pp. 1742–50.

Travell, J. S. and Simons, D. G. (1986) *Myofascial Pain and Dysfunction: the Trigger Point Manual*, Williams & Wilkins, Baltimore.

Turk, D. C. and Flor, H. (1984) Etiological theories and treatments for chronic back pain. *Pain*, **19**, 209–33.

Turk, D. C. and Flor, H. (1987) Pain and pain behaviors: the utility and limitations of the pain behavior construct. *Pain*, **31**, 277–95.

Turk, D. C. and Matyas, T. A. (1992) Pain-related behaviors: communication of pain. *American Pain Society Journal*, **1**, 109–11.

Turk, D. C., Meichenbaum, D. and Genest, M. (1983) *Pain and Behavioral Medicine: A Cognitive-Behavioral Perspective*, Guildford Press, New York.

Turk, D. C. and Rudy, T. E. (1987) Towards a comprehensive assessment of chronic pain patients. *Behaviour Research and Therapy*, **25**, 237–49.

Turk, D. C. and Rudy, T. E. (1991) Neglected topics in the treatment of chronic pain patients – relapse, noncompliance, and adherence enhancement. *Pain*, **44**, 5–28.

Turk, D. C. and Fernandez, E. (1991) Pain: A Cognitive Behavioural Perspective, Cambridge University Press, Cambridge.

Turner, J. A. and Chapman, C. R. (1982) Psychological Interventions for chronic pain: a critical review. II. Operant conditioning, hypnosis, cognitive-behavioral therapy. *Pain*, **12**, 23–46.

Waddell, G. (1992) Understanding the patient with back pain, in *The Lumbar Spine and Back Pain*, 4th edn, (ed M.I.V. Jayson), Churchill Livingstone, Edinburgh, pp. 469–85.

Waddell, G., Bircher, M., Finlayson, D., *et al.* (1984) Symptoms and signs: physical disease or illness behaviour? *British Medical Journal*, 289, 739–41.

Waddell, G., Somerville, D., Henderson, I., *et al.* (1992) Objective clinical evaluation of physical impairment in chronic low back pain. *Spine*, 17, 617–28.

Wall, P. D. and Melzack, R. (1989) *Textbook of Pain*, 2nd edn, Churchill Livingstone, Edinburgh.

Weiner, B. (1988) Attributional theory and attributional therapy: some theoretical observations and suggestions. *British Journal of Clinical Psychology*, **27**, 93–104.

Wessler, R. A. and Wessler, R. L. (1980) *The Principles and Practice of Rational-emotive Therapy*, Jossey-Bass, San Francisco.

Wolpe, J. (1969) *The Practice of Behavior Therapy*, Pergamon Press, Elmsford, New York.

CHAPTER 3

Recent advances in the treatment of chronic pain

Keith Budd and Pam Price

3.1 INTRODUCTION

During the last two decades, the management of pain has emerged from the dark ages into, if not the light, at least a lightening area. Significant changes have been wrought not only in the methods of providing analgesia but also in the way these are provided and, above all, the concepts surrounding pain and pain management.

Even the name has changed as it has been realized that relief was not always possible and so the word management emerged to indicate that more often than not we must consider providing for each patient a personalized programme to aid them rather than a single item of treatment applied once only.

In addition, there has been the growing awareness that doctors are not the only ones able to help the person in pain. This has led to the development of true interdisciplinary teams comprising nurses, psychologists, physiotherapists and others, with the doctor only part of this team rather than its dictator as of right. Consequently, a much more integrated approach to problem solving has evolved with the patient benefiting significantly. Now this is being seen in the management of acute pain whereas before it had not emerged beyond chronic and cancer pain therapy.

To examine the recent advances in the management of the chronic aspect of pain it is probably necessary to divide them into their component parts.

- Drug therapy
- Primary analgesics
- Opioids
- Non-steroidals
- Specific antagonists

- Secondary analgesics
- Psychoactive agents
- Adrenergic agents
- Serotonin agonists
- Diphosphonates
- Drug delivery systems
- External
- Internal
- Interventional methods
- Neuroablation
- Neurostimulation
- Psychological methodology
- Complementary therapy
- The role of the nurse

3.2 DRUG THERAPY

3.2.1 Opoids

In the field of opioid analgesics, advances have been slow to show. There was hope of both kappa and delta agonists being brought from the research into the clinical areas, but so far nothing has appeared.

Kappa agonists were shown to have clear aversive action in animals and in man sedation and psychomimetic reactions proved problematical (Pfeiffer and Brantl, 1986). In addition with U 50, 488H tolerance and receptor down regulation was seen to occur (Bhargava, Romarao and Gulati, 1989).

The high affinity site delta, the enkephalin receptor, shows marked selectivity for peptide structures compared with mu site which interacts preferentially with naturally occurring and synthetic opioids.

Although a series of potent and selective agonists have been produced (Belleney and Gacel,[1] 1989) and peptide bonds can be stabilized so that prolonged duration of action is achieved, the problems of brain penetration and absorption from the gastrointestinal tract still remain to be solved. However, more recently derivatives of oxycodone have been shown to have some degree of delta selectivity but it remains to be seen whether this will be of clinical use.

Agents with multiple modes of action are always of interest. Tramadol hydrochloride shows not only mu opioid activity but also exerts analgesic effects via monoamine re-uptake inhibition. In addition there is no respiratory depressant effect, a unique aspect of an agent with opioid activity and the side-effect profile appears limited to minor problems such as drowsiness and nausea. The latter can be readily prevented or treated with dopamine antagonists e.g. prochlorperazine, and drowsiness frequently becomes less noticeable after persisting with therapy for a week or two.

There is a major advantage in the use of an agent with multiple modes of activity. Many patients' pain is due to a mixed picture of nociceptive, neuropathic and/or sympathetically mediated and, therefore, an agent with opioid and monoaminergic activity will be able to cope with most of the variations of pain type seen in clinical practice as opposed to an agent with only one mode of activity which will only be able to treat one variety of pain.

In addition, tramadol has several formulations allowing a variety of routes of administration to be used, and hence can be used in both acute and chronic pain situations with ease and efficacy. Tramadol probably indicates the way for further research in that the majority of clinical pain syndromes are of mixed pathology rather than of a pure nociceptive, neuropathic or sympathopathic derivation. Consequently, an agent with the ability to cope with each variety of pain in a single molecule will signficantly reduce the need for polypharmacy and decrease the likelihood of serious side-effects and drug interactions.

The endogenous opioids, particularly the enkephalins, have been a potential target for manipulation to produce analgesic agents with clinical value. Both leu- and met-enkephalin are rapidly degraded in the body having half-lives of less than two minutes. The more attractive strategies would be either to develop receptor specific agonists with good bioavailability, or to protect the enkephalins from enzymatic biodegradation with inhibitors capable of crossing the blood–brain barrier in significant amounts (Hughes and Smith, 1975).

The enkephalins are metabolized by cleavage of the molecule at the GLY^3-PHE^4 linkage or at the TYR^1-GLY^2 site (Figure 3.1) the former by a peptidase originally designated enkephalinase but now shown to be a neutral metalloendopeptidase (NEP) and the latter by aminopeptidase N (APN). Both enzymes belong to a family of zinc metallopeptidases and therefore the possibility of producing a mixed inhibitor of both NEP and APN is being actively pursued (Table 3.1).

$TYR^1 - GLY^2 - GLY^3 - PHE^4 - MET$

Methionine enkephalin

$TRY^1 - GLY^2 - GLY^3 - PHE^4 - LEU$

Leucine enkephalin

Fig. 3.1 Methionine and leucine enkephalins: amino acid sequences.

Table 3.1 Enkephalinase inhibitors

APN selective	NEP selective	Mixed
Bestatin	Thiorphan	Kelatorphan
Leucinethiol	Retrothorphan	RB38A
	Acetorphan	PC12
	RB38B	PC19

The first inhibitors introduced were poor analgesics even after intra-cerebroventricular injection. More recently produced agents such as kelatorphan and RB38A show much greater activity whilst agents with the property of crossing the blood–brain barrier in adequate concentration have also been isolated, PC12, PC19 (Noble and Coric, 1990). A comparable analgesic effect between morphine and endogenous opioids could be induced, provided that their synaptic concentrations and receptor occupancy were the same, but it has been disappointing to see that even at high concentrations, RB38A was not able to show a maximum analgesic effect equivalent to that of morphine.

Nevertheless, RB38A at high dose produces low tolerance and dependence, whilst other NEP inhibitors show an analgesic effect greater than aspirin, glafenine, etc. In addition, kelatorphan has not shown any degree of respiratory depressant effect.

In terms of 'physiological analgesia', it becomes increasingly evident that only complete inhibition of enkephalin metabolism can produce a strong antinociceptive response and early results now need confirmation with agents chronically administered (Chipkin *et al.*, 1987; Foong and Nakagawa, 1990).

3.2.2   Non-steroidal and anti-inflammatory agents

The large group of drugs collectively known as the non-steroidal anti-inflammatory drugs (Figure 3.2) exert a number of clinically useful properties including analgesia, anti-inflammatory and anti-pyrexial effects.

The main mode of action of these agents appears to be by incorporation into the lipid bilayer of the cell membrane where they inhibit, at sufficiently high concentrations, the metabolic conversion of fatty acids into prostaglandins by the cyclo-oxygenase enzyme system (Brune, 1982; Brune and Lanz, 1984). Whilst prostaglandins are not considered as primary nociceptive agents, they do sensitize tissue to the algesic action of certain chemicals including bradykinin, 5HT, etc, and do precipitate the release of some of these algesic agents.

Prostacyclin is considered as the most important algesic mediator at sites of inflammation and tissue damage, other arachidonic acid metabolites contributing to lesser degress.

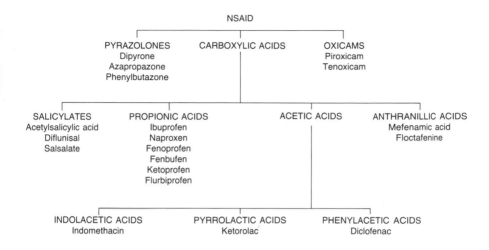

Fig. 3.2 Chemical groupings of NSAIDs.

Whilst there are comprehensive data to support the relationship between the degree of efficacy as anti-inflammatory agents and the degree of cyclo-oxygenase activity, the NSAID's mode of action as analgesics is less well defined. In addition to cyclo-oxygenase inhibition, analgesic activity may also be generated by:

- activation of the descending spinal inhibitory pathway;
- direct effect upon spinal receptors;
- indirect reduction of neurotransmitter release;
- free radical scavenging.

(Piomelli and Grengard, 1990; Lunec and Halloran, 1981; Bjorkman and Hedner, 1990; Vescovi and Passeri, 1987).

Because of this probable multimodal analgesic activity, the selection of NSAIDs for pain reduction should not be by cyclo-oxygenase inhibitory efficacy. There is evidence that analgesic effect is inversely proportional to such enzymatic inhibition (Table 3.2). The naloxone reversibility of the analgesic effect of certain of the NSAIDs does indicate that direct or indirect opioid mechanisms do play an important role.

The NSAIDs' value can be severely limited by their propensity to cause side-effects particularly involving gastrointestinal and renal systems. However, certain of the newer agents produce fewer effects upon certain systems, sulindac and etodolac having low toxicity on the renal

Table 3.2 Comparison of analgesic efficacy of NSAIDs with cyclo-oxygenase inhibition

NSAID	Analgesic efficacy	Cyclo-oxygenase inhibition μ/mol/L
Ketorolac	High	0.5
Tenoxicam		1.2
Diclofenac		1.6
Piroxicam		2.3
Naproxen		5.7
Ibuprofen		39.0
Phenylbutazone		490.0
Acetyl salicylic acid	Low	3300.0

tract and ketorolac and etodolac being less likely than others to affect the gastrointestinal system (Mandel and Herbert, 1990).

In addition, the gastrointestinal tract may be protected by the use of agents such as misoprostol, a prostaglandin analogue, or omeprazole, a proton pump inhibitor, both of which will protect against the effects of NSAIDs upon stomach and duodenum.

When the appropriate NSAID has to be chosen for use, consideration must be given to whether the analgesic or anti-inflammatory aspect is needed, the potential side-effect profile of the agent and whether the patient may be prone to existing pathology of renal or gastrointestinal tract, and to the formulations available for several NSAIDs that are now supplied in a single daily dose presentation.

3.2.3 Specific antagonists

In the generation and transmission of the nociceptive impulse from the damaged periphery to the central nervous system, a number of important chemicals are involved. These may be amino acids, catecholamines or peptides and in contemporary pharmacology agonists and antagonists have been produced to affect their action.

(a) Amino acids

Rapid excitatory events are transmitted within the dorsal horn of the spinal cord by the release of glutamic and aspartic acid. These excitatory amino acids act at N-methyl-D-aspartate (NMDA) receptor sites activating dorsal horn nociceptive neurons. Antagonists at NMDA receptors, therefore, have a potential for inducing analgesia and it is known that the dissociative anaesthetic agent, ketamine, which is also an analgesic even at low doses, is an NMDA antagonist (Bristow and Orlikowski, 1989; Grant, Nimmo and Clements, 1981).

NMDA receptors are also involved with spinal cord plasticity and hyperexcitability, both of which are ultimately involved with the perpetuation of chronic pain. Blockade by competitive (D-CPP) and non-competitive agents (Dizocilpine, MK801) will reverse these states and may well indicate an alternative approach to analgesia in the near future.

NMDA antagonists differ from conventional opioid analgesics in that the dose required to prevent the establishment of central sensitization is the same as that which abolishes it once it has been induced. NMDA antagonists, therefore, could be effective in reducing central sensitization whilst leaving normal physiological responses intact (Woolf and Thompson, 1991).

(b) Purines

Purinergic receptor modulation of afferent processing has recently been brought into prominence.

Adenosine exerts its effect at specific A_1 or A_2 receptors, inhibiting or stimulating adenylate cyclase. By this mechanism, spinal adenosine receptors are involved in the mediation of the antinociceptive effects of antagonists at both A_1 and A_2 receptors.

In animals, adenosine analogues have a powerful modifying effect even at low dosage on strychnine induced hyperaesthesia. This contrasts with opioids which only have a poor effect. The characteristics of strychnine hyperaesthesia appear to mimic the clinical phenomenon observed in man after nerve injury and suggest a role for adenosine analogues in practice (Sosnowski and Yaksh, 1989).

(c) Peptides

Substance P (SP), an eleven amino acid peptide, is thought to be one of the primary noniceptive transmitters responsible for the slow component of pain, the deep, burning aspect of the more prolonged response to injury. SP is found in small cell bodies in the dorsal root ganglion and in central terminals in the superficial dorsal horn. In the former location, it is frequently co-localized with glutamate.

The peripheral 'flare and weal' following tissue damage is due to the release of histamine mediated by SP and other peptides, notably calcitonin gene related peptide (CGRP).

SP antagonists have been found to exert an analgesic effect especially in neuropathic conditions. Capsaicin (trans–8-methyl-N-vanillyl–6-nonenamide) selectivity blocks small diameter, unmyelinated nociceptive sensory afferents from skin and mucous membrane, many of which utilize SP, but also somatostatin and other neuropeptides (Jessel, Inversen and Cuello, 1978). Clinical studies have indicated the value of topically applied capsaicin in the treatment of post herpetic neuralgia and other neuropathic states producing pain (Bernstein and Bickers, 1987; Watson *et al.*, 1988). Analogues of capsaicin are now available that are antinociceptive without the initial stimulation of capsaicin and may be extremely valuable in treating painful states triggered by C fibre input (Lynn, 1990; Dray, 1990).

Bradykinin (BK) is a nonapeptide mediator of inflammation and activates sensory nerve endings and sensory neurones. In sensory neurones, BK may act through a G-protein-coupled receptor to activate a number of intracellular second messengers. As BK antagonists have been shown to have activity in a number of pain and inflammation models (Steranka and Manning, 1988), development of clinically applicable agents will develop (Burch, Farmer and Steranka, 1990). Current usefulness is limited by rapid *in vivo* breakdown by enzymatic degradation, but this problem will no doubt be solvable.

Cholecystokinin (CCK) is an important neuropeptide distributed throughout critical and periaqueductal areas, the ventromedial thalamus and the spinal dorsal horn; all areas associated with pain modulation. CCK is a neuroexcitatory agent and is seen to potentiate the activity of many neurotransmitters. CCK antagonists, particularly of the CCK-B receptors, will both enhance morphine analgesia and exert antinociceptive effects. L365260 in addition will obtund panic attacks and is currently being evaluated clinically for this purpose (Dourish, 1990).

Somatostatin is another small peptide concerned with neuronal transmission and the perpetuation of chronic pain states. Somatostain exerts modulatory effects, usually inhibitory, on transmission mediated by SP, hormones and CAMP. Its major clinical drawback is its very short half-life and, therefore, the development of a long acting analogue, octreotide, has been beneficial in the treatment of the hyperaesthesia associated with acute injury and headache associated with acromegaly (Ellis, 1990).

3.2.4 Psychoactive agents

It has long been recognized that psychoactive agents have a valuable anti-nociceptive action. There is good evidence to suggest that this analgesic activity is independent of any effect upon mood (Monks and Merskey, 1989). Although the mode of action remains to be elucidated, it would appear to be via effects upon central neurotransmitter function. These may be of an inhibitory nature such as the blockade of the reuptake of 5HT and noradrenaline (NA) from intersynaptic clefts by antidepressants or the facilitatory mode of certain GABA agonist anticonvulsants which augment GABA-mediated inhibitory neuronal transmission (Budd and Hill, 1991).

Psychoactive agents may be used to treat a wide variety of pain

Table 3.3 Neurotransmitters influenced by various groups of drugs with secondary analgesic effect

Type of agent	Affected neurotransmitter
Mono-amine oxidase inhibitor	5HT, NA, DA
Tricyclic antidepressant	5HT, NA, DA, ACh, H
Phenothiazine derivative	DA, GABA, H, NA, A
Anticonvulsant	GABA, DA
Butyrophenone	DA, NA
Benzodiazepine	GABA, NA

Table 3.4 Effect of some antidepressants upon neurotransmitters involved in nociception

Drug	Transmitter effect					
	NA	DA	H	$5HT_1$	$5HT_2$	ACh
Amitriptyline	++	+	+++	+++	++	+++
Clomipramine	+++	++	++	−	++	++
Desipramine	++	+	++	−	++	++
Fluoxetine	−	−	−	−	+	+
Fluvoxamine	+	−	−	−	−	−

syndromes and will be beneficial in all three varieties of pain types. In the majority of cases it would appear that to engender effective analgesia, several neurotransmitters must be influenced and hence the older agents are more successful, or a combination of agents must be used to allow a wide spectrum of transmitter effect. Most commonly used combinations are antidepressant with phenothiazine derivative or anticonvulsant.

It is also seen that it is not only which transmitters are affected but also the degree to which that effect is exerted. Consequently, as this aspect still remains unclear, combination therapy is somewhat inaccurate and this may be one reason why the analgesic effect is not always consistent even within a single pathology. More recently, agents which have a specific effect on only one neurotransmitter, have been shown to have analgesic activity in diabetic neuropathy. Paroxetine, fluoxetine and fluvoxamine are three of the newer antidepressants with such activity (Sinrup et al., 1990, Theesen and Marsh, 1989).

Anticonvulsants have found favour in the treatment of neuropathic pain, and whilst they are all considered as GABA-A agonists, each has a different site of action from the others, and in selecting the optimal agent for any patient more than one drug may have to be tried. The newer anticonvulsants such as vigabatrin and lamotrigin have yet to be evaluated in pain control but as their modes of action differ again from the established agents, they may bring further facility to a notoriously difficult clinical area.

Certain benzodiazepine anxiolytics have been shown to have anagesic effect in neuropathic and atypical facial pain. Clonazepam and clobazam have been successfully used in both indications and appear to be agents of choice for many of the facial neuralgias. The use of another benzodiazepine, midazolam, has indicated clinically significant anti-nociception when administered intrathecially: no analgesia is evident when administered orally in standard doses (Serrao *et al.*, 1992). It would appear that the analgesic effect is mediated via spinal GABA-A receptors (Edwards *et al.*, 1990). In man, intrathecal midazolam has been used to treat back pain and spinal metastatic tumour deposits, and its clinical value is still being further evaluated. With the introduction of new and selective agents, there is gradually being built up adequate information to allow accurate selection of the optimal agent for each pain type. However, there remains the need for careful clinical observation to feed back the appropriate guidance.

3.2.5 Adrenergic agents

The use of adrenergic agents administered by the intrathecal route has been shown to generate effective analgesia in a number of species including man, when tested against thermal, mechanical and chemical stimuli (Coombs *et al.*, 1984).

Clonidine is the best known example of such agents which exert a direct agonist effect upon dorsal horn α_2 adrenoceptors. Clinically, clonidine may produce severe hypotension as well as analgesia and therefore has to be used with care (Nagasaka and Yaksh, 1990), although once an analgesic effect has been produced by intrathecal administration, the oral route can be used for maintenance.

Medetomidine is a new, highly selective and potent α_2 agonist, significantly more effective than clonidine although its value might well be greater in the treatment of neuropathic rather than nocigenic pain (Kauppila *et al.*, 1991).

3.2.6 Serotonin agonists

5HT is an important neurotransmitter and ligand binding studies have enabled four major classes of 5HT receptors to be delineated (5HT 1–4), and for some of these to be subdivided (5HT$_1$ A–D).

5HT$_{1A}$ receptors produce their response by stimulation of adenylate cyclase, unlike the other 5HT$_1$ subtypes. This delineation of receptor subtypes has enabled the site of action of migraine prophylactic agents to be identified (Fozzard, 1990).

The introduction of a 5HT$_{1A}$ agonist, sumatriptan, has given a novel therapeutic agent for rapid relief of the migraine attack. It is a specific and selective agonist of 5HT$_{1A}$ receptors of cranial blood vessels causing vasoconstriction (Humphrey and Feniuk, 1991). Sumatriptan has little effect on other 5HT or on adrenergic or dopaminergic receptors, and does not penetrate the blood-brain barriers. The agent may be given either subcutaneously or orally (Pearce, 1992).

3.2.7 Biphosphonates

Biphosphonates are pyrophosphate analogues resistant to rapid break-down by endogenous phosphatases. The main benefit is derived from the inhibition of osteoclast-mediated bone resorption by a direct effect upon the osteoclasts. Biphosphonates alter the morphology of these cells suggesting an effect upon the activity (Body *et al.*, 1987).

This family of drugs is successful in the treatment of tumour-induced osteolysis (Paget's disease) leading to impressive pain relief, and may have a role in the prevention and treatment of osteoporosis (Elomaa *et al.*, 1992).

3.3 DRUG DELIVERY SYSTEMS

The rationale of drug delivery systems is to deliver the active component to the site of action as quickly and effectively as possible. Provision should be made for the duration of action of the agent to be as close to optimal as possible.

Three concepts that have significantly altered clinical practice in the last decade have been the introduction and wide use of sustained release oral preparations, the use of the intraspinal route for drug delivery and the introduction of reservoirs and pumps, either external or internal, to deliver agents on a continuous basis.

Whilst sustained release formulations are not new, the availability of the continuous formulation and its application to the prolonged delivery of morphine has without doubt made a significant contribution to the treatment of pain, particularly that due to malignant disease (Leslie, 1981). The same technique is being applied to other opioids but the conceptual breakthrough has already been made (Wotherspoon, Henny and McArdle, 1992).

The discovery that opioids applied in the epidural space produced prolonged analgesia opened up a further avenue for pain control (Behar *et al.*, 1979). Since then, most opioid analgesics have been given both epidurally and intrathecally with varied success. There has, overall, been a positive effect but not all opioids are kinetically suitable for this technique and side-effect problems have, on occasions, been difficult to combat.

In addition to opioids, other agents have been used to not only achieve analgesia (midazolam, clonidine, medetomidine) but also to

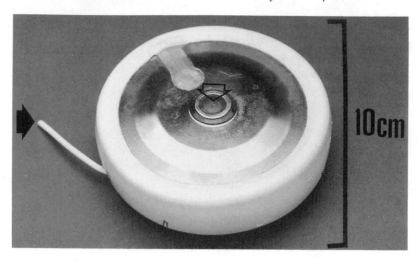

Fig. 3.3 Infusaid Pump. Filling port indicated by open arrow, spinal lead by closed arrow. (Reproduced by permission – Infusaid Corporation).

treat spasticity (buprenophine, baclofen) (Glynn, McQuay and Lloyd, 1984).

To avoid the necessity of intermittent injections of analgesic drugs into muscle or intraspinal spaces, the use of catheters linked to small pumps has become a valuable technique. For short term use, the pump may be of the syringe driven variety delivering intermittent boluses of drug either subcutaneously or to the intraspinal catheter. For longer term use, the pump-catheter system can be completely inplantable, with the pump being refilled at regular intervals percutaneously via the port seen in the centre of the body (Figure 3.3). Variations on this device include a multidose reservoir which enables the patient to self administer a predetermined aliquot by pressing a button on the surface of the infuser. Services of these types are normally implanted in the subcutaneous tissue of the abdominal wall for ease of use and refilling.

As well as the high technological and expensive methods of drug delivery, much work is being done on formulating analgesic drugs for simple application. Transdermal and intrapleural routes of analgesic administration are now well tried and seem to be effective (Duthie, Rowbotham and Wyld, 1988; Caplan, Ready and Oden, 1989). The buccal and intranasal routes are successful for some agents and are well used with sublingual buprenorphine and phenazocine. Buccal morphine appears difficult to formulate whilst intranasal opioids will soon be clinically available (Hoskin *et al.*, 1989; Striebel, Koenigs and Kramer, 1992).

The application of extrapleural intercostal block in the long term may mirror its success in the treatment of pain following thoracic and abdominal surgery (Berrisford *et al.*, 1990; Sabanathan *et al.*, 1990).

3.4 INTERVENTIONAL METHODS

3.4.1 Neuroablation

The concept of cutting a sensory nerve to remove the pain experienced in its locus of peripheral distribution has long been held. However, the frequent failure of techniques designed to do this has led to a significant reduction in the exposure of patients to neuroablative techniques.

Discoveries leading to a better understanding of the pathophysiology of the nervous system, the concept of plasticity and that the best way to treat pain is to prevent the occurrence of central nervous system changes leading to plasticity, has all but delivered the *coup de grâce* to neuroablation (Woolf, 1989). The only procedures which may produce lasting benefit are those designed to ablate sensory ganglion cells in either trigeminal or dorsal root ganglia by the use of radiofrequency lesioning or the injection of glycerine.

3.4.2 Neurostimulation

In direct contrast to neuroablation, there has been a significant increase in the use of neurostimulation in the treatment of pain. Transcutaneous Electrical Neural Stimulation (TENS) is widely used (Figure 3.4). The reduction in price per unit together with improvements in electrode technology has meant that availability is within the reach of every patient, and compliance in use is enhanced. The use in cancer related pain has also increased with improved knowledge of efficacy.

The use of Dorsal Column Stimulation (DCS) is a burgeoning area, especially with the increased areas of value being seen. Not only is it of value in the treatment of post traumatic pain (De La Porte and Siegfried, 1983; Shatin, Mullett and Hults, 1986) but for patients with intractable angina (Mannheimer *et al.*, 1988) and peripheral vascular disease (Miles, 1992) the cost effectiveness has been well proven.

Positioning of the electrode so that it is in the midline of the posterior epidural space (Figure 3.5a, b) can be performed at open operation or percutaneously. The stimulator may be either buried in the abdominal wall (Figure 3.6) or an aerial may be buried beneath the skin and an external stimulator may be placed over this to induce current in the implanted system.

The modes of action of the different stimulation techniques are thought to differ: TENS has a predominantly segmental effect within the spine whilst DCS induces activity in the anterior pretectal nucleus

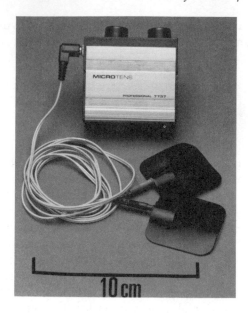

Fig. 3.4   TENS Apparatus.

in the midbrain via stimulating the dorsal spinal columns. The activity will produce descending impulses in the bulbo-spinal tract which is inhibitory to the dorsal horn cells, blocking the onward transmission of afferent nociceptive impulses.

3.5   PSYCHOLOGICAL METHODOLOGY

It is now quite clear that the psychological aspects of painful conditions cannot be separated from the physical in diagnosis, treatment or maintenance. Psychological factors play a major role in the manner in which patients will tolerate, describe and cope with their pain, how they will relate to the therapeutic team and how they will respond, or not, to the treatment. In a separate, yet inter-related area, are the socio-economic factors which may also play an important and varying role in the patients' attitudes and responses. The main advances have come through the acceptance of the importance of the psychological aspect of pain and the reliance now laid on the use of psychologically orientated treatment.

   In spite of the many psychological inventories and questionnaires, there is still no conclusive way in which the degree of psychological involvement in a painful process can be measured. Certain guides can be obtained about personality, version, etc. but nothing more than an

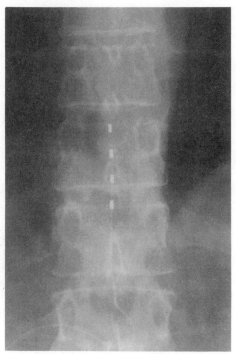

Fig. 3.5 (a) AP X-ray spine. Electrode in the mid line with tip at T_{11}.
(b) Lateral X-ray spine. Electrode in the posterior epidural space with tip at T_{11}.

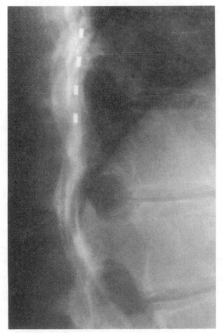

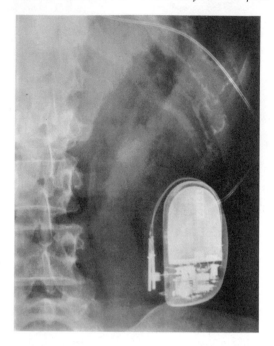

Fig. 3.6 Itrel DCS stimulator implanted in the left iliac fossa.

adequate in-depth interview can obtain. This can be performed effectively only by a trained psychologist or psychiatrist.

It should be observed that one major recent advance has been the increase in the number of clinical psychologists involved in pain management as part of the interdisciplinary team. The other important advance has been the growing institution of pain management programmes which deal with behavioural, physical and pharmacological aspects in a controlled environment either out-patient or in-patient. The ultimate spin-off from such programmes are those which the patients organize and run for themselves (Flor, Fydrich and Turk, 1992).

3.6 COMPLEMENTARY THERAPY

Complementary medicine has always been with us and only recently has the establishment of traditional medical practice accepted the role, often a very important one, that such therapy has to play in the treatment of the whole patient. It is this realization and the willingness to incorporate such diverse aspects as osteopathy, hypnosis and aroma therapy into therapeutic schedules alongside surgical and drug treatment that has advanced the cause of the patient so much in the last decade. As with so many other aspects of patient care, the real advances have been conceptual every bit as much as technological.

3.7 THE ROLE OF THE NURSE

Traditionally the management of pain has been left to nursing staff. At first sight this seems entirely reasonable, since nurses spend more time dealing directly with the patient than any other health-care professional. Unfortunately the lack of education given to student nurses in the basic principles of pain manifestations and management, results in nurses dealing out analgesics in a misconceived and ritualistic manner. Without knowledge nurses and doctors make subjective judgements of their patients' pain: they are unaware of the individual variations in cause, response and nature of display of the effects of pain. Nurses are not alone in perpetuating such errors. Doctors still prescribe standard doses and intervals for analgesia, which are often based only on the type of operation or disease, and not on the individual's needs. Fear of addiction is still cited by both doctors and nurses as a reason to withhold opioid analgesia. Fortunately this situation is beginning to change, albeit slowly. Nursing has changed, with more emphasis given to individual patient care. No longer is nursing task-orientated with patients having to conform to strict ward routines. It is recognized that patients are individuals, with their own set of beliefs and unique past experiences which must be respected. This more holistic view of the patient has led to a greater understanding.

Many nurses wish to extend their knowledge and understanding of the subject of pain. They wish to be better able to help and relieve the suffering. To facilitate this progression some hospitals are now employing specialist nurses in pain management. Many of these nurses were drawn into pain therapy not only by recognizing their own limited knowledge of the subject, but also by consultants specializing in the management of pain. In turn the consultants found that nurses added an entirely different and unexpected dimension to pain management.

By contact with patients attending out-patients' clinics, the nurse became knowledgeable of the different origins of pain, and the variations between an individual's degree and response to pain. The nurse became aware of the host of ancillary factors affecting patient response. Patients find it easier to talk to a nurse, and ask questions relating to their condition and treatment. Many patients still wish to please the doctor!

Concurrently, in the management of acute post-operative pain, which employs techniques of regional anaesthesia, continuous epidural and, more recently, patient controlled analgesia, nursing interest and involvement has been refocused from the standard regimes of the past on to the active management of individuals. The nurses have become educated and have influenced the clinicians. The conjunction of these two areas, chronic pain management and acute post-operative pain control, place an enormous workload on the clinical nurse specialist. Additionally, from beginning as a self-educating speciality, by way of enlisting the collaboration of many disciplines, progression has led to nurse education programmes, to which doctors are welcome.

Because of the nurse specialist's ability to enter into close collaboration with the patients, she cannot avoid developing a great deal of expertise in the management and results of various forms of pain therapy. She can discover areas where physical, psychological, social, environmental and marital factors have a bearing on the patients' perceived problems. Because of their attention to the minutiae of detail, in individual cases the nurse pain-specialist is able to distil the essential disturbance of the patient and proffer it to the health-care team. There is no doubt that the clinical nurse specialist's role has expanded. This is demonstrated by the increasing numbers of articles appearing in both nursing and medical journals, and the national press. Patients themselves are becoming better informed of the newer ways of relieving pain.

Many more referrals are being made to the nurse-specialist. She is asked to assist the primary nurse in the assessment of their patients' pain, and to offer advice about pain-relieving techniques. Co-operation in this way ensures that the primary nurse extends her own knowledge. Many nurses are no longer prepared to accept that there is no more that can be done to alleviate their patients' suffering.

The employment of nurse specialist in this vastly expanding field is at first sight costly. Many studies have shown that a pain-free patient recovers mobility more quickly, has fewer complications post-operatively and can leave hospital earlier. This economic advantage is not always supported. Resistance to change and the inability to see hidden benefits, shackles pain management services by starving them of their resources.

The potential for nurses to contribute to the control of pain is enormous. It is unrealistic for a single nurse specialist in each hospital to take responsibility for all patients with pain, and for all the education needs of the nursing staff. The nurse specialist is a facilitator to be used for her expertise and help with the management of difficult pain symptoms, and particularly to educate staff in the wards and clinics to appreciate the importance of pain in the patients' lives.

It is imperative that the basic principles of pain-management be incorporated into the student nurse curriculum. A foundation course encompassing the principles of physiology, psychology, pharmacology, the social, emotional and spiritual components of pain along with pain assessment and a knowledge of complementary therapies are essential.

Without this knowledge nurses will continue to deal only with those pains they feel can be dealt with.

Because of their 'wide angle' approach to pain management, clinical nurse specialists are well placed to draw together many professions into educational activities. Particularly effective are one-day symposia where modern understanding of the nature of pain can be promulgated and comparisons made between different organizations. In practice such activity needs to be repeated several times a year.

It is also an important part of the nurse specialist's role to promote and participate in research. It follows that it is equally and probably more important that she promote the conclusions of research studies insofar as carers are led to adopt more rational methods of management.

Many areas of nursing are ritualistic and demonstrably of no value. People carry fixed assumptions about the way things are or should be. It is this personal commitment to beliefs that leads to resistance to change, even to viewing change as threatening their very selves.

Prior to 1970 nursing was based on notions of subservience to medicine, and an oral tradition of beliefs passed from sister to student. There was no sense of professional knowledge unique to nursing. The work of researchers in the last twenty years has been frustrated because their findings are challenging beliefs.

While it is difficult to change such attitudes by argument alone, the nurse specialist in the clinical setting can demonstrate that research modifications do result in improved patient care. If we hold an attitude that something will not work, and we then operate that something for a while and experience shows that it does work, we have a problem in reconciling our knowledge with our own beliefs. This reconciliation often leads to a change in beliefs. (The key to unlocking the door to change is known as 'cognitive dissonance' theory.)

In the context of acute pain services the advocation of pain assessment documentation (e.g. visual analogue scales) would be expected to provoke resistance by ward nurses. The value of such tools in the modification of therapy regimes was soon apparent. Disbelievers became converted to advocates for their use. Superior pain-control has been practically demonstrated in the wards, to relieve nurses of the load imposed in caring for more serious illness which results, from a higher incidence of complications.

REFERENCES

Behar, M., Olshwang, D., Magora, F. *et al.* (1979) Epidural Morphine in the treatment of pain *Lancet*, **1**, 527.

Belleney, J. and Gacel, G. (1989) Delta opioid receptor selectivity induced by conformational constraints in linear enkephaline related peptides: 1H 400Hz NMR study and theoretical calculation. *Biochemistry*, **28**, 7392–400.

Bernstein, J. E. and Bickers, D. R. (1987) Treatment of chronic post-herpetic neuralgia with topical capsaicin. *Journal of the American Academy of Dermatology*, **17**, 93–6.

Berrisford R. G., Sabanathan S. S., and Mearns, A. J. *et al.* (1990) Pulmonary complications after lung resection: the effect of continuous extrapleural intercostal nerve block *European Journal of Cardio-thoracic Surgery*, **4**, 407–11.

Bhargava, H. N., Romarao, P. and Gulati, A. (1989) Effects of morphine in rats treated chonically with U50, 488H, a kappa opioid receptor agonist. *European Journal of Pharmacology*, **16**, 257–64.

Bjorkman, R. and Hedner, J. (1990) Central naloxone-reversible antinociception by diclofenac in the rat. *Naunyn-Schmiedebergs Archives of Pharmacology*, **342**, 171–6.

Body, J. J., Pot, M., Borkowski, A. *et al.* (1987) Dose response study of aminohydroxyproplyidene biphosphonate in tumour associated hypercalcaemia. *American Journal of Medicine*, **82**, 957–63.

Bristow, A. and Orlikowski, C. (1989) Subcutaneous Ketamine analgesia: post-operative analgesia using subcutaneous infusion of ketamine and morphine. *Annals of the Royal College of Surgeons of England*, **71**, 64–6.

Brune K. (1982) Prostaglandins, inflammation and anti-inflammatory drugs. *European Journal of Rhematology and Inflammation*, **5**, 335–49.

Brune, K. and Lanz, R. (1984) Non opioid analgesics, in *Analgesia; Neurochemical, Behavioural and Clinical Perspectives*, (eds. M. J. Kuhar, G. W. Pasternak), Raven Press, New York, pp 149–73.

Budd, K. and Hill, R. G. (1991) Mechanisms of transmitter block, in *Conductive Blockade for Post-Operative Analgesia* (eds J. A. W. Wildsmith, J. McClure) Edward Arnold, London, pp. 55–77.

Burch, R. M., Farmer, G. S. and Steranka, L. R. (1990) Bradykinin receptor antagonists. *Medical Research Review*, **10**, 143–75.

Caplan, R. A., Ready, L. B. and Oden, R. V. (1989) Transdermal fentanyl for postoperative pain management. *Journal of the American Medical Association*, **261**, 1036–9.

Chipkin, R. E., Berger, J. G., Peters, M. *et al.* (1987) SCH 34826. The first orally active enkephalinase inhibitor. *Pain* **54**, S254.

Coombs, D. W., Saunders, R. *et al.* (1984) Clinical trial of intrathecal clonidine in cancer pain. *Journal of Regional Anaesthesia*, **9**, 34–5.

De La Porte, C. and Siegfried, J. (1983) Lumbo sacral spinal fibrosis. Its diagnosis and treatment by spinal cord stimulation. *Spine*, **8**, 593–603.

Dourish, C. T. (1990) The selective CCK-B receptor antagonist L365260 enhances morphine analgesia and prevents morphine tolerance in rat. *European Journal of Pharmacology*, **176**, 35–44.

Dray, A. (1990) NE 19550 and NE21610 antinociceptive capsaicin analogues: a study on nociceptive fibres of the neonatal rat tail in vitro. *European Journal of Pharmacology*, **181**, 289–93.

Duthie, D. J. R., Rowbotham, D. J. and Wyld, R. (1988) Plasma fentanyl concentrations during transdermal delivery of fentanyl to surgical patients. *British Journal of Anaesthesia* **60**, 614–18.

Edwards, M., Serrao, J. M., Gent, J. P., *et al.* (1990) On the mechanism by which midazolam causes spinally mediated analgesia. *Anaesthesiology*, **73**, 273–7.

Ellis, W. V. (1990) Octreotide, a small peptide, alleviates burning pain and hyperaesthesia: a preliminary study. *The Pain Clinic*, **3**, 239–42.

Elomaa, I., Kylmalat, Tammelat, *et al.* (1992) Effect of oral Clodronate on bone pain. *International Urology and Nephrology*, **24**, 159–66.

Flor, H., Fydrich, T. and Turk, D. C. (1992) Efficacy of multidisciplinary pain treatment centres: a meta-analytic review. *Pain* **49**, 221–30.

Foong, F. W. and Nakagawa, N. (1990) A novel enkephalinase inhibitor as an orally active analgesic. *Pain*, **35**, 5198.

Fozzard, J. (1990) 5HT in migraine – evidence from 5HT receptor antagonists for a neuronal aetiology, in *Migraine: a Spectrum of Ideas*, (eds M. Sandler and G Collins), Oxford University Press, London, pp. 154–32.

Glynn, C. G., McQuay, J. J. and Lloyd, J. W. (1984) Intrathecal buprenorphine for painful muscle spasms in paraplegic patients. *Pain* **52**, 5341.

Grant, I. S., Nimmo, W. S. and Clements J. A. (1981) Pharmacokinetics and analgesic effects of I M and oral ketamine. *British Journal of Anaesthesia*, **53**, 805–9.

Hoskin, P. J., Hanks, G. W., Aherne, G. W. *et al.* (1989) The bioavailability and pharmacokinetics of morphine after intravenous, oral and buccal administration in healthy volunteers. *British Journal of Clinical Pharmacology*, **27**, 499–505.

Hughes, J. and Smith H. W. (1975) Identification of two related pentapeptide enkephalins with potent opioid agonist activity. *Nature*, **258**, 577–9.

Humphrey, P. P. A., and Feniuk, W. (1991) Mode of action of the anti-migraine drug Sumatriptan. *Trends in Pharmacological Science*, **12**, 444–6.

Jessel, T. M., Inversen, L. L. and Cuello, A. C. (1978) Capsaicin induced depletion of SP from primary sensory neurons. *Brain Research*, **152**, 132–88.

Kauppila, T., Kemppainene, P., Tanila, H. *et al.* (1991) Effect of systemic medetomidine, an alpha 2 adrenoreceptor agonist, on experimental pain in man. *Anaesthesiology*, **74**, 3–8.

Leslie, S. T. (1981) Continuous controlled release preparations. *British Journal of Clinical Practice*, **10**, 5–8.

Lunec, J. and Halloran, S. P. (1981) Free radical oxidation products in serum and synovial fluid in rheumatoid arthritis. *Journal of Rheumatology*, **8**, 233–3.

Lynn, B. (1990) Capsaicin: actions on nociceptive C fibres on therapeutic potential. *Pain*, **41**, 61–9.

Mandel, A. K. and Herbert, L. A. (1990) Renal diseases. *Medical Clinics of North America*, **74**, 909–17.

Mannheimer, C., Augustinsson, L. E., Carlsson, C. A. *et al.* (1988) Epidural spinal electrical stimulation in severe angina pectoris. *European Heart Journal*, **59**, 56–61.

Miles, J. B. (1992) Electrical stimulation of the spinal cord in peripheral vascular disease. *British Medical Journal*, **304**, 1313.

Monks, R. and Merskey, H. (1989) Psychotropic drugs, in *Textbook of Pain*, 2nd Edition (eds P. D. Wall and R. Melzack) Churchill Livingstone, London, pp. 702–21.

Nagaska, H. and Yaksh, T. L. (1990) Pharmacology of intrathecal adrenergic agonists. *Anesthesiology*, **73**, 1198–207.

Noble, F. and Coric, P. (1990) Analgesic properties of systematically active mixed enkephaline-degrading enzyme inhibitors, in *New Leads in Opioid Research* (ed. J. M. Van Rec), Exerpta Medica, Amsterdam, pp. 83–6.

Pearce, J. M. S. (1992) Sumatriptan: efficacy and contribution to migraine mechanisms. *Journal of Neurology, Neurosurgery and Psychiatry*, **55**, 1103–5.

Pfeiffer, A. and Brantl. V. (1986) Psychotomimesis mediated by the K receptor. *Science*, **233**, 774–6.

Piomelli, D. and Grengard, P. (1990) Lipoxygenase metabolites of arachidonic acid in neurone transmembrane signalling. *Trends in Neuro Sciences* **11**, 367–73.

Sabanathan, S. S., Mearns, A. J., Bickford-Smith, P. J. *et al.* (1990) Efficacy of continuous extrapleural intercostal block on post thoracotomy pain and pulmonary mechanisms. *British Journal of Surgery*, **77**, 221–5.

Serrado, J. M., Marks, R. L., Morley, P. J. *et al.* (1992) Intrathecal Midazolam for the treatment of chronic mechanical low back pain. *Pain*, **48**, 5–11.

Shatin, D., Mullett, K., and Hults, G. (1986) Totally implantable spinal cord stimulation for chronic pain: design and efficacy. *Pace*, **9**, 577–83.

Sinrup, S. H., Gram, L. F., Brusen, K. *et al.* (1990) The selective serotonin reuptake inhibitor paroxetine is effective in the treatment of diabetic neuropathy symptoms. *Pain*, **42**, 135–44.

Sosnowski, M. and Yaksh, T. L. (1989) Role of spinal adenosine receptors in modulating the hyperaesthesia produced by spinal glycine receptor antagonism. *Anesthesia and Analgesia* **69**, 587–92.

Steranka, L. P. and Manning, D. C. (1988) Bradykinin as a pain mediator: receptors are localized to sensory neurons and antagonists have analgesic action. *Proceedings of the National Academy of Science USA*, **85**, 3245–9.

Striebel, H. W., Koenigs, D., Kramer, J. (1992) Postoperative pain management by intranasal demand – adapted fentanyl titration. *Anesthesiology*, **77**, 281–5.

Theesen, K. A. and Marsh, W. F. (1989) Relief of diabetic neuropathy with fluoxetine. *The Annals of Pharmacotherapy*, **23**, 572–4.

Vescovi, P. and Passeri, M. (1987) Naloxone inhibits the early phase of diclofenac analgesia in man. *The Pain Clinic*, **1**, 151–5.

Watson, C. P. N., Evans, R. J. and Wath, V. R. (1988) Post herpetic neuralgia and topical capsaicin. *Pain*, **33**, 333–40.

Woolf, C. J. and Thompson, S. W. N. (1991) The induction and maintenance of central sensitization is dependent on NMDA receptor activation: implications for the treatment of post injury pain hypersensitivity states. *Pain*, **44**, 293–9.

Woolf, C. J. (1989) Recent advances in the pathophysiology of pain. *British Journal of Anaesthesia*, **63**, 139–46.

Wotherspoon, H. A., Henny, G. N. C. and McArdle, C. S. (1992) Analgesic efficacy of controlled release dihydrocodeine. *Anaesthesia*, **46**, 915–17.

CHAPTER 4

Pain assessment, management and research: the nurse's role

Laurel Archer Copp

The pain grew intense again, like some huge grizzly bear taking me between its paws. I screamed from the sheer shock of its sudden violence. But there was nothing I could do to stop myself shrieking, feeling that if I bore the agony a moment longer it would split my skin.

Denton Welch (De-la-Noy, 1986)

4.1 THE PAIN EXPERIENCE

It is the nature and context of the pain experience itself that must be understood before roles, reactions, and responses of physicians, dentists, nurses, and family members can become therapeutic. How can pain behaviours be interpreted unless we have studied non-pain behaviours? How can we properly interpret the pain experience if there is no working knowledge of illness behaviours and health behaviours?

Since pain is a subjective experience, and only the experiencer can translate and interpret it, we seek the repositories of that knowledge. In effect, it is 'going to school' to the pain patient through a deeper understanding of self-image, coping strategies, self-report, and the individual's search for meaning of this experience.

4.2 SELF-IMAGE

4.2.1 Victim

Many persons see pain as all-powerful, and themselves as at the mercy of this overwhelming force. They describe the pain as merciless, irrational, continuous, and overwhelming. They report their self-situ-

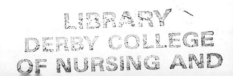

ation as fragile, helpless, dread-filled, abandoned, and suffering (Copp, 1985). Coping consists of scepticism, fate, ritual, and magical thinking.

What is wanted of the staff? As with all responses to the pain experience, the patients want the staff to 'make the pain go away'. But they are sceptical that anything or anyone can actually help. What is needed is hope, empowerment, and learning more effective coping strategies. But since pain is omnipotent in the judgement of some patients, they often turn away the help offered. Until the staff can prove themselves as equally powerful as pain itself and imbue the pain patient with that power, some patients sink into disillusionment and even depression.

4.2.2 Soldier

The pain experience for some is one of seeing pain as strong, sharp, dominating, episodic, and testing. As a result they themselves become a soldier. These individuals say they must 'fight it', and they resolve, 'I am going to beat it this time!' They see themselves as fighter, coper, survivor, soldier, and confronter. They cope through muscle language, counter-pain, and aligning themselves with an armamentorium which can be used to make their fight against pain more effective.

What do persons having this pain experience expect of staff? Action. It is clear to them that the pain is coming. They wonder how can the staff 'stand around' and not mobilize to this personal emergency when pain is on the way or at hand. Soldiers give orders and estimate the exact time of pain's arrival. The staff may respond to the emergency for which the soldier is relieved and appreciative. The staff may balk at being told what to do, or even to be told to 'do something!' Negative-minded staff respond by being resentful, punishing, and withholding. The soldier fights harder – fighting both pain and staff.

4.2.3 Seeker/thinker

For this group of pain patients, the pain may be a reality, the power of which is put on a life–death significance continuum. For these individuals pain seems to be testing, demanding, hidden, mysterious, cosmic. They see themselves as confronting, suffering, and enduring. Their pain experience requires coping through focusing, meditating, and searching for meaning. That experience continues long after the pain has abated. Expression of the pain experience is compelling and these individuals often attempt to put their pain into words, art, music, written diaries, and poetry. These individuals particularly dwell on the 'why questions'. Why me? Why now? Why? They may describe pain as a turning point in their lives, or continue to capture insight from their pain experience.

4.2.4 Watcher/waiter

The pain experience for some individuals is a vigil waiting for pain which they believe may invade them at any time. They see pain as cunning, and they must be on duty to intercept it. What do they expect of staff? They cannot trust them to keep the vigil and ward off pain. Taking hypnotics, tranquillizers, or analgesics might help the pain but it would cloud their vigilance and put them at a disadvantage with sneaking, stealthy pain. Therefore, they do not ask for analgesics, which is interpreted by staff that they have no pain. For them, pain is hidden, faceless, and sly. It is degrading and may invade at any time. Therefore, they must monitor, wait, watch, and be ready. Their coping consists of pain anticipation, rehearsal, looking for early warning signals. They wait for pain to come, go, and come again. They prefer not to risk, and their fear compels them to suffer the same way in subsequent pain experiences.

4.2.5 Consumer

For these individuals the pain is demanding and they must put themselves in an environment in which pain relief is a service provided by the staff and is part of the belief system. Sometimes this is advertised, sometimes not, but the consumer expects the staff to stand by him or her and provide the relief promised. He sees pain as intense, persistent, sharp, ill-tempered, and treacherous. But he sees himself as a reasonable person: cooperator, collaborator, communicator, and one able to make contracts with the staff for pain control. What does he expect from staff? He copes through bonding with staff, setting limits, arranging for contractual agreements, and he expects to play by the rules if the staff will do the same. He doesn't suffer fools easily, and discharges himself from settings where his pain needs are not met. But when he and staff members provide service of pain-reduction, and do it on time, he bonds with the staff, and advertises their skills to others.

There are many sub-sets in the pain typologies in which these are only a few and the most recurring. Pain is a personal response. Each person in pain has a right to his own experience. He does not wish to counter stories from other patients or staff about 'his pain' or 'their operations'. Pain has left a mark on him. It does not fade immediately or easily.

4.3 Pain assessment in adults

Artist and writer, Denton Welch, could assess his own pain and communicate its urgency in exquisite words now in print. But at the time the pain overwhelmed him even into wordlessness.

Pain assessment, part of everyone's responsibility, often critically falls to the nurse who may be doing the initial pain assessment. 'The nurse may be the first health-care provider to encounter the person experiencing pain as well as to identify the problem of uncontrolled pain.' The Consensus Conference defined the role of the nurse in these ways: Examples of the types of interventions that should be provided by the generalist nurse include: (a) preoperative patient education to lessen postoperative pain; (b) nursing care plans that reflect individual medication based on individual preference and activity schedules; and (c) implementation of nonpharmacological methods during acutely painful events such as childbirth, burn wound debridement and diagnostic tests. The role of the nurse with advanced preparation should include: (a) clinical management responsibilities such as titration of analgesics within a protocol according to the patient's level of analgesia, assessment, and participation in the use of both pharmacological and non-pharmacological modalities; (b) provision of consultation and education services to other members of the nursing staff, other providers, and community groups; and (c) active participation in research (National Institutes of Health 1987). Perhaps for this reason there is much research activity in the area of pain assessment. And because verbal and non-verbal communication of pain cues are open to a variety of interpretations, the community of professionals strives for some reliable method of pain assessment in which words and concepts are used in the same way repeated amongst and between persons in pain. The nurse needs to be making and recording an initial pain assessment on the order developed by Johnson which includes characteristics of pain, pain responses, pain communication, coping techniques, factors that can affect pain, and sources that should be used in assessing pain (Johnson, 1977).

Copp urges both a pain history and a pain coping history be used in initial assessments in order to augment already developed sustaining inner resources as well as to help staff members understand the individuality of the patient's own pain experience. Congruent with the pain history is the necessity of a pain-coping history. In learning how patients explicate their pain, verbally, non-verbally, using extrinsic coping mechanisms, or internal coping mechanisms, provides insight into how the pain experience is being negotiated, psychologically. When working with the patient to develop a pain-journal or diary, the enormity of the invasion of pain into the person's life becomes apparent, as do the patterns of pain recurrence. This is especially pragmatic when interacting with persons in episodic pain or the chronic pain patient with multiple hospital admission (Copp, 1990a).

In many settings the McGill Pain Questionnaire is the tool of choice for both research and pain management. It is used by professional nurses in pain research as well as in pain management. Chapman, *et al*. (1985) and others, encourage its use for obtaining both qualitative and quantitative pain data. As the literature substantiates, it is used for research and therapy goals, and assists in the bridging of understanding by the selection of sensory, evaluative, and effective words (Melzack, 1987). In reviewing research in the official publication of the International Association for the Study of Pain, the McGill pain questionnaire appears most consistently. Nurse Mary Ellen Jeans, Melzack, and colleagues studied a new method of scoring which better addresses chronic pain (Melzack, Katz and Jeans, 1985).

Nursing pain assessment was comprehensively researched by Meinhart and McCaffery (1983) who posed general guidelines to the assessment process. They include

- An overall assessment of the patient's pain problem, subjective and objective, identifying how these characteristics affect the patient.
- The pain of intervention including specific pain measures is then formulated.
- After implementation an evaluation points to ongoing assessment or reassessment.

Many of the assessment tools as well as those which measure various aspects of pain are abandoned by health-care providers in the pressure of the clinical setting but L. McGuire's Pain Assessment Tool, a brief one-page assessment, enables pain data to be gathered in a systematic manner, even in a busy hospital (McGuire, 1981). McGuire (1984) like other nurses–researchers has both researched clinical pain management, and developed a tool for assessing the patient's pain, including larger dimensions of setting and circumstance.

Of vital importance is the practice of all staff members agreeing upon and using at least one pain measurement tool. For this reason such tools as the Memorial Pain Assessment Card, developed by and for Memorial Sloan-Kettering Cancer Center, have proven successful. It is easy to administer, and provides such data as a pain adjective rating scale, pain intensity, pain relief and mood rating scale. The use of a universal or hospital-wide tool, enhances pain communication between patient and staff as well as amongst staff members.

Visual analogue scales are being used more consistently and comprehensively in all settings. By simply putting his finger on a horizontal or vertical line ranging from no pain to most pain, the patient can quantify his pain. When the line is numerically calibrated from 1 to 10, he also assigns a number to his pain which can be compared to numbers in other assessments by nurses at various times of the day or night. Some scales also use a spectrum of colours coinciding with each numerical gradation. In some cases this simple tool is used alone, and in other it is but one of several pain-assessment tools given together.

McCaffery and Beebe (1989), in their considerable work on pain and practice, have developed a pain flow sheet. The value of this document on the patient's chart is that it provides a record and monitoring mechanism of the patient's pain over time. It is available for staff on all shifts. For reference by any staff member are the following data: time, pain rating (number on the visual analogue scale or the number associated with the patient's self-report of his pain), analgesics, respiration, pulse, blood pressure, level of arousal, other (aspects of greatest concern such as vomiting, constipation, clouded sensorium) and plan (actions to be taken).

Such formalization of the assessment process provides documentation to compare pain trends, note patterns of episodic pain, and pain trajectories which may be traced.

Donovan (1987) targets nursing research and management by emphasizing clinial assessment of cancer pain. Disquietingly, she states that all too often, doctors and nurses not only omit using the most simple of assessment tools, but they may not even ask the patient if he or she is in pain! (Donovan, 1989). Therefore opportunities for pain monitoring are lost and bases for comparisons and calculation of pain trajectories are also overlooked.

Pain assessment is inextricably related to quality of life. Therefore, in the Ferrell questionnaire, patients in pain may also give staff insight into their personal world. In asking items about physical well-being and psychosocial well-being, patients in pain may provide the nurse with a wider scope of insight into the ways pain impacts their total life (Ferrell, Wisdon and Wenzl, 1989).

4.4 ASSESSMENT OF CHILDREN'S PAIN

'Don't Bump My Bed!
Don't Touch My Feet.'

(Caswell and Eland, 1989)

The pain experience in children is only now being understood. Professionals denied that children could and did have pain, and some studies have shown that children receive but a small fraction of analgesics compared to adults with the same surgeries. In the past children often received no pain medications.

Eland and Anderson were the first nurse researchers in the USA to develop pain tools for children (Eland and Anderson, 1977). Eland's colour tool is a technique where the child in pain not only colours in a drawing of a child's body where the pain is, but is provided with an opportunity to communicate the intensity of the pain by standardized use of the colour crayons selected to 'colour the pain'. Associated work by Stewart (1977), provided colour choices and wheels in the Stewart Pain Colour Scale.

Beyer copyrighted 'the Oucher Scale' in which older children can select the pain facial characteristics with which to indicate their own pain intensity (Beyer, 1989).

In her nursing research Hester developed assessment tools which are used with children. Hester's Poker Chip Tool instructs children to rate their own pain by thinking of the chips as 'pieces of hurt' (Hester, 1990).

Part of the initial pain assessment is taking a pain history. Too often we think of the patient as representing a *tabula rasa* when in fact there may have been a long history of 'this pain,' or 'other pains' or 'recurring pain' or, in fact, of multiple problems which produce multiple pain phenomena. It is rare to have a single problem patient. What is more common is for a patient to have both acute and chronic pain even simultaneously. Examples include a person with long-term rheumatoid arthritis suddenly having acute pain indicative of kidney stone. Or, conversely, a patient with acute appendicitis identified as a young person with sickle cell anaemia and its attendant painful episodes.

Assessment tools can themselves be thought of as researchable. However, the assessment tool in management of care is a communication bridge btween the patient's pain experience and the effort made by nurses, doctors, and other staff to meet his pain needs (Eland, 1988).

4.5 PAIN MANAGEMENT

Pain is a bond between nurse and patient. Pain management is a pact between them. All too often the physician does not hear the pleading as he exercises his option to leave the scene. The patient and nurse cannot leave – as much as both may like to do so. How they work out pain management agreeable to both is the essence of nursing care.'

(Copp, 1990b)

The role of the nurse as assessor of the patient's pain is paramount to care. Perceptions by others of the patient's pain present professional and social 'filters' which often contribute to poor care and poor prescribing. The physician depends on the nurse's assessment. If the patient cries 'this is the worst pain I have ever endured' and the nurse reports it as 'the patient seems to be somewhat uncomfortable', every juncture of the decision tree in diagnosis and treatment is affected.

Furthermore, the physician, knowingly or unknowingly, may be sending wrong signals to the staff through his practice of prescribing analgesics. When he or she orders very little pain medication, the nursing staff may assume the patient is not in pain or 'shouldn't' be in pain. If the physician orders opioid analgesics, the nursing staff may be alerted to the patient's pain potential, but the patient still may not be achieving adequate pain control and is therefore mismanaged.

In the insightful original study and its eventual follow-up and replication, Marks and Sachar (1973) described the consistent under-prescribing of analgesia by physicians. In researching colleague nurses, Cohen (1980) learned that of these already too few medications, nurses gave only a portion of analgesics they were authorized to administer.

Why is pain medication withheld when it is not only in our power to reduce the patient's pain, but in most cases it is also possible to alleviate pain and to prevent pain? One answer is that health-professionals hold an uneducated opinion about the risk of addiction. Their irrational fears are unsubstantiated by many studies showing the addiction risk is less than 1% of pain patients unless they were previous drug abusers (Porter and Jick, 1980). Referring to Melzack, 'Contrary to popular belief', the author says, 'morphine taken solely to control pain is not addictive. Yet patients worldwide continue to be undertreated and to suffer unnecessary agony' (Melzack, 1990).

In two follow-up studies, it was confirmed that the average dose of narcotics was still below therapeutic levels, and that the average dose taken by the patient was from one-fourth to one-third of that which was ordered (Donovan, Dillion and McGuire, 1987). Only close monitoring and improved communication and practice between the triad of nurse, physician, and patient, can reverse this negligence. It is particularly troublesome that a few physicians and nurses who are responsible for pain management of hospitalized patients have neither commitment nor insight into pain alleviation practices so available by today's varied methods. But those with hospice experience or holding hospice beliefs about basic pain relief often assist hospital staff to risk change and demonstrate that it is only when the pain is reduced that the patient can communicate, rest, and heal effectively.

Practices of PRN administration of analgesics have many unfortunate effects. There are many reasons to avoid the roller-coaster trajectory of recurring pain. (By this is meant the build-up of pain to an intolerable level, getting relief with an analgesic injection, followed by the build up of pain to an intolerable level again.) One is the failure to attain a proper blood level of medication which can be achieved by even modest analgesics if titrated (Sofear, 1992). Another is to avoid a pain-anxiety cycle (Jones, 1987).

In the management of the patient's pain, the nurse must correct his or her nursing practice related to 'PRN' analgesics. As is needed, according to whom? When there is no anticipation of continuing pain and continual reassessment, the patient is required to wait for pain to return, and must make a demand for medication. The practices of 'on demand' puts the patient in a supplicant role unnecessarily. Guilt is added to his anxiety and his pain.

He often admits he 'stood it as long as he could' before asking. The patient often apologizes for his pain, for his need of relief, and 'doesn't want to bother the busy nurses.' Fagerhaugh and Strauss (1977) describe that part of the politics of pain as an overvaluing of 'ward work' which is given precedence over pain work and accountability. Some patients will never ask, because of a stoic philosophy or cultural conditioning. Many patients go home not having had pain medications because no nurse ever inquired about their pain nor informed them there was a pain medication ordered for them. Pain management is one of the many services the patient pays for and has the right to expect.

Patient-controlled analgesia is practised in increasingly wide settings, using a variety of modes. This can range from patients taking their own oral analgesics at the bedside after surgery (Jones, 1987) or through PCA pumps, and it is the area of study for some nurse researchers (King, *et al.*, 1987). Patient controlled analgesia should not be thought of as a way to lessen responsible nursing care or patient supervision. The nurse is alert for signs of tolerance or break-through pain. Vigilance must be exercised by the professional nurse to assess if the dose is correct, if the drug is effective, and if the route of administration is the most desirable. There must be instruction and reassurance ready for both patient and family. The nurse is also responsible for documentation of these estimates, using a pain flow chart or similar tool, thus assessment and nursing care are inextricable in proper pain management.

The role of the nurse in pain management is certainly not confined to administration of analgesics. Other roles include nurse as: intervenor, patient-educator, therapist or implementor of therapy, evaluator of therapy, negotiator, advocate, care planner/giver, and pain communicator (Copp, 1987).

Walker and Campbell (1988) remind us of holistic approaches to pain assessment and the nursing process. Akinsanya asserts that 'pain and nursing are inextricably linked because the assessment and management of the pain process is one of the many functions of the nurse' (Akinsanya, 1980).

4.6   WHEN DOES PAIN BECOME SUFFERING?

As one moves through stages of pain research, what is discovered are basic false assumptions. Simplistically, one supposes that a little pain is 'hurt'. Moving into greater pain one might suppose that 'pain is pain'. Next, one might suppose that 'great pain is suffering'. Suffering persons teach us that although it may be, it is not necessarily so.

Therefore, some patients in great pain agree they are suffering. Yet, others in similar situations deny suffering. Suffering becomes a construct, formed by a number of vital concepts, each of which have valences of varying power depending on the individual life experiences of the sufferer.

Experientially, suffering seems to be made up of (at least) some ten concepts. These include: pain, vulnerability, dehumanization, self-concept, coping, mind-body relationships, outcome, time, space, and stress (Copp, 1990c). That is to say that when pain is superimposed on any of these other conditions, it exacerbates the condition into ultimate suffering. And in every case the sufferer wears cultural, philosophical, and religious 'glasses' through which he sees his own human condition.

Contrary to popular democratic opinion, all men are not born equal. Vulnerability of babies *in utero*, by virtue of genetic problems, AIDS, or crack cocaine, meant that nurses can see children born with pain or into pain. Other sources of vulnerability, such as trauma, disease, ageing, or death, combine with pain to exhibit great suffering.

Dehumanization such as in concentration camps flourishes today. Furthermore, pain and torture are used today for political ends, in a variety of countries, even as this sentence is being read (Scarry, 1985).

Self-Concept and coping we have dealt with, though very briefly. One speculates about the power of Cartesian dualism which seems to fuse with time and space reinforcers, making it unfortunately real to us some decades later. We speak of patients' physical needs, psychological needs, cognitive needs, etc., with only occasional concern for interaction of the whole person.

Outcome has a power of its own. If the pain of labour produces a healthy child, pain is minimized retrospectively in halo vision. But, conversely, if the pathology tests prove cancer, the suffering of dread may propel us more surely towards ultimate suffering and death, depending on our conception of ourselves and that which is real.

Time is perhaps the greatest exacerbator of suffering – moving pain towards suffering with such a rush that it is easily seen in the waiting room or in the coronary care unit. The pain patient soon learns the difference between chronological time, psychological time, linear time, and the suffering of waiting (Dossey, 1982).

Space, inner and outer, gives us a kind of spatial reality with pain. Pain comes and goes, the nurse brings pain with him/her, or pushes the patient towards or away from pain, literally and symbolically. As patients have reported to this writer, 'I am exhausted from having pain chase me around all day – I want so much to rest'. Or, 'It isn't until I go through pain and come out the other side, that I get any relief from my suffering.'

Autton urges us to values and states 'a patient in pain needs to be helped to create his own *personal meaning* and to integrate his suffering with his personal goals and values (Autton, 1986).

Cassell urges us to compassion and speaks of four ways in which suffering can be altered. They include:

- living entirely in the present because suffering requires anticipating a feared future;
- suffering can be altered by development of total indifference to what is happening;
- denial is a third strategy that permits people not to suffer in circumstances where they might otherwise live in misery;
- that suffering can be relieved or prevented, also highlights how individual differences in the nature of persons are crucial in determining whether suffering will occur (Cassell, 1991).

The voice of nursing related to suffering comes through the writings of Starck and McGovern (1992) and Kahn and Steeves (1986) who urge us to the meaning of suffering. Of course we cannot forget the foundation of understanding given us by Frankl (1959) about suffering, and through his own suffering. This is the meaning of self-transcendence.

4.7 COMMITMENT TO PAIN CONTROL

Some improvement in attention to the pain-needs of all persons is being documented. The American Pain Society and the International Association For the Study of Pain have been striving for pain management practice guidelines for accredited hospitals/medical centres by Hospital Quality Assurances Committee (American Pain Society, 1990). Some correction factors for the astonishing dearth of pain-management content in the curricula of Schools of Medicine and Schools of Nursing in North America and the United Kingdom have also been documented. Recent publications on acute pain management have been disseminated throughout the USA by the Department of Health and Human Services (Agency for Health Care Policy and Research, 1992).

The commitment seems more established in bringing comfort to cancer patients. The World Health Organization accepted a commitment to cancer pain-management as one of their major initiatives as is reflected in their action and literature (World Health Organization, 1986). Additionally, individual states have followed the historic Wisconsin Initiative For Improving Cancer Pain Management (Joranson and Engber, 1986).

The position paper of the Oncology Nursing Society reflects a resolve of cancer nurses to incorporate pain control, reduction, and alleviation as a primary part of their nursing care (Oncology Nursing Society, 1991).

Pain control is a professional responsibility, be it in acute or chronic pain, in the unaddressed pain related to diagnostic procedures, or iatrogenic practices. But we also have an ethical responsibility for pain management. All health-science professionals acknowledge some alignment with the ethical principles of non-malfeasance and beneficence, responsibility and judgement, autonomy, competence, veracity, justice, and patient advocacy (Copp, 1993). However, to have the ability, science, and opportunity to control a patient's pain and to choose (by omission or commission) not to do so, places responsbility for unethical practice on the person and licence of most health-professionals. Unfortunately the ethics of practice seem not as compelling as potential fear of litigation, an unfortunate endstage of some persons' pain experience.

4.8 THE PAIN RESEARCH AGENDA

A refreshing diversity of approaches to pain inquiry is being pursued in research and clinical settings by nurses and others. Those posing researchable questions seem to dwell on certain areas, enhancing the quest for a critical mass of data. However, conversely, the under-represented areas lie dormant with uneven and unaddressed problems which seem to be cyclically discovered and forgotten in the research agenda.

To be specific and to provide context, these domains of inquiry (Copp, 1987) are in part reviewed and listed below:

- Pain specifics
  Pain cognition and transmission mechanisms;
  Pain and organ or body part;
  Pain and disease;
  Pain and trauma;
  Pain and body systems.

- Pain theory and measurement
  Pain theories;
  Cause and effect;
  Mind-body relationships;
  Pain assessment;
  Pain measurement.

- Pain management
  Pain assessment and reassessment;
  Pharmacological interventions;
  Non-pharmacological interventions;
  Multidisciplinary approaches;
  Diagnostic pain;
  Pain associated with treatment.

- Quality assessment
  Quality of care;
  Efficacy of care settings;
  Pain policies.

- Human responses to pain
  Pain coping;
  Pain in Special populations (age, need, circumstance);
  Suffering;
  Pain behaviours;
  Pain and gender;
  Pain expression in the humanities.

- Pain and values
  Anthropological indicators;
  Sociological Indicators;
  Pain, values, ethics, and belief systems;
  Pain purposes and meaning;
  Pain policy and litigation;
  Pain politics;
  Pain economics.

- Prevention of pain
  Pain prevention strategies;
  Pain and education;
  Epidemiology of pain;
  Pain and those at special risk.

- Pain and social responsibility
  Iatrogenic pain;
  Pain caused by environment;
  Pain caused by natural events and disasters;
  Pain caused by man-made error;
  Pain caused by intent (war and torture);
  Pain advocacy and social action.

In reviewing the many approaches to pain research, one is aware of the diversity of investigators, as well as the wealth of backgrounds they bring to problems in pain. They have been educated in different disciplines, read a variety of professional journals, negotiate pain language, yet have at least one thing in common: they are striving to know more about pain and the human condition. For these reasons there are more productive approaches to pain research which free scholars from disciplinary roles and stereotypes, and join them conceptually. There are nurses working in all of the categories listed above, some alone, some in teams of nurse researchers, others in multidisciplinary research. But these research efforts enhance the communication of the sole experiencer of pain, the patient. Through these diverse approaches to pain research, the person in pain has a better chance of gaining our understanding.

REFERENCES

Agency For Health Care Policy and Research (1992) *Clinical Practice Guidelines for Acute Pain Management: Operative or Medical Procedures and Trauma*, Department of Human Services Public Health Service, 1, Rockville, Maryland.

Akinsanya, J.A. (1980) The biological sciences in nursing education. *Nursing Times*, March 6, 427–32.

American Pain Society Subcommittee on Quality Assurance Standards (1990) *Oncology Nursing Forum*, **17**(6), 952–4.

Autton, N. (1986) *Pain, An Exploration*, Darton, Longman and Todd, London, pp. 130–1.

Beyer, J. E. (1989) The Oucher Scale: a pain intensity scale for children, in *Key Aspects of Comfort*, (eds S.G. Funk, E.M. Tornquist, M.P. Champagne *et al.*), Springer Co., New York, pp. 65–71.

Cassell, E. J. (1991) *The Nature of Suffering and the Goals Of Medicine*, Oxford University Press, Oxford, pp. 59–61.

Caswell, J. L. and Eland J.M. (1989) Don't bump my bed, don't touch my feet. *Journal of Pediatric Oncology Nursing*, **6**(4), 111–20.

Chapman, D. D., Casey, K.L., Dubner, R. *et al.* (1985) Pain Measurement: An Overview. *Pain*, **22**, 1–31.

Cohen, F. L. (1980) Postsurgical pain relief: patients' status and nurses' medication choices. *Pain*, **9**(2), 265–74.

Copp, L. A. (1985) Pain coping, in *Perspectives on Pain*, (ed L. Copp), Churchill Livingstone, Edinburgh, pp. 3–16, 49.

Copp, L. A. (1987) The role of the nurse in chronic pain management, in *Handbook of Chronic Pain Management*, (eds G. D. Burrows, D. Elton, and G. V. Stanley), Elsevier, Amsterdam, pp. 227–39.

Copp, L. A. (1990 a) Pain diaries, journals, and logs. *Orthopedic Nursing*, **9**(2), 37–9.

Copp, L. A. (1990 b) The patient in pain: USA Nursing Research, in *Nursing Research for Nursing Practice: An International Perspective*, (ed. R. Bergman), Croom Helm, London, pp. 131, 125.

Copp, L. A. (1990 c) The nature and prevention of suffering. *Journal of Professional Nursing*, **6**(5), 247–9.

Copp, L. A. (1993) An ethical responsibility for pain management. *Journal of Advanced Nursing*, **18**(1), 1–2.

De-la-Noy, S. Y. (1986) *The Making of a Writer*, Penguin Books, London, p. 98.

Donovan, M. I. (1987) Clinical assessment of cancer pain, in *Cancer Pain Management*. (eds. D.B. McGuire and C.H. Yarboro), Grune and Stratton Co., New York, pp. 105–31.

Donovan, M.I. (1989) Relieving the pain: the current bases for practice, in *Key Aspects of Comfort*, (eds, S.G. Funk, E.M. Tornquist, M.P. Champagne, *et al.*), Springer Co., New York, pp. 25–31.

Donovan, M.I., Dillion, P. and McGuire, D. (1987) Incidents and characteristics of pain in a sample of medical-surgical inpatients. *Pain*, 30, 69–78.

Dossey, L. (1982). *Space, Time, and Medicine*. Shambhala Co., Boulder, Colorado, pp. 45–55.

Eland, J. and Anderson, A. (1977) The experience of pain in children, in *Pain: A Source Book For Nurses and Other Health Professionals*, (ed A. Jacox), Brown Co., Boston, pp. 453–73.

Eland, J. (1988) Persistence in pediatric pain research: One nurse researcher's efforts. *Recent Advances In Nursing*, Churchill Livingstone, Edinburgh, pp. 43–62.

Fagerhaugh, S. Y. and Strauss, A. (1977) *Politics of Pain Management: Staff-Patient Interaction*. Addison-Wesley Co., Menlo Park, California, p. 244.

Ferrell, B., Wisdon, C. and Wenzl, C. (1989) Quality of life as an outcome variable in management of cancer pain. *Cancer*, **63**, 2321–9.

Frankl, V. E. (1959) *Man's Search For Meaning: An Introduction*, Beacon Press, New York, pp. 3–10.

Hester, N. O. (1990) Measuring children's pain: The convergent and discriminant validity of the pain ladder and the poker chip tool. *Journal of Pain and Symptom Management*, **4**, S6.

Johnson, M. (1977) Assessment of clinical pain, in *Pain: A Source Book For Nurses and Other Health Professionals* (ed A. Jacox), Little, Brown, Co., Boston, pp. 139–66.

Jones, L. (1987) Patient-controlled oral analgesia. *Nursing Research*, **6**(1), 38–41.

Joranson, D. E. and Engber, D. (1986) Wisconsin Initiative For Improving Cancer Pain Management: Progress Report. *Journal of Pain and Symptom Management*, **4**, 246.

Kahn, D. L. and Steeves, R. H. (1986) The experience of suffering: conceptual clarification and theoretical definition. *Journal of Advanced Nursing*, **11**, 623–31.

King, K. B., Norsen, L. G., Robertson, R. K. and Hicks, G. L. (1987) Patient management of pain medication after cardiac surgery, *Nursing Research*, 36 (3), 145–50.

Marks, R. M. and Sachar, E. J. (1973) Undertreatment of medical inpatients with narcotic analgesics. *Annals of Internal Medicine*, **78**, 173–81.

McCafferey, M. and Beebe, A. (1989) *Pain: Clinical Manual For Nursing Practice*, Mosby Co., St. Louis, pp. 27–32.

McGuire, D. (1984) The measurement of clinical pain. *Nursing Research*, **33**, 153–256.

McGuire, L. (1981) A short, simple tool for assessing your patient's pain, *Nursing 81*, **11**, 48–9.

Meinhart, N.T. and McCaffery, M. (1983) *Pain: A Nursing Approach To Assessment and Analysis*. Appleton-Century Crofts Co., Norwalk, Conn. pp. 350–60.

Melzack, R. (1987) The McGill pain questionnaire: major properties and scoring methods. *Pain*, **1**, 275–99.

Melzack, R. (1990) The tragedy of needless pain. *Scientific American* **262** (2), 27–33.

Melzack, R., Katz, J. and Jeans, M.E. (1985) The role of compensation in chronic pain: analysis using a new method of scoring the McGill pain questionnaire. *Pain*. 23, 101–12.

National Institutes of Health (1987) The integrated approach to the management of pain. National Institutes of Health consensus development conference. *Journal of Pain and Symptom Management*, **2**(1), 35–44.

Oncology Nursing Society (1991) For position paper write to Oncology Nursing Society, 501 Holiday Drive, Pittsburgh, Pa 15220–2749.

Porter, J. and Jick, H. (1980) Addiction rare in patients treated with narcotics. *New England Journal of Medicine*, **302**, 123.

Scarry, E. (1985) *The Body in Pain. The Making and Unmaking of the World*. Oxford University Press, Oxford. pp. 3–23.

Sofear, B. (1992) *Pain: A Handbook for Nurses*. Chapman and Hall Co., London, p. 49.

Stark, P. L. and McGovern J. P. (eds) (1992) *The Hidden Dimensions of Illness: Human Suffering*. National League for Nursing, New York. pp. 25–42.

Stewart, Mary L. (1977) Measurement of clinical pain, in *A Source Book for Nurses and Other Health Professionals*, (ed. A. Jacox), Little, Brown, Co., Boston, pp. 107–37.

Walker, J. and Campbell, S. (1988) Pain assessment and the nursing process, *Senior Nurse*, 28–31.

World Health Organization (1986) *Cancer Pain Relief*, (World Health Organization Guidelines), Geneva, Switzerland.

CHAPTER 5

The treatment of pain by placebos and unorthodox techniques

Hamilton B. Gibson

5.1 INTRODUCTION

This chapter describes some unorthodox techniques for the control of pain, not as mere examples of medical curiosities and 'alternative therapy', but for the purpose of elucidating the basic mechanisms of pain. An understanding of such mechanisms is necessary for the development of all effective means of treating both acute and chronic painful conditions. At the end of this chapter the principles of placebo action will be discussed.

In pre-scientific times a variety of methods, often bizarre and dependent on sympathetic magic, were used in attempts to control pain. That they were sometimes effective, although lacking in any scientific rationale, should cause us no surprise, for with our modern understanding of the placebo reaction, we realize how powerfully psychological factors can affect physiology and subjective experience. The greater insight into the mechanisms of pain that has been achieved over the past 30 years has produced quite a revolution in our attitudes to therapeutic procedures.

If we go back no further than the last two centuries when medicine has been trying to achieve the status of a scientific discipline, several unorthodox procedures for the control of pain commend themselves for study, as they illustrate principles that still apply today.

5.2 METALLOTHERAPY

Interest in metallotherapy reached its peak in the middle of the nineteenth century (Burq, 1853; Dingwall, 1957). In the previous century the newly discovered wonders of electricity and magnetism had greatly excited the scientific world, and furthered the study of metals and their supposed influences. Because metals proved to be conductors of the electric 'fluid', and ferrous metals could be magnetized, they played an important part in therapy and the treatment of painful conditions.

Franz Mesmer, working with Father Hell in Vienna in the 1780s, experimented with magnetized iron, which was supposed to have the power of drawing out pain. Mesmer proved to have a more scientific outlook than his Jesuit colleague, and discovered that equally good results could be obtained with wooden objects that were painted to resemble magnets, and thus he came to realize that success depended upon the patients' imagination, and not on any magnetic force (Ellenberger, 1970). Mesmer was dishonest enough to conceal his knowledge from both patients and colleagues, and when he came to set up his *baquet* in his famous salon in Paris, he included iron filings and conducting iron rods among the other flummery that was to impress those who sought treatment there, and he claimed that he was influencing their 'animal magnetism'. Because of the prevailing belief in the virtues of metals and magnetism, psychosomatic and painful conditions were relieved, and sometimes cured by Mesmer's methods, which incorporated an elaborate ritual (Tinterow, 1970).

Another interesting use of metallotherapy was in Perkins' Tractors, that came into use in the 1780s. Dingwall (1957) refers to the American physician, Elisha Perkins, who developed an instrument that consisted essentially of two rods of different metals joined together in parallel. This was drawn repeatedly over painful areas, and it was alleged to have an analgesic effect and to benefit a variety of disorders. These beneficial results were achieved not only with naive and unsophisticated people who commonly resort to quacks and faith-healers, and Perkins was able to publish a list of over 5000 patients who had benefited from his treatment, including eight professors, 21 physicians, 19 surgeons, and 30 clergymen. Langworthy (1798) relates how Perkins' son Benjamin set up a Perkins Institute in London, where he sold the Tractors for five guineas, a considerable sum of money at the time, and published a treatise on the subject (Perkins, 1799).

Quite obviously, the Tractors were not in the same class as the many quack remedies that were sold by mountebanks in the markets; they differed in that they carried the great prestige that attached to Elisha Perkins' name in both the USA and in Britain. A widespread emancipation from religious superstition had been achieved by the Enlightenment of the eighteenth century. People no longer sought pieces of the True Cross or the bones of saints with which to treat their ills; they sought to understand pain and disease in scientific terms, and the Tractors, like Mesmer's *baquet*, supposedly operated on scientific principles. Perkins was fully aware that critics might attribute his successes simply to the imaginative capacity of his patients, and so he experimented with various animal species, and reported on the benefits they received. While horses and cows were supposed to be favourably affected, sheep did not appear to respond, and this he attributed to the greasiness of their skins, a finding that suggested that electric conductivity was a factor in the successful operation of the Tractors.

The Tractors came in for sceptical criticism soon after their introduction. The roots of such criticism were twofold. First, some people tried them on themselves and their friends, and obtained no benefit whatsoever, so empirical trials indicated that, with some individuals, they were useless. Second, Perkins and his followers gave no scientific rationale for the Tractors' supposed action. Langworthy (1798) mentions that Elisha Perkins himself never attempted to advance any theory of the function of his Tractors, but an explanation by Vaughan, an American physician, is quoted. First, Galvani's experiments on the influence of electricity on animal nervous and muscular tissue are discussed, and then the hypothesis is advanced that, 'Pain or super-sensation, tumefaction, inflammation, etc. are occasioned by *an extra degree or superabundance of it collected in the part affected.*'

Vaughan's suggestion was that the metals attracted excess energy from the afflicted part, and thus relieved painful and pathological conditions. His explanation was even less convincing than Mesmer's account of how he manipulated the disordered 'animal magnetism' of afflicted patients. Indeed, advocates of Perkins' Tractors were soon to be accused of merely re-hashing Mesmer's claims as to the existence and utility of his postulated 'fluid' of 'animal magnetism'. Such claims were held to be discredited since the Franklin Commission of 1784 which, after a well-conducted investigation of the mesmeric system, as practised by Mesmer's colleague Deslon, pronounced that, 'the existence of the fluid is absolutely destitute of truth, and that the fluid, having no existence, can consequently have no use' (Franklin *et al.*, 1785, p. 126).

One critic, Dr Haygarth (1801), demonstrated that imitation tractors made of such non-metallic materials as wood, but painted to represent the genuine article, were equally effective in producing the desired effect in some patients provided that they did not know that they were being deceived. There was, in fact, quite a good deal of scepticism about the utility of the Tractors at the end of the eighteenth century. An article in the *Monthly Review* (April, 1799. 28, 463–4) discussed the whole question of metallotherapy, and came to very adverse conclusions. Perkins's Tractors became the object of popular derision and satirical verse, but neither scientific demonstration nor the popular derision, put an end to the trade in these instruments. Serious though somewhat deluded writers such as Deleuze (1813) continued to argue for their utility, and such champions continued to support the mesmeric practices of the time also, pointing out the undeniable fact that pain and certain disordered conditions could be relieved or cured by these methods, whatever the scientists might say. We have the same situation today in the late twentieth century; 'alternative therapy' continues to flourish alongside of orthodox medicine. The difference is that whereas today most 'alternative' practitioners disdain the whole scientific outlook and methods of procedure, in the late eighteenth century practitioners such as Mesmer, Perkins, Deleuze and their followers tried to justify their methods on scientific grounds, however absurd their pretentions may appear to us today.

It is noteworthy that faith in various forms of metallotherapy persisted throughout the nineteenth century among otherwise sophisticated people, including the great neurologist Charcot, and is still active among the more credulous of the population. We read advertisements for metal bracelets as a specific against pain and many forms of ill-health; such bracelets are sometimes plated with silver or gold and sold at astonishingly high prices. A contemporary advertisement claims that one such product:

> consists of non-allergic metals, which create through their particular combination a continuous electro-magnetic field. It has long been recognized in Eastern cultures that many bodily illnesses derive from a disturbance to the electro-magnetic field. The ********* appears to effortlessly deal with stress and rheumatism as well as allergies.

An accompanying illustration indicates that when worn on the left wrist it is associated with 'Beta waves', and worn on the right wrist, with 'Alpha waves'. If some people derive any benefit from the bracelets, then it is undoubtedly the same sort of benefit that was obtained through Perkin's Tractors.

5.3   ANALGESIA THROUGH THE STIMULATION OF SENSORY CHANNELS

Some genuine researchers into the control of pain have occasionally been misled into false beliefs about the power of various forms of sensory input to counteract pain, and elaborated unsound techniques based upon chance findings. No-one denies that sensory input can attenuate the experience of pain, but without a fairly sophisticated understanding of the mechanisms of pain, such has been achieved in the last thirty years, empiricism undirected by theory has led to some quite absurd practices that have been widely used by a number of orthodox therapists.

5.3.1 Visual stimulation

Camille Redard carried out valuable research into pain control by means of ethyl chloride and cocaine, and was appointed to a Chair in the Academy of Dentistry at Geneva in 1881. He then began to experiment with various types of non-pharmacological techniques, and found that he could produce a degree of analgesia when engaged on dental operations by the following method, as described in the *British Medical Journal* (Editorial Comment, 1905).

Prior to the operation, the patient's head was put into a large mask in which there was a source of intense blue light, and after about 30 seconds' exposure to this stimulation, the mask was removed and the operation began. The analgesic effect was alleged to persist for some minutes, long enough for a simple dental operation to proceed. Redard reported that he had tried both yellow and red light but found them to be ineffective, and therefore concluded that the colour blue somehow had a soothing effect. Without giving any details of his experiments with different colours, he used the failure of the yellow and red light to produce analgesia as an argument to prove that the analgesic phenomenon was not the result of the patient staring fixedly at a light and going into a hypnotic trance, as had been demonstrated by Braid (1843). This did not dispel the suspicion that some sort of hypnotic phenomenon was involved. Hilliard (1905a; 1905b) reported considerable success with using Redard's method of producing analgesia, and although he doubted whether such a high proportion of people in the population would be sufficiently susceptible to hypnosis to benefit, he concluded that:

> From so limited an experience I am unable to form any opinion as to whether the patients are merely hypnotised, or whether they are actually rendered analgesic by the chemical action of blue light rays, acting through the optic nerve on the central nervous system, as suggested by Professor Redard.
>
> (*Hilliard, 1905a, p. 273*)

This new analgesic technique was seriously taken up by the dental profession at the beginning of this century, although they had several pharmacological methods at their disposal. A contemporary dental journal carries the following report:

> Blue light rays, as a new surgical anaesthetic, have been introduced into the Dental Department of the London Hospital with great success. Six cases were treated, and all the patients stated that they felt no pain, although from two to five extractions were performed in four of the cases. In one case, in which only one tooth was extracted, the patient was so pleased with the anaesthetic that he asked to have two more molars removed, and this was done quite

painlessly. Most of the patients stated that they were conscious of something being done, but they felt no pain. In a further series of fifteen patients at the Royal Dental Hospital, the method was in ten cases successful. . . . In the five remaining cases the patients were conscious of what was going on, but the doctor doubted whether they felt more than the others. They were the sort of persons who scream whether they are hurt or not.

(Editorial Report, 1904, pp. 544–5)

Redard's early successes persuaded him that he had discovered an important analgesic technique. He did not proceed to investigate the matter scientifically by the use of experimental controls, such as the dental surgeon being unaware as to whether the light had been on or off before deciding whether analgesia had been achieved, and he advanced no coherent hypothesis as to *why* exposure to blue light might induce analgesia. This is surely the stumbling block for all those who adopt unorthodox methods and proceed entirely empirically, and we still have examples of it in current medical and para-medical practice today. Various dentists in Britain and on the Continent continued to use Redard's method for some years in the earlier part of this century, as noted in successive editions of Johnson's *Textbook of Operative Dentistry*. In the 4th Edition, Buckley was still describing the technique, and his final comment was, 'Whether the blue light acts locally, or affects the vision and thus the general nervous system, has yet to be demonstrated. The result of the author's experience with this agent has not been encouraging' (Buckley, 1923). The technique appears to have been abandoned during the 1920s.

5.3.2 Auditory stimulation

It has been known since the earliest times that a loud noise may inhibit pain, and the travelling tooth-pullers who operated at country fairs used to have a source of loud music outside the booths in which they operated. The purpose of the music was to drown any cries of pain that might come from within, as the tooth-puller claimed to operate 'painlessly', but in many cases the blaring sound had the effect of attenuating the pain, for as discussed in the review by Bolles and Fanselow (1980), any powerful and exciting stimulus will tend to inhibit acute pain temporarily.

Gardner and Licklider (1959) referred to their discovery of the analgesic properties of a loud sound as 'serendipitous'. Their various papers described how they came to inaugurate a short-lived era in which audio analgesia became popular, particularly in dentistry. The procedure, as described by Licklider (1961), is as follows. The patient wears earphones, and controls by means of two knobs the volume of the sound he receives; these two controls are for music and white noise (noise delivered at all frequencies). At the beginning of the session the patient sets the intensity of the music at a comfortable level. When the dental operation begins, or when it starts to feel uncomfortable, the patient turns up the volume of the music, and as soon as any pain is felt, the level of the white noise can be increased. Licklider claimed that 'The intense noise drowns out or suppresses the pain in the great majority of cases.' He goes on to state that in his opinion there is no longer any question of the efficacy of the procedure in dental operations.

Licklider reported that his colleague, Dr Gardner, used audio-analgesia with more than 1000 patients who had previously required chemical analgesics, and that it was completely effective in 65% of cases. In a further 25% it was effective enough that no other agent was required, and on subsequent visits the patients preferred the procedure to other analgesic methods. At the time of his writing, ten other dentists had had fairly extensive experience with the use of audio analgesia, and their success had been similar to that of Dr Gardner. Over 5000 patients had been treated by it.

The popularity of audio analgesia during the 1960s can be gauged by the number of papers dealing with its use that are reported in the *Index Medicus* for that period. Its popularity then waned in the early 1970s, and although one may still see occasional reference to its use for dentistry and obstetrics in Italian and Eastern European journals, English-language journals mention it very seldom.

Licklider lists seven factors in 'explanation' of the success of audio analgesia:

(1) direct suppression of the pain sensation;
(2) the production of relaxation;
(3) distraction of attention from the pain;
(4) masking of the sound of the dentist's drill, when that is in use;
(5) improved communication with the dentist, who also wears earphones and hence can monitor the patient's experience;
(6) providing an active role for the patient;
(7) suggestion.

He adds, 'This kind of "explanation" seems unsatisfactory, but it is about all that can be achieved without resource to hypotheses that involve the neurophysiological substratum of behavior.' With hindsight after 30 years of progress in pain research, and the new neurophysiological insights that have been gained, particularly through the gate control hypothesis first advanced by Melzack and Wall (1965), we can indeed criticize Licklider's factors as being inadequate. In the first, pain is regarded according to the old and discredited specificity theory as though it were a simple sensation, like hearing, whereas now we regard it as a complex experience that is both physiological and psychological;

(2) may be criticized in that while music may be relaxing, listening to a loud blast of white noise will produce high arousal, which itself can attenuate the experience of acute pain, as in the model of Bolles and Fanselow (1980); (3) is certainly valid, as distraction has been shown to inhibit pain under certain circumstances (McCaul and Mallott, 1984); (4) is also valid, and Licklider points out that patients may have formed a conditioned anxiety to the sound of the drill through earlier painful experiences; (5) and (6) are valid because the feeling of helplessness is removed and the patient now has an active role to play; (7) is probably the most important factor of them all, as the patient has been told and led to expect that pain will be removed by the whole elaborate procedure, and the experiment described below confirms this conclusion.

Melzack, Weisz and Sprague (1963) designed an experiment to investigate just what factors were responsible for the attenuation of pain in the procedure that Gardner and Licklider had developed. We must view the results of any laboratory experiment that sets out to investigate pain with caution, because as Beecher (1959) has pointed out, the pain that is administered to willing subjects in the experimental laboratory is very different from that experienced unwillingly in real life. However, in this experiment it was possible to supply a form of pain that is very like that experienced in the dental chair, although the experimental subjects do not have the same degree of anxiety which frequently exacerbates it.

Volunteers were all subjected to the cold pressor test (a procedure in which a hand is immersed in circulating ice water, which induces a steadily mounting pain) and provided with the audioanalgesia apparatus. The subjects were divided into three groups; group (a) were given the usual procedure but were not told that the purpose of the auditory stimulation was to reduce pain; they received the music and noise at full intensity and were simply told to turn the intensity knobs to maintain equivalence between music and noise. When the pain became too bad to bear they were to say 'stop'. Group (b) were treated in the same way, except that they were led to expect that the noise they listened to would abolish the experience of pain. Group (c) were not given the music and loud sound through their earphones, but were told that they were being exposed to 'ultrasonic sound' which would certainly prevent them from feeling pain. Thus group (a) received the sound stimulus only; (b) the sound plus strong suggestion for analgesia; (c) strong suggestion only. The results were quite clear; only group (b) achieved a significant increase in their tolerance of pain, compared with the level reached in previous testing. The other groups showed no significant improvement.

This experiment demonstrated that the procedure of audio analgesia, as it had been administered by the dentists, was only effective if they strongly suggested to their patients that little pain would be felt. A pain-free outcome depended on a combination of several of the seven factors mentioned earlier by Licklider with the strong suggestion that pain would be avoided. Failure would occur with people who are naturally low in suggestibility, a matter that will be discussed later, or where the dentist had not given suggestions forcefully enough.

Thus when audio analgesia was effective, it worked for the same reason that Redard's blue light treatment was sometimes successful. A strong stimulus was given, and the patient's suggestibility, following the dentist's assurances, operated to interpret the neural signals benignly, and prevented the build-up of a perception of pain.

5.3.3 Stimulation of cutaneous and subcutaneous senses

One of the most ancient and well-known methods of attempting to attenuate pain is acupuncture. It is unnecessary here to deal with this enormous subject in general; we will simply be concerned to discuss whether acupuncture really can inhibit pain, and if it does, why. There is a vast literature on the subject, and specialists are strongly divided in their views about it. Felix Mann's book *Acupuncture: The Ancient Chinese Art of Healing* (Mann, 1962) attracted some attention in the 1960s, but it was in the early 1970s that the medical profession began to take a serious interest in acupuncture. Two factors precipitated this interest. First, Ronald Melzack, who was recognized internationally as a very distinguished research worker in the study of pain, realized that the gate control theory of pain, referred to above, could find some confirmation in acupuncture analgesia, and he and his colleagues instituted an impressive programme of research in this field. In his popular book, *The Puzzle of Pain* he was willing to accept that, 'The available evidence (Brown 1972) suggests that a much higher proportion of patients in China, perhaps as high as 90 per cent, undergo surgery with the acupuncture procedure' (Malzack 1973a, pp. 187–8). Few people nowadays would accept the evidence advanced by Brown (1972) as presenting a true picture of what really went on in hospitals in Maoist China. In a series of quite enthusiastic articles in both the popular and scientific press, Melzack gave the impression it was well established that, whatever the merits or demerits of acupuncture in promoting general health were, it could certainly be relied upon to produce analgesia (Melzack, 1973a; 1973b; 1973c).

The second factor leading to the widespread interest in acupuncture analgesia rather later, was the discovery of the mechanisms responsible for opioid analgesia and the enkephalins and endorphins (Bloom, 1983). Here clinical and experimental researchers with human beings may have been misled by the animal studies, for it was overlooked that animals' reaction to pain is essentially different from the human response as far as acupuncture goes. For whereas human patients look upon the needling as a benign procedure and anticipate relief from pain as a result, animals are generally made anxious by the procedure. As is well known, their fear may bring on the tonic immobility reaction which confers analgesia (Gallup *et al.*, 1970), and is associated with the release of endorphins (Carli, 1978). Galeano *et al.* (1979) performed an important experiment with rabbits, and demonstrated very clearly that when they were treated gently and rendered unanxious, acupuncture conferred no analgesia on them whatsoever.

In contrast to the enthusiastic acceptance of acupuncture analgesia as a valid field for study by scientists such as Melzack and his colleagues, and by many clinicians who were less scientifically orientated, there was outright rejection of it by others. In the USA Sweet (1981), after a careful review of the available evidence, dismissed acupuncture as clinically worthless. Skrabanek launched an outright attack on acupuncture, stating:

> By 'rediscovering' the five vital principles of Chinese medicine (equivalent to the four humours of the ancient Greeks) and Chinese acupuncture (equivalent to European bloodletting) we degrade medicine to shamanism. If we can now treat obesity or smoking addiction with a 'staple' in the ear, why not a copper bracelet or red flannel for rheumatism next? Let us leave quackupuncture to quacks and let us tell the misinformed patient the truth, so that he or she can choose.
>
> *(Skrabanek, 1984, p. 1171)*

It should be noted that Skrabanek is not denying that acupuncture can sometimes produce analgesia; he is inveighing against members of his profession using the whole mystique of acupuncture in the treatment of a huge range of diseases and disorders in defiance of the principles of scientific medicine. Regarding the practice of treating painful conditions by needling, he has this to say in the earlier part of his article:

> Many investigators use the neutral term 'transcutaneous electric stimulation' for one of the acupuncture equivalents. Similar descriptive terms could be employed for other acupuncture equivalents to avoid obfuscation. There is nothing mystical about claiming pain relief by distractive sensory stimuli: for example, the effect of needling in acute pain, particularly in lumbago, has been observed and described by many medical practitioners who did not care for 'Oriental' practice – e.g. Osler, who learned the technique from Ringer.
>
> *(Skrabanek 1984, p. 1170)*

Here Skrabanek is referring to Osler (1901). The term 'transcutaneous electric stimulation' is used by Melzack and Wall (1982) in a book that is really an enlarged and modified edition of *The Puzzle of Pain*. In the later book they discuss it under the general heading of 'Hyperstimulation Analgesia', along with ice massage and needling, as well as acupuncture. These other methods will not be described or discussed here as they are orthodox medical treatments, and therefore not within the scope of this chapter.

It is apparent then, that there is no particular mystery about acupuncture. Shorn of its trappings of Chinese folk-medicine it is a simple technique which, when it produces analgesia, does so for the same reasons that audio analgesia and Redard's blue light treatment do, and in addition it may sometimes stimulate the large-diameter non-nociceptive sensory nerve fibres that serve to close the 'gates' of pain (Fields, 1984). Such treatments provide an impressive physical stimulus, which, combined with adequate suggestibility on the part of the patient, alter the perception of pain in a manner largely explicable in terms of gate control theory. Whether or not there is an involvement of opioid peptides in such analgesia is a matter that has not yet been fully clarified, and is not crucial to the issue of hyperstimulation analgesia.

Perhaps most surprising of all in the voluminous literature on acupuncture analgesia is the final admission of Felix Mann, who was so influential in reviving the interest of the medical profession in the subject thirty years ago. He finally came round to the following view:

Acupuncture anaesthesia (really analgesia) works only, in my experience (though others who are experts disagree) in the hyper-strong reactor. In 1974 I reported the results of a hundred experiments in acupuncture analgesia and came to the conclusion that it worked reasonably, though not perfectly, in 10% of patients. Since then I have come to the conclusion that the criteria I used were a little optimistic, and the figure should be revised to a mere 5%. Some experiments were performed which showed that the acupuncture analgesia was an objective and not a psychosomatic phenomenon, in the few in which it worked.

(*Mann, 1983, pp. 44–5*)

Although acupuncture continues to be practised all over the world by some medically qualified doctors (partly, some say, so that it should not be entirely in the hands of unqualified quacks), a sort of epitaph on it was recently published in *The Lancet*:

Whilst careful scientific research can never entirely exclude the possibility that a dwarf is hiding in the corner of the room, many western researchers may now conclude that the existence of the dwarf approaches asymptotically to zero.

(*Editorial, 1990*)

5.4 MESMERISM

The term mesmerism originated in the work of the eighteenth century physician, Franz Mesmer, who was referred to earlier in this chapter in relation to metallotherapy. But the use of magnets and metals formed only part of his elaborate system which was based upon his contention that there was an invisible fluid which he termed 'animal magnetism' which could be manipulated by skilled practitioners. Derangement of this mysterious fluid was supposed to be responsible for all manner of physical and emotional ills, and the ministrations of Mesmer and his colleagues sometimes proved quite effective in alleviating or curing various disorders. The commissioners who investigated the mesmeric practices attributed the successes of the treatment to the 'imagination' of the patients, and in doing so tended to dismiss it as valueless, without taking note of what a very powerful and therapeutically valuable force 'imagination' had been shown to be.

The later followers and imitators of Mesmer did not adhere closely to his practices, and various schools of mesmerism developed. Buranelli (1975) describes, 'scientific', 'occult' and 'political' mesmerism, the last dying out with the French revolution. The mesmerists could be further divided between the 'fluidists' (who took Mesmer's theory of the invisible fluid of 'animal magnetism' quite literally), and the 'animists' (who were more interested in the psychological phenomena of mesmerism). In the course of time an intermediate theory became more general among mesmerists, but even when trying to be scientific all mesmerists embraced a good deal of pseudo-scientific nonsense.

Whatever benefits mesmerism may have conferred in the way of suggestive therapy and placebo action, especially with disorders of a psychosomatic and hysterical nature, the one area in which they were undoubtedly successful in certain cases was in the attenuation or prevention of pain in surgical operations. The form of mesmerism that was used to secure the 'mesmeric trance' has been described by writers such as Deleuze (1813) and Esdaile (1846). The method was to immobilize the patient, generally in a prone position, and then to make repeated 'passes' down the body, either above it or in light contact, this process being continued for hours, if necessary, until the patient went into a sleep-like trance and did not react to noxious stimuli.

The mesmeric trance strongly resembled the condition of tonic immobility which can easily be induced in many small mammals and birds by immobilizing them and, in some cases, simply by turning them upside-down. The condition of tonic immobility is potentiated by fear, and has been referred to as 'death-feigning'. It is generally accepted that in this state their non-response to noxious stimuli is due to a general condition of analgesia which may be mediated by endorphins, as hypothesized by Carli on the basis of his experimental work (Carli,

1978). It has been postulated elsewhere (Gibson, 1982) that tonic immobility in animals and the mesmeric trance can meaningfully be compared. It is quite natural that patients awaiting surgery in the preanaesthetic period of the nineteenth century would be suffering from extreme fear, and this may well have potentiated the immobile and analgesic trance that has been described by Esdaile and those who witnessed his operations, and by the observers of other mesmeric surgeons (Elliotson (1843). While we may dismiss the claims of people like Elliotson as being too partial to be reliable, more weight must be attached to the opinions of sceptics like Sir John Forbes who poured scorn on the occult pretentions of the mesmerists, but acknowledged the reality of their painless surgery (Forbes, 1845).

It is unfortunate that we are unable to investigate the true nature of the mesmeric trance scientifically, because it would be unethical to induce extreme fear in human beings, such as has been done by Gallup and his colleagues with chickens in the investigation of tonic immobility (Gallup *et al.*, 1970). From contemporary accounts it is evident that all patients did not react favourably to mesmerism, and it was impossible to depend on inducing analgesia by this means reliably. It remains one of the scientific curiosities in the history of analgesia. The medical profession as a whole rejected it as humbug for the very good reason that mesmerists mixed their practice with a great deal of occult nonsense, and while doctors were trying to get their profession recognized as being scientifically respectable they could not afford to associate with quacks. It came at a time when the more enlightened members of the profession were trying to get chemical anaesthesia accepted by their more conservative colleagues (some of whom maintained that pain was beneficial). When the American surgeon John Warren permitted the dentist, William Morton, to anaesthetize a surgical patient with ether, at the end of this successful operation that was painless he said, 'Gentlemen, this is no humbug,' thus dissociating chemical anaesthesia from the alleged 'humbug' of mesmeric surgery (Keys, 1963).

5.5 HYPNOSIS

Hypnotism must be distinguished from mesmerism, although many modern writers assume that the two terms are interchangeable. Mesmerism is essentially a process whereby a physiological condition is produced in which the experience of pain is attenuated or abolished; the basis of this derangement of normal function is uncertain. As mentioned above, it is possible that it is mediated by the endorphin system; this is comparable to the tonic immobility that can be induced in animal species. It is also probable that this change can only take place under conditions of fear and high arousal, and those who are susceptible to it are in some way abnormal. What is meant by hypnotism nowadays is quite different. Hypnosis is a psychological phenomenon which can be induced in most normal people by verbal suggestion, and is strongly related to the individual's capacity for imaginative involvement. There are considerable differences between individuals in their capacity to experience hypnosis, and this has been the subject of extensive experimental investigation (Fromm and Shor, 1979; E. R. Hilgard, 1965; J. R. Hilgard, 1970; Tellegen and Atkinson, 1974; Wilson and Barber, 1983).

Because of the confusion between mesmerism and hypnotism there is a widespread belief that a state of hypnosis automatically confers a measure of analgesia, which is certainly not the case. The point is made quite forcibly by those who have investigated hypnosis in relation to pain:

> [We] can report that hypnosis alone, without analgesia suggestions, does not reduce pain any more than it reduces other sensory functions. Through suggestions, the hypnotic subject can be made deaf and blind also, but without special suggestions he hears and sees as well within hypnosis as when not hypnotized. The same thing has been repeatedly found for the experience of pain.
>
> (*Hilgard and Hilgard, 1983, p. 71*)

The above reference to hypnotic deafness and blindness introduces us to one of the most striking of the hypnotic phenomena, the alteration of the perceptual processes of the hypnotized subject. Such induced deafness and blindness is purely functional and operates at only one level of consciousness. Hypnotically deaf subjects can be made to hear again simply by being told by the hypnotist that they can hear, which shows that all the time there is communication via the auditory modality, although at one level of consciousness the subject is subjectively deaf (Malmo, Boag and Raginsky, 1954). Similarly, the nature of hypnotically induced analgesia occurs at only one level of consciousness. While a patient in whom analgesia has been induced by hypnotic suggestion may endure with equanimity an operation that would normally be excruciatingly painful, there is evidence that pain is being experienced at another level of consciousness. This phenomenon was reported by Chertok and his colleagues (Chertok, Michaux and Doin, 1977) working with two women undergoing surgery with no analgesia other than that which was induced hypnotically. Reports of the patients' experience were obtained by interrogation later after re-hypnosis. They reported that during the operation they were not conscious of any pain, although they felt that 'some other person' was suffering pain.

Ernest Hilgard has investigated this phenomenon with experimental subjects undergoing the cold pressor test mentioned above. He found that some experimental subjects could endure what would have been an extremely painful ordeal without suffering pain; but when they were interrogated under hypnosis with the suggestion that at another level of consciousness there was more awareness of their total experience, a report might be obtained indicating consciousness at another level of awareness. Interestingly, the intensity of pain reported on a pre-arranged scale was rather less than that reported on base-line testing in a fully awake condition (Hilgard *et al.*, 1975).

This procedure may seem somewhat preposterous to the sceptic, who will find it difficult to believe that there may be independent and isolated systems of consciousness, between which some people may alternate at will when hypnotized. Nevertheless, the reality of this, which is referred to as the 'hidden observer' phenomenon, has been accepted as genuine by serious researchers in the field of pain. A number of research studies by independent laboratories have confirmed the original findings about the 'hidden observer' effect (Laurence and Perry, 1981; Laurence, Perry and Kihlstrom, 1983; Laurence *et al.*, 1986; Nogrady *et al.*, 1983). One of the important features of it is that while it is possible to elicit the phenomenon only with subjects who are highly susceptible to hypnosis, not all hypnotic virtuosos respond in this manner. This strange finding appears to relate to the fact that people vary as to the extent to which their consciousness *dissociates* in hypnosis, a matter that is still the subject of experimental investigation (Nadon *et al.*, 1988). The whole area of multiple consciousness is the subject of a book by Hilgard, which of course deals with the inhibition of pain by hypnotic suggestion (Hilgard, 1986).

It should be noted that when a negative hallucination for pain is induced by hypnotic suggestion the phenomenon is entirely *psychological* and may have little effect on the physiological indices of pain, such as heart-rate and blood pressure, although these may be somewhat reduced because anxiety is lowered (Hilgard *et al.*, 1974). When the phenomenon of hypnotically induced analgesia was investigated experimentally it was natural that the possibility of the involvement of endorphins was scrutinized, but Nasrallah, Holley and Janowsky (1979) found that this was not the case in their own study, and in several which they reviewed.

Because pain is a complex phenomenon involving a suffering component as well as a sensory experience, it may be attenuated to some extent by anti-anxiety drugs such as diazepam which have been shown to have no chemically analgesic properties (Chapman and Feather, 1973). The question therefore arises as to whether hypnotic suggestion for analgesia acts principally through reducing anxiety. Experimental work by Greene and Reyher (1972) indicates that hypnotic suggestion acts principally by blocking the perception of pain, rather than by reducing anxiety as a tranquillizing drug would do. Similar conclusions may be drawn from the work of Stern *et al.* (1977); they compared the efficiency of hypnotic suggestion for analgesia with that of the analgesic drugs morphine and aspirin, and the tranquillizer diazepam. They also used acupuncture and two kinds of placebo. Hypnotic suggestion proved to give the greatest relief from pain engendered by the cold pressor test and by induced ischaemia; morphine was second, and acupuncture third. Aspirin, diazepam and placebo did not produce a significant reduction in pain.

The fact that hypnotically induced analgesia, both in a clinical and experimental context, has been shown to be more than a placebo, has led to some debate among clinicians and experimentalists. In all therapeutic treatments, whether by drugs, surgery, or psychological measures, *some* placebo component is involved; therefore, if the ritual of a hypnotic induction is carried out even with patients who are utterly insusceptible to hypnosis, there may be some therapeutic gain, including a lessening of pain. This had led to the belief among some clinicians that they can 'hypnotize' anyone, and that individual differences in susceptibility are irrelevant.

An important review by Wadden and Anderton (1982) revealed, perhaps to many clinicians' surprise, that hypnotic suggestion in treatment was not very effective in cases of addiction to smoking, drugs, alcohol, and over-eating. Where there was some improvement it was probably due to the placebo value of the whole treatment. The authors characterized such conditions as being 'self-rewarding'. By contrast, hypnotic treatment of conditions such as pain, asthma, and skin diseases was often effective, but success was correlated with the degree of susceptibility of the patients. This imposes an obvious limitation on the clinical usefulness of hypnotic suggestion in dealing with pain patients. Although we know something about the personality correlates of susceptibility to hypnosis, so far no-one has evolved a reliable method for increasing hypnotic susceptibility; it appears to be a very fundamental personality trait that is little changed over the years. According to Bowers (1983, p. 128) 'It is becoming increasingly clear that hypnotic susceptibility and its correlates are deeply imbedded in a person's biological organization. This is undoubtedly one reason for the relative stability of hypnotic stability in mature people.' Some social psychologists who are reluctant to acknowledge the biological basis for hypnotic responsiveness, have been initiating experimental programmes to increase measured susceptibility in the psychological laboratory. This endeavour has necessitated the creation of a new scale of susceptibility which tends to re-define susceptibility in terms of compliance (Spanos *et al.*, 1983), and coaching experimental subjects in how to respond to it. Gibson and Heap (1989, p. 36) discuss the matter and comment, 'The exercise seems rather like drilling subjects in the correct answers to an I.Q. test, and if this were done, we might wonder whether the increased score truly reflected an increase in intelligence.'

Many studies have been cited from the 1970s because during that decade there was considerable rapprochement between workers in hypnosis and in pain. Previously, research in pain had not paid much attention to hypnosis, and Melzack, in his earlier thinking, had believed that there was, 'no reliable evidence from controlled clinical studies to show that (hypnosis) is effective for any form of chronic pain' (Melzack, 1980, p. 149).

It is surprising that Melzack should continue to publish his earlier thinking on this matter as late as 1980, because he had already participated in a study which included the successful treatment of chronic pain patients by hypnosis, which was later described as follows:

> Melzack and Perry (1975) found that EEG biofeedback alone had no demonstrable effect on chronic pain compared to the level of pain relief obtained in 'placebo' baseline sessions. In contrast they found that hypnotic training instructions produced substantial relief of pain – significantly greater than biofeedback. . . . However, when the hypnotic training instructions were presented together with biofeedback the pain relief was significantly greater than produced by baseline placebo sessions.
>
> (*Melzack and Wall, 1982, p. 349*).

This study by Melzack and Perry (1975) was something of a milestone in clinical research, as it pointed the way forward, indicating that the successful treatment of both chronic and acute pain frequently involved the combining of hypnotic suggestion with other techniques such as biofeedback, as described in an excellent review by Hart (1991).

As the decade of the 1980s progressed, more and more attention to the use of hypnotic suggestion in the treatment of pain was increasingly manifest in published studies, such as those referred to by Gibson and Heap (1991, Chapter 8), most of them appearing in the prestigious journal *Pain*. However, the considerable attention to hypnotic procedures that has been given in this chapter is not because of its clinical effectiveness that has been recognized in rather recent years, but because of the light it shines upon the mechanisms of the experience of pain. Unlike the techniques mentioned in the earlier part of this chapter, hypnotic treatment involves something over and above the inevitable placebo component inherent in all forms of treatment.

5.6   THE PLACEBO EFFECT

Shapiro (1960) notes that there was a sudden increase in the number of papers concerning placebo action published in the four years 1954–1957 (35 papers), whereas only 25 relevant papers had been published in the previous half-century. He notes that the placebo effect was not unknown in the nineteenth century, and even before, but that it became

a matter of comment only in the 1950s when a great number of new drugs came into use in medicine – drugs that were not only new, but, for the first time in the history of medicine, many of them were effective.

> When one considers that the normative history of medical treatment, until relatively recently, has been the history of the placebo effect, one is amazed to find a veritable curtain of silence about it.
>
> (*Shapiro, 1960, p. 114*)

A more cynical view would be that the curtain of silence was entirely to be expected, and that most doctors simply did not want to know that many of the medicines and treatments that they prescribed were, in themselves, wholly neutral, their success depending entirely on the patients' faith. Indeed, Pepper (1945) pointed to the stubborn resistance of the medical profession to acknowledge the existence of the placebo effect that had really been known throughout the ages. Elisha Perkins, Camille Redard, Gardener and Liklider, and more recently, many acupuncturists and hypnotherapists, have enjoyed their success because of the medical profession's less than frank acceptance of the placebo effect.

It was in the area of pain research that the placebo effect first came into prominence. The seminal work of Beecher (1959) and his colleagues had the double effect of alerting the scientific community to the inadequacy of current conceptions of the nature of pain, and of the necessity for admitting the enormous part that placebo action played in the operation of even powerful drugs like morphine. Evidence that morphine, even in large doses, will relieve severe pain in only 75 per cent of patients, was certainly surprising at the time it was published. Quite obviously, a huge and variable component of active analgesics was simply due to the placebo effect, and important questions then began to be raised. Was there a discernible type of patient who was a placebo responder? What kinds of pain could and could not be alleviated by analgesic drugs and procedures? Under what circumstances can pain be relieved by placebo action?

5.6.1   The question of 'suggestibility'

It was natural that authors should write of placebo action being associated with the patient's 'suggestibility', without being too concerned about the precise meaning of the latter term. Suggestibility had acquired a specialized meaning since the time of Bernheim (1886/1973) as being associated with susceptibility to hypnosis, and no-one was troubled by the imprecision of the term until experimental psychologists began to investigate just what sort of people were more and less suggestible. Psychologists in the earlier part of this century had devised a wide range of tests of suggestibility without really establishing whether people who scored highly on one such test would respond equally well on other tests alleged to measure suggestibility. A series of investigations were carried out by Eysenck and Furneaux to investigate this matter (Eysenck, 1943; Eysenck and Furneaux, 1945; Furneaux, 1946), and they discovered that while some well-known tests of suggestibility were strongly predictive of hypnotizability, others proved to be quite unrelated. They referred to the former group as measuring 'primary' suggestibility, and the latter 'secondary' suggestibility. Those in the latter group were not strongly related to one another, and did not predict susceptibility to hypnosis. This work was taken up by other psychologists, notably Stukat (1958) and Duke (1964) who confirmed the earlier findings.

One of the important findings that became clear from this series of psychological investigations was that while 'primary' suggestibility was a meaningful concept in relation to hypnotizability, all the tests in the 'secondary' category were merely a rag-bag collection of action tendencies that had little relation to one another, and had no relevance to hypnotizability. An individual might be highly 'suggestible' in one context but not at all in another. This has a bearing upon reactivity to placebos. The postulated relationship of the placebo effect to the inhibition of experimental pain by hypnotic suggestion was taken up by McGlashan, Evans and Orne (1969). The conditions of the experiment included a normal control without hypnosis, hypnotic suggestion of analgesia, and a placebo condition. The results of this rather complex study are as follows:

1. For subjects insusceptible to hypnosis, some pain reduction may be achieved through hypnotically suggested analgesia, but it will correspond to a reduction by placebo.
2. For subjects highly susceptible to hypnosis, pain reduction through hypnotically suggested analgesia is far greater than by placebo. For these subjects, the average placebo response is negligible or even negative (Hilgard and Hilgard, 1983, p. 74).

When considering such results it is important to bear in mind that the placebo effect in experimental work differs in significant ways from placebo action in the clinical field, where the anxiety component of pain is likely to be much higher. However, the above-mentioned experimental study does indicate that the term 'suggestibility' which has been loosely applied in this chapter in relation to various examples of placebo action is not the same as the more technical term of 'primary' suggestibility applied to hypnotic susceptibility. The latter has been shown to be a fairly stable personality trait, whereas responding to a placebo is an *ad hoc* reaction depending on a person's needs at a particular time, in a particular situation. The independence of the placebo response and hypnotizability has been established in a number of more recent studies, as reviewed by Evans (1989).

5.6.2   The mechanisms of placebo action

There is quite an extensive literature dealing with the search for the personality characteristics of the 'placebo reactor'. A review of such literature is given by Spiro (1986) and reveals that in more recent years it has become generally accepted that there is no such personality type. However, although we can safely say that the great majority of people will react to placebos in appropriate circumstances, it has been possible to identify a minority of people who are 'non-reactors': that is they show an atypical response in circumstances where most normal people would react positively. Such non-responders are not only peculiar in respect to placebos; when given ordinary medicines they do not respond typically; it is as though they give a physiological response comparable to the Ganser syndrome, reacting negatively where a positive response is normal. Such people have been characterized as being somewhat paranoid and afraid of having their equilibrium influenced by others (Brody, 1980). Having now given various examples of the inhibition of pain by a variety of techniques, some of them most certainly depending wholly on placebo action, (such as Perkins' tractors), and others in which placebo action does not account for the whole of the analgesic effect, (like hypnotic suggestion), it is necessary to discuss the mechanisms responsible for the placebo effect. There are two main theories of placebo action, the verbal expectancy model (Kirsh, 1985), and the conditioned response model (Wikramasekera, 1980).

In the expectancy model the patient, or experimental subject, is led to expect a certain outcome from the treatment that is about to be given, and consequently, all subsequent experience is interpreted in the light of that expectation. Thus if a patient is told firmly that he will have no dental pain following the application of Redard's blue light, and he truly believes this, he may be unwilling to regard as painful whatever sensations he experiences afterwards, either in his own self-perception or in his report to the dentist. The number of people who achieved a good deal of analgesia when this means of treatment was being used may not have been very great, but their analgesic experience is explicable in terms of modern pain theory. Fields (1981) would go further, and suggest that the expectation of immunity from pain activates the endorphin-mediated system, but the evidence for this has not been confirmed.

The conditioned-response model derives from the classic work of Pavlov (1927). He noticed that dogs began to salivate before they could see or smell their food, as when the technician or the food-container was visible, and he realized that when a stimulus that was completely neutral in itself was repeatedly presented before one (food) that naturally produced the response, the normal physiological reaction of salivation would take place. He then began his well-known experiments in which a bell became the conditioned stimulus to produce salivation. When we apply this model to the placebo phenomenon, it is apparent that the neutral stimulus (such as a dummy tablet looking like aspirin) can give real relief from pain because the patient has been conditioned over the years to experience analgesia following the swallowing of aspirin.

It should be noted that in most of the examples cited earlier, a stimulus that is definite and strong – a blue light, a loud sound, needles in the skin – is needed to produce the conditioned response of pain reduction; this parallels the sound of the bell, or an electric shock, that was used in Pavlov's experiments. Interestingly enough, different individuals react to one sort of placebo stimulus and not to others. Some people respond well to substances they swallow, others to impressive apparatus with flashing lights, and still others to procedures that are a little painful. The origins of these individual differences in placebo reactivity relate to the past history of the people concerned. Painful conditions, and indeed many types of disorder, are typically variable, disappearing or noticeably lessening sometimes for no obvious reason. Thus if a chronic pain patient finds that being the object of solicitous attention lessens pain, any sort of ministration that involves social interaction, such as the ritual of acupuncture, or being stroked with Perkins' Tractors, may become a conditioned stimulus that abolishes the pain of this individual. The placebo reaction has been discussed above in terms of the classical conditioning theory of Pavlov, but it might be more appropriate in many cases to refer it to the operant conditioning theory of Skinner (1938). In the latter body of work it was shown that quite accidental features in the environment might become the conditioned stimuli for a certain response; thus in a fluctuating painful condition, relief from pain might become associated with certain environmental factors quite fortuitously. This would explain why some people will respond favourably to one class of stimuli (say, swallowing various substances) and other people to quite a different class of placebos (say, social stimuli). Conditioning theory also explains negative placebo effects, such as pain rising in intensity when the sufferer fails to get an expected degree of attention from his family.

Most of the early work to test the applicability of the conditioning model to the placebo response was carried out with animals, but later work has extended experimental inquiries to humans (Lang and Rand, 1969; Voudouris, Peck and Coleman, 1989, 1990). In the latter study an attempt was made to compare the relative effectiveness of a placebo procedure based on the verbal expectancy model with one employing the conditioning model. This involved volunteer subjects undergoing experimental pain. In this experiment the conditioning procedure proved to be the more effective, but it must be remarked that in most clinical situations both expectancy and conditioning mechanisms are involved when pain is reduced by the placebo effect. Because pain is such a subjective phenomenon in which the individual's attitude and mental state is so strongly involved, it is difficult to conceive of any situation in which pain is relieved by the placebo effect where the sufferer has not a strongly positive attitude to the therapeutic procedure, and expectancy that it will bring relief.

REFERENCES

Beecher, H. K. (1959) *Measurement of Subjective Responses*, Oxford University Press, London.

Bernheim, H. (1886/1973) *Hypnosis and Suggestion in Psychotherapy*, (Trans. C. A. Herter), Jason Aron, New York.

Bloom, F. E. (1983) The endorphins: a growing family of pharmacological peptides. *Annual Review of Pharmacology and Toxicology*, **23**, 151–70.

Bolles, R. C. and Faneslow, M. S. (1980) A perceptual-defensive-recuperative model of fear and pain. *The Behavioral and Brain Sciences*, **3**, 291–323.

Bowers, K. S. (1983) *Hypnosis for the Seriously Curious*, W. W. Norton & Co., New York.

Braid, J. (1843) *Neurypnology: Or the Rationale of Nervous Sleep Considered in Relation with Animal Magnetism*, John Churchill, London.

Brody, H. (1980) *Placebos and the Philosophy of Medicine*, University of Chicago Press, Chicago.

Brown, P. E. (1972) Use of acupuncture in major surgery. *Lancet*, i, 1328–30.

Buckley, J. P. (1923) The treatment of sensitive dentine, in *A Textbook of Operative Dentistry*, 4th edn, (ed. C. N. Johnson), P. Blackiston Sons & Co., Philadelphia, pp. 201–9.

Buranelli, V. (1975) *The Wizard from Vienna*, Peter Owen, London.

Burq, V. (1853) *Metalotherapie*. Paris.

Carli, G. (1978) Animal hypnosis and pain, in *Hypnosis at its Bicentennial*, (eds F. H. Frankel and H. S. Zamanski), Plenum Press, New York, pp. 69–77.

Chapman, C. R. and Feather, B. W. (1973) Effects of diazepam on human pain tolerance and human sensitivity. *Psychosomatic Medicine* **35**, 330–40.

Chertok, L., Michaux, D. and Doin, M. C. (1977) Dynamics of hypnotic analgesia: some new data. *Journal of Mental and Nervous Disease*, **64**, 88–96.

Deleuze, J. P. F. (1813) *Histoire Critique du Magnetisme Animale*, Schoelle, Paris.

Dingwall, E. J. (1957) *Abnormal Hypnotic Phenomena*. Vol. I. J & A Churchill, London.

Duke, J. D. (1964) Intercorrelational status of suggestibility tests and hypnotizability. *Psychological Record*, **14**, 71–80.

Editorial Comment (1905) Blue light as an anaesthetic. *British Medical Journal*, i, 1290.

Editorial Report (1905) A new anaesthetic. *British Journal of Dental Science*, 544–5.

Editorial Comment (1990) Many points to needle. *Lancet* 335, 20–1.

Ellenberger, H. F. (1970) *The Discovery of the Unconscious*, Basic Books, New York.

Elliotson, J. (1843) *Numerous Cases of Surgical Operations Without Pain in the Mesmeric State*, H. Bailliere, London.

Esdaile, J. (1846) *Mesmerism in India and its Practical Application in Surgery and Medicine*. Longmans, Brown, Green and Longmans, London.

Evans, F. J. (1989) The independence of suggestibility, placebo response, and hypnotizability, in *Suggestion and Suggestibility. Theory and Research*, (eds V. A. Gheorghiu, P. Netter, H. J. Eysenck and R. Rosenthal), Springer Verlag, Berlin.

Eysenck, H. J. (1943) Suggestibility and hypnosis – an experimental analysis. *Proceedings of the Royal Society of Medicine*, **36**, 349–54.

Eysenck, H. J. and Furneaux, W. D. (1945) Primary and secondary suggestibility: an experimental and statistical study. *Journal of Experimental Psychology*, **35**, 485–503.

Fields, H. L. (1981) Pain II: New approaches to management. *Annals of Neurology*, **9**, 101–6.

Fields, H. L. (1984) Neurophysiology of pain and pain modulation. *American Journal of Medicine*, **77**, 2–8.

Forbes, J. (1845) *Mesmerism True – Mesmerism False*, J. Churchill, London.

Franklin, B. *et al*. (1785/1970) Report on Animal Magnetism, (trans. W. Godwin), in *Foundations of Hypnosis*, (ed. M. M. Tinterow), C. C. Thomas, Springfield, Ill., pp. 82–128.

Fromm, E. and Shor, R. E. (eds) (1979) *Hypnosis: Developments in Research and New Perspectives*, Revised 2nd Edn. Aldine: New York.

Furneaux, W. D. (1946) The prediction of susceptibility to hypnosis. *Journal of Personality*, **14**, 281–94.

Galeano, C., Leung, C. Y., Robitaillie, R. and Roy-Chabot, T. (1979) Acupuncture analgesia in rabbits. *Pain*, **6**, 71–81.

Gallup, G. G., Nash, R. F., Potter, R. J. and Donnegan, N. H. (1970) Effects of varying conditions of fear on immobility reactions in domestic chickens. *Journal of Comparative Physiology and Psychology*, **73**, 442–5.

Gardner, W. J. and Licklider, J. C. R. (1959) Audio analgesia. *Journal of the American Dental Society*, **59**, 1144–9.

Gibson, H. B. (1982) *Pain and its Conquest*, Peter Owen, London.

Gibson, H. B. and Heap, M. (1991) *Hypnosis in Therapy*, Lawrence Erlbaum Associates, Hove.

Greene, R. J. and Reyher, J. (1972) Pain tolerance in hypnotic analgesia and imagination states. *Journal of Abnormal Psychology*, **79**, 29–38.

Hart, B. (1991) Hypnosis and pain, in *Hypnotherapy: A Handbook*, (eds M. Heap and W. Dryden), Open University Press: Milton Keynes, pp. 87–107.

Haygarth, J. (1801) *The Imagination as a Cause and Cure of Disorders of the Body*, Bath.

Hilgard, E. R. (1965) *Hypnotic Susceptibility*, Harcourt, Brace and World, New York.

Hilgard, J. R. (1970) *Personality and Hypnosis: A study in Imaginative Involvement*. University of Chicago Press: Chicago.

Hilgard, E. R. (1986) *Divided Consciousness: Multiple Controls in Human Thought and Action*, J. Wiley, New York.

Hilgard, E. R. and Hilgard J. R (1983) *Hypnosis in the Relief of Pain*, W. Kaufmann, Inc.: Los Altos, Calif.

Hilgard, E. R., Morgan, A. H. and McDonald, H. (1975) Pain and dissociation in the cold pressor test: A study of hypnotic analgesia with 'Hidden reports' through automatic key pressing and automatic talking. *Journal of Abnormal Psychology*, **84**, 280–9.

Hilgard, E. R. Ruch, J. C., Lange A. F. *et al*. (1974) The psychophysics of cold pressor pain and its modification through hypnotic suggestion. *American Journal of Psychology*, **87**, 17–31.

Hilliard, H. (1905a) Note on the anaesthetic effect of blue light rays. *Medical Times and Hospital Gazette*, **33**, 273.

Hilliard, H. (1905b) Blue light as an anaesthetic. *British Medical Journal*, i, 1405.

Keys, T. E. (1963) *The History of Surgical Anaesthesia*, Dover Publications, New York.

Kirsch, I. (1985) Response expectancy as a determinant of experience and behavior. *American Psychologist*, 1189–1202.

Lang, W. and Rand, M. (1969) A placebo response as a conditional reflex to glyceryl trinitrate. *Medical Journal of Australia*, 1, 912–14.

Langworthy, C. C. (1798) *A View of Perkinean Electricity*, Bath.

Laurence, J-R., Nadon, R. Nogrady, H. and Perry, C. (1986) Duality, dissociation, and memory creation in highly hypnotizable subjects. *International Journal of Clinical and Experimental Hypnosis*, **34**, 295–310.

Laurence, J-R. and Perry C. (1981) The 'hidden observer' phenomenon in hypnosis: some additional findings. *Journal of Abnormal Psychology*, **90**, 334–44.

Laurence, J-R., Perry, C. and Kihlstrom, J. (1983) "Hidden observer" phenomena in hypnosis: an experimental creation? *Journal of Personality and Social Psychology*, **44**, 163–9.

Licklider, J.C.R. (1961) On psychological models, in *Sensory Communication: Contributions to the Symposium on the Principles of Sensory Communications*, (ed. W. A. Rosenbluth), MIT Press: Cambridge, Mass., pp. 49–72.

McCaul, K. D. and Mallott, J. M. (1984) Distraction coping with pain. *Psychological Bulletin*, 95, 516–633.

McGlashan, T. H., Evans, F. J. and Orne, M. T. (1969) The nature of hypnotic analgesia and the placebo response to experimental pain. *Psychosomatic Medicine*, **31**, 227–46.

Malmo, B., Boag, T. J. and Raginsky, B. B. (1954) Electomyographic study of hypnotic deafness. *Journal of Experimental and Clinical Hypnosis*, 2, 305–17.

Mann, F. (1962) *Acupuncture: The Ancient Chinese Art of Healing*, Heinemann, London.

Mann, F. (1983) *The Scientific Aspects of Acupuncture*, Heinemann, London.

Melzack, R. (1973a) *The Puzzle of Pain*, Penguin Books, Harmondsworth.

Melzack, R. (1973b) How acupuncture can block pain. *Impact of Science on Society*, **23**, 65–75.

Melzack, R. (1973c) Why acupuncture works. *Psychology Today*, **7**, 28–37.

Melzack, R. (1980) Psychological aspects of pain, in *Pain* (ed. J. J. Bonica), Raven Press, New York.

Melzack, R. and Perry (1975) Self regulation of pain: the use of alpha biofeedback and hypnotic training for the control of chronic pain. *Experimental Neurology*, 46, 452–69.

Melzack, R. and Wall, P. D. (1965) Pain mechanisms: a new theory. *Science* 150, 971–9.

Melzack, R. and Wall, P. D. (1982) *The Challenge of Pain*, Penguin Books, Harmondsworth.

Melzack, R., Weisz, A. Z. and Sprague, T. (1963) Strategies for controlling pain: contributions of auditory stimulation and suggestion. *Experimental Neurology*, **8**, 239–47.

Nadon, R., D'Eon, J., McConkey, K. M. *et al.* (1988) Posthypnotic amnesia, the hidden observer effect and duality during hypnotic age regression. *International Journal of Clinical and Experimental Hypnosis*, **36**, 19–37.

Nasrallah, H. A., Holley, T. and Janowsky, D. S. (1979) Opiate antagonism fails to reverse hypnotic-induced analgesia. *Lancet*, i, 1355.

Nogrady, H., McConkey, K. M., Laurence, J-R. *et al.* (1983) Dissociation, duality and demand characteristics in hypnosis. *Journal of Abnormal Psychology*, **92**, 223–35.

Osler, W. (1901) *The Principles and Practice of Medicine*, 4th edn, K. Kimpton, London.

Pavlov, I. P. (1927) *Conditioned Reflexes*, (Trans. G. V. Anrep) Oxford University Press, London.

Pepper, O. H. (1945) A note on the placebo. *American Journal of Pharmacology*, 117, 409.

Perkins, B. D. (1799) *The Influence of Metallic Tractors on the Human Body*, Ogilvy and Son, London.

Shapiro, A. K. (1960) A contribution to the theory of the placebo effect. *Behavioral Science*, **5**, 109–35.

Skinner, B. F. (1938) *The Behavior of Organisms*, Appleton-Century-Crofts, New York.

Skrabanek, P. (1984) Acupuncture and the age of unreason. *Lancet*, **i**, 1169–71.

Spanos, N. P., Radke, H. L., Hodgins, D. C. *et al.* (1983) The Carleton University Responsiveness to Suggestions Scale. *Psychological Reports*, **53**, 523–35.

Spiro, H. M. (1986) *Doctors, Patients and Placebos*, Yale University Press, New Haven.

Stern, J. A., Brown, M., Ulett, G. A. *et al.* (1977) A comparison of hypnosis, acupuncture, morphine, valium, aspirin, and placebo in the management of experimentally induced pain. *Annals of New York Academy of Science*, **296**, 175–93.

Stukat, K-G. (1958) *Suggestibility: A Factorial and Experimental Analysis*, Almkquist & Wiksell, Stockholm.

Sweet, W. H. (1981) Some current problems in pain research and therapy (including needle puncture acupuncture). *Pain*, **10**, 297–309.

Tellegen, A. and Atkinson, G. (1974) Openness to absorbency and self-altering experiences (absorption): a trait relating to hypnotic susceptibility. *Journal of Abnormal Psychology*, **83**, 268–77.

Tinterow, M. M. (1970) *Foundations of Hypnosis*, C. C. Thomas, Springfield, Ill.

Voudouris, N. J., Peck, C. L. and Coleman, G. J. (1989) Conditioned response models of placebo phenomena: Further support. *Pain*, **38**, 109–16.

Voudouris, N. J., Peck, C. L. and Coleman, G. J., (1990) The role of conditioning and verbal expectancy in the placebo response. *Pain*, **43**, 121–8.

Wadden, T. A. and Anderton, C. H. (1982) The clinical use of hypnosis. *Psychological Bulletin*, **91**, 215–43.

Wikramasekera, I. (1980) A conditioned-response model of the placebo effect: predictions from the model. *Biofeedback and Self-Regulation* **5**, 5–18.

Wilson, S. C. and Barber, T. X. (1983) The fantasy-prone personality. Implications for understanding imagery, hypnosis, and parapsychological phenomena, in *Imagery: Current Theory, Research and Application*, (ed. A. A. Sheikh) J. Wiley & Sons: New York, pp. 340–87.

CHAPTER 6

Hypnotic techniques in the control of pain

Barry B. Hart and P. A. Alden

6.1 INTRODUCTION

This chapter is divided into sections on assessment of pain, strategies of pain control, and hypnotic techniques used in the management of both acute and chronic pain. Although our focus is on the use of hypnosis to ameliorate pain, we feel that it is clinically indefensible to apply hypnotic techniques indiscriminately without a clear understanding of how the client experiences pain, the meaning of it and the effect on the client of the pain, pre-existing coping strategies and the type of pain experienced. We therefore begin with a brief description of various assessment strategies, and direct the reader to Copp (1993) for a more detailed analysis of this area.

In order to assist the reader in effectively applying hypnotic techniques for pain control, we then offer a section on general strategies to consider when treating pain. We suggest that it is of great assistance to both clinician and patient for the former to think strategically before commencing treatment rather than simply to try out various hypnotic techniques. Finally, hypnotic techniques are described as a function of visual, sensory and cognitive categories with case studies offered to demonstrate their appliction.

6.2 ASSESSMENT

The initial interview is critical in establishing rapport and obtaining important information on the patient and his/her pain. The clinician needs to gather the following information:

- the patient's attitude to the referral (especially if this is to a non-physician);

- the patient's hopes, expectations and goals of treatment (e.g. decreasing pain or pain behaviours);
- the type of pain experienced or anticipated (i.e. acute vs. chronic; episodic vs continuous; related to injury, medical procedure or of unknown cause);
- a description of the sensory, affective, and overall evaluative (distressing) aspects of the pain;
- the meaning of the pain for the patient (e.g. emotional significance);
- frequency, duration and intensity of pain and the consequent restrictions on the patient's life;
- previous treatments for pain (and why they have failed);
- pre-existing coping strategies;
- what makes the pain better or worse (e.g. cold vs. warmth);
- potential pain control methods;
- with children, the child's developmental level; social and environmental factors maintaining pain behaviour, and constitutional factors;
- why the patient is presenting now for treatment;
- the patient's attitudes and preconceptions about, and capacity for, hypnosis.

Brown and Fromm (1987) advise that patients self-monitor their pain and recommend, as a supplement to the interview, the administration of the McGill Pain Questionnaire (Melzack, 1975) for the purpose of assessing the sensory, affective and overall evaluative aspects of pain. Although the McGill Pain Questionnaire can be used with adolescents, the Varni/Thompson Paediatric Pain Questionnaire (Varni *et al.*, 1987) and the Children's Comprehensive Pain Questionnaire (McGrath, 1990) are more suited to assess pain in younger children.

To the extent that hypnotizability is more related to the sensory aspects of pain control (Price and Barber, 1987) these questionnaires can also indicate the pain experiences that will be most influenced by the client's hypnotic capacity. By this point in the interview it is hoped that the client will feel that the pain is being taken seriously and acknowledged as being real. This critical aspect of rapport building will help ensure that the client remains in therapy and that the intervention strategies will be credible.

Having the client describe the colour, size and 'shape' of the pain also provide useful indicators of the kind of pain control techniques which are appropriate. Mills and Crowley (1986) have children draw how the pain looks 'right now'; how the pain looks 'all better,' and what will help 'picture one' change into 'picture two'. This is thus both an assessment and treatment strategy.

Part of the assessment of affect will be to evaluate the expression of anxiety and depression. The Beck Anxiety Inventory (Beck *et al.*, 1988) and the Beck Depression Inventory (Beck, 1967) are useful adjuncts to the clinical interview for this purpose. Acute and chronic pain often differ in the expression of anxiety and depression and this can suggest a differential emphasis in treatment (Vingoe, 1993). That is, clients with acute pain, which we conceptualize as being predictable, transient, having signal value and often responsive to medical treatment, often suffer from greater anxiety than those with chronic pain. This is probably due to its more predictable nature, which creates an anticipation of discomfort. Examples are pain associated with childbirth, dysmenorrhoea, and medical and dental procedures such as injections, venipunctures, bone marrow aspirations, lumbar punctures, IUD insertion and surgery.

Chronic and recurrent pain is conceptualized here as being unpredictable, lasting at least six months, having no signal value, usually being unresponsive to medical intervention and greatly affecting psychological health and lifestyle. Examples are pain from spinal injury, low back pain, tension headache, migraine, irritable bowel, atypical facial pain, arthritic and rheumatic pain and pain associated with cancer. Depression and demoralization are common owing to the unremitting nature of chronic pain, the disappointing outcome of therapy, and the losses involved (e.g. in employment, general activity, socializing, hope and self-esteem) (Axelrad, 1990 and 1992).

The importance of assessing pre-existing coping strategies in adults and children is emphasized by Chaves and Brown (1987) and Siegel and Smith (1989), respectively. Chaves and Brown (1987) found that 44% of 75 adult patients undergoing dental procedures employed their own (i.e. spontaneous) pain coping strategies, most notably attention diversion and positive self-statements. Of equal interest was the finding that 37% of the patients studied engaged in catastrophic thinking, which exaggerated the fearful aspects of their experience. Similarly, Siegel and Smith (1989) report on an earlier study by Siegel (1983) where 80 hospitalized children, 8–14 years old, were found to differ in their ability to cope with several potentially stressful and painful procedures as a function of self-generated coping strategies.

Chaves (in press) concludes that, 'The hypnotic subject typically does not present the clinician with a *tabula rasa* on which suggestions can be inscribed without regard for what is already present.' The implication is that if clinicians know of existing strategies used by their patients for managing pain these can be enhanced within a hypnotic context. While a process approach is advocated by Siegel and Smith (1989) with children, the Pain Coping Questionnaire (Brown, 1984) can be a useful adjunct to the interview with adults.

Chaves and Brown (1987) admit to the possibility, however, that it may be equally or more effective to broaden the spectrum of coping skills by introducing new and perhaps unfamiliar strategies to clients.

In order to determine which coping strategies might be most effective, Brown and Fromm (1987) carry out a waking assessment of coping strategies for pain control using the pinching method of pain induction (Spiegel and Spiegel, 1978). Acute neural pain is induced by pinching the webbing of one hand between the thumb and index finger and having the client rate the subsequent discomfort on a 0–5 scale. Pain coping strategies (see column 1, Table 6.1, p.130) are consecutively introduced to determine which is most effective. This is then kept in mind when the focus shifts on to the clinical pain.

In reviewing pain management with children, Dolgin and Jay (1989) suggest that the initial assessment should include an examination of the child's likes, dislikes and fears. Other areas of focus include the child's cognitive and affective status (i.e. developmental level, degree of anxiety/depression, expectations and past coping experience); the amount of positive/negative reinforcement and sociocultural and familial demands for pain expression or suppression; and constitutional factors (e.g. differences in age and pain threshold). The authors believe that this assessment strategy both generates information to allow for hypnosis to be tailored to the child and makes clear its limitations. Interested readers are recommended to see O'Grady (1991) and Olness and Gardner (1988), who provide excellent reviews of hypnosis in the management of childhood pain.

Lastly, some authors (e.g. Hilgard and Hilgard, 1985) believe that the client's capacity for hypnosis (i.e. their hypnotizability) is a crucial and stable determinant in predicting responsiveness to hypnoanaesthesia and thus deserves early measurement. This view is quite contentious, however, with 'non-state' theorists claiming that hypnotizability is best viewed as a modifiable skill (e.g. Gorassini and Spanos, 1986). A third group of more 'Ericksonian-influenced' clinicians (e.g. Barber, 1980) believe that hypnotic scales measure response to only direct suggestion and are thus of little use in pain control when indirect and more conversational methods are used.

Brown & Fromm (1987) prefer a graded difficulty scale (of their own design) to allow a positive yet realistic initial experience with hypnosis to correct patient attitudes about it and its potential use to decrease pain. They acknowledge the disadvantage that this is not a standard test of hypnotizability but claim that it is more likely to foster a sense of self-efficacy in their clients. An interesting variation in assessing clients' capacity to engage in hypnotic phenomena relevant to pain control is the 'Is it possible?' protocol (Margolis, Byrne and Holst-Goltra, 1992). This is similar to Brown and Fromm's (1987) graded difficulty scale but provides more useful information on what the client is able to experience in different sensory modalities that can later be utilized for pain control. Margolis and her colleagues therefore find this 'awareness exercise' far more useful than results from standard hypnotizability scales. As it is so potentially useful, and somewhat difficult to obtain, it is reproduced below, with the authors' permission:

RELAXATION BY SENSORY AWARENESS

Just sit comfortably in the chair and pay attention to what I am going to be saying to you. I am going to ask you a series of questions. Each question could be answered by 'yes' or 'no' but you will not have to say 'yes' or 'no' out loud, or perhaps even to yourself. You can let your answer to the question be whatever your internal response is. Just let yourself respond internally to whatever the particular question is. There is no right or wrong way to respond. I will ask you afterwards how you felt and what you noticed as we went along. Are you ready? Any questions? Remember, you don't have to answer out loud or make any 'yes' or 'no' signs as we go along.

(Allow 5-second pauses between each question)

Is it possible for you to allow your eyes to close?

If they are not closed yet you may close them now.

Is it possible for you to be aware of the area of your back that is in maximum contact with the back of the chair (or with the bed)?

Is it possible for you to think of the chair (bed) as strong, and let it support you?

Is it possible to feel the floor beneath your feet?

Is it possible to be aware of all the sounds that you can hear?

Is it possible to feel the coolness of air in your nose and throat as you inhale?

Is it possible to notice the settling down of your chest and upper body as you exhale?

Is it possible to notice any changes in temperature of any part of your body as you relax?

Is it possible to feel yourself floating, as if on a cloud?

Or are you feeling much too heavy for that?

Is it possible to notice a warm, heavy feeling in your arms and hands?

Is it possible to feel any tingling in your hands . . . or feet?

Is it possible to be aware of the space within your mouth? And can you be aware of the position of your tongue inside your mouth?

Is it possible to notice patterns of light and movement behind your closed eyelids?

Is it possible to feel your face getting very soft?

Is it possible to hear the sound of music in your mind?

Is it possible to imagine a beautiful color in the eye of your mind?

Is it possible to imagine the smell and taste of a food which you like?

Is it possible to imagine yourself in a peaceful, relaxing place?

To look all around in this place and notice details of what you can see, or touch, or hear? (Longer pause)

Is it possible to be aware again of your body in the chair (bed) . . . your feet on the floor . . . the sounds you can hear?

And is it possible to bring yourself back slowly to being awake and alert? You can open your eyes and then take a few more moments to give yourself time to feel completely awake, alert and refreshed, wide awake and comfortable.

Inquiry follows, regarding:

. . . what was noticed

. . . what was felt

. . . which questions were easiest to respond to

. . . which questions were least comfortable or natural to respond to

. . . an estimate of how much time elapsed during the exercise.

In summary, the assessment phase focuses on the clients' description and experiences of their pain as well as pre-existing and potential coping strategies in order to tailor hypnotic pain control techniques to their unique circumstances.

6.3 STRATEGIES FOR PAIN CONTROL

The need for a long-term plan to achieve goals with pain patients is perhaps best summed up by Olness and Gardner (1988): 'Hypnotherapists sometimes approach the problem of pain (in children) in a trial and error fashion, randomly trying hypnoanalgesic techniques with which they are most familiar, with little thought as to why one method might be preferable to another in a particular instance' (p. 175).

A number of strategies can be employed, however, to assist clinicians in rationally selecting pain relief techniques. For example, Spiegel and Spiegel (1990) advocate using different pain control techniques for different levels of hypnotizability. Highly hypnotizable clients are taught self-hypnosis for directly suggesting numbness or body dissociation; mid-range subjects are taught sensory alteration or fantasy techniques; and low hypnotizables are encouraged to use distraction techniques. The authors claim that all of these approaches focus on decreasing the unpleasant aspects of pain while at the same time producing a sense of relaxation. Unfortunately, this approach makes no attempt to make use of existing coping strategies that clients bring with them and thus has limited appeal.

Hammond (1990) suggests that therapists first establish by means of ideomotor signalling whether unconscious factors or past events (e.g. self-punishment or incest) contribute to patient's pain. If no unconscious dynamic is found, 'straightforward' suggestive hypnotic techniques are advocated (e.g. direct suggestion for anaesthesia or imagery modification). He advises against trying to eliminate 100% of the pain except in certain situations such as dental or surgical procedures, terminal illness, phantom limb pain and childbirth. He also advocates having a realistic goal and retaining the signalling function of pain while decreasing the suffering and incapacitating aspects.

If these initial suggestions do not have the desired effect, Hammond (1990) recommends using more complex techniques such as symptom substitution, displacement or time distortion. He claims these latter approaches are particularly useful with chronic or multi-sited pain. He recommends working in a multi-disciplinary team with chronic pain and, like Brown and Fromm (1987) suggests working initially with the least difficult or intense pain first, where success is most likely. Hammond's (1990) approach is somewhat more appealing than Spiegel and Spiegel's (1990), as some effort is made to understand the aetiology of the client's pain prior to the administration of anaesthetic type suggestions.

Similarly, Rossi and Cheek (1990) offer guidelines for treating chronic pain that start with an examination of unconscious motives and early memories of the pain (i.e. 'points of origin') by means of ideomotor signalling. They then suggest that in an hypnotic state the patient turn off all pain at an 'unconscious level' (*sic*), and give a conscious verbal report to confirm this has been done. The patient is then asked to bring back the pain at twice its original strength, followed by its decrease associated with a cue word, to be used as a posthypnotic suggestion. This is rehearsed several times in the office, followed by a future pacing to a time when the patient can see himself/herself in good health and totally free from pain. Ideomotor signalling is used throughout to confirm, at an unconscious level, that all this is occurring just as the therapist suggests. Lastly, Rossi and Cheek advise that patients practise self-hypnosis for relaxation two or three minutes, four times each day.

An impressive strategy for treating chronic pain is the multimodal approach described by Brown and Fromm (1987). They rely heavily on Bandura's (1977) concept of self-efficacy as it relates to decreasing pain and anxiety; that is, the extent to which the belief exists that one has the skills to achieve a desired outcome.

Brown and Fromm (1987) suggest always starting with a symptomatic approach to pain control and using either a lack of response or the response plateau as the criterion for referral on for dynamic hypnotherapy. Approximately 33% of their patients require exploratory methods, either because they do not respond to suggestive hypnosis or because they reach a plateau in response.

According to Brown and Fromm (1987), the initial choice of hypnotic coping strategies is dictated by an interest in enhancing a sense of self-efficacy in their patients. These strategies are then used for the initial phase of treatment of chronic pain in a way that the authors believe undermines the client's sense of despair. That is, they advise against working initially with the primary or target pain; rather they focus on building the client's sense of mastery by exposure to a hierarchy of pain experiences in hypnosis that are progressively difficult to master. They start with induced acute, nonclinical pain and then move on to acute clinical pain (if experienced). Secondary chronic postural pain is next worked on and lastly, the target pain.

In an hypnotic state, the client is given suggestions to lessen induced pain, using the previously chosen coping strategies from the pinching method described above. Ideomotor signalling is used to indicate which coping strategy the client expects to be the most effective. The immediate goal is to have a positive experience in reducing (nonclinical) pain distress and then, if possible, the intensity of the pain sensation, though more important than the latter, is increasing the client's self-efficacy. If successful, suggestions are then given to use the same strategy for coping with pain higher on the hierarchy (i.e. peripheral clinical pain). The strategy continues from the least intense and most peripheral pain and progresses to the target pain only after the client is confident in his/her ability to cope with this pain.

In the next phase of treatment, the client is encouraged to explore a full range of pain-coping strategies, spending increasing time focusing on the pain. Brown and Fromm (1987) believe that this undermines pain-avoidance strategies to escape the pain and alters the perception of pain as unchanging. They find that with experience, patients move from strategies of avoidance and alleviation of pain to turning awareness to the full pain experience by strategies of alteration and awareness of pain (see Table 6.1, p.130). Daily half-hour self-hypnosis sessions are recommended, with or without audiotapes.

The eventual aim is to prevent pain by using coping strategies automatically as soon as any pain is noticed, without having to carry out a ritualized hypnotic procedure. Posthypnotic suggestions are given that as soon as the client notices any pain he/she will automatically use pain coping strategies. The goal is to replace formal hypnotic and self-hypnotic inductions with strategies that work automatically. A pain challenge is then carried out by inducing pain in hypnosis and having the client use hypnotic strategies to decrease it. This is followed by exposure to situations that typically were associated with pain and the client rehearses dealing with them.

For those patients who do not respond to the above protocol, Brown and Fromm (1987) recommend a conflict-resolution approach, such as dynamic psychotherapy/hypnotherapy or family therapy, followed by pain coping strategies. Lastly, the authors describe how hypnosis can be used in the rehabilitation and remobilization phase of treatment and the interested reader is directed to the original source for further details of this.

Melander and Finer (1986) and Finer (1987) describe the use of group hypnosis with chronic pain patients as part of a multi-disciplinary team approach. They acknowledge some disadvantages of a group format but conclude that the advantages of working with groups far outweigh them. Finer suggests having a co-therapist, who, in his clinic, is a female psychologist who also has a chronic pain condition. Three to five in-patients, or eight out-patients, are seen in the group format. All patients are viewed as having an 'inherent trance ability'. Finer's approach is a slow, progressive relaxation induction followed by encouragement to imagine reduced symptoms, constructive attitudes and improved social abilities. There is an emphasis on self-hypnosis, which is taught as soon as possible, and may be tailored to the patient's needs if necessary.

Finer and Melander (1985) admit that treating chronic pain patients is very difficult, and report that from 1978–83 the results from a ten-item questionnaire showed that 35–40% of their patients had less negative symptoms, 50% were unchanged and 10–15% had worsened.

Finally, various other strategic tips are offered by Barber (1982), Ewin (1986), Soskis (1986), Olness and Gardner (1988); Wester and O'Grady (1991), Axelrad (1990 and 1992), Chaves (1992 and in press) and Dane and Brown (1992) for pain control:

- If the patient has difficulty believing that hypnotic pain control is possible, it may be helpful initially to demonstrate other forms of altered body sensation (e.g. hand catalepsy or arm levitation).
- Describe hypnosis as a skill that will develop with time.
- To avoid losing credibility, do not be too specific about when and how the pain will go away.
- Hypnosis tapes tailored to the patient often appear to be more effective than self-hypnosis.
- Administer suggestions for acute pain control prior to its onset.
- Use a combination of strategies when more is learned about the client's experience with pain and his/her coping mechanisms and response to previous hypnotic procedures.
- For maximum effectiveness combine the client's attitudes, expectations, beliefs and contextual and cognitive factors that can modulate the experience of pain.
- Include suggestions for both analgesia and relaxation, as the intensity of pain seems to respond better to the former but the 'unpleasantness' of pain responds better to the latter. With acute pain it is particularly important to offer anxiety reduction suggestions.

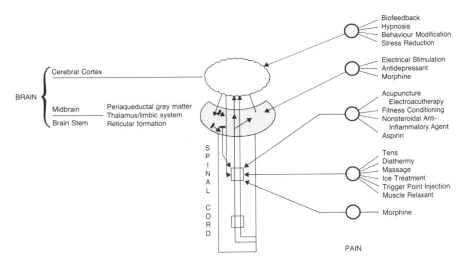

Fig. 6.1 Multi convergent pain management (Axelrad, 1992).

- When seeing children of up to at least 8 years of age, involve their parents from the outset to remind the child of the strategies to use.
- As chronically ill patients can experience all categories of pain (e.g. chronic episodic, benign or malignant, and acute) hypnosis can be useful in different ways at different times in their illness.
- Hypnosis for chronic pain should be applied within a multiple convergent framework, including both physical and psychological interventions (see Figure 6.1).
- Work from the premise that all pain is real but not all pain is useful.
- Inhibiting catastrophizing can be as effective as facilitating coping.
- A direct assault on pain by contradicting the client's experience (e.g. '. . . it doesn't hurt that much . . .') undermines the establishment of rapport and leads to ineffective treatment. Instead, the acknowledgement of pain and hurt and matching the client's experience build rapport. Once this is established, the therapist can then lead the client into comfort with appropriate suggestions.
- With chronic pain, be clear at the outset whether you plan to adopt a 'pain perception' or a 'pain management' model. In the former, a decrease or change in pain sensation will be attempted. In the latter, the goal will be to alter pain behaviours, medication and activity.

Table 6.1 Classifying hypnotic suggestions for pain relief

Brown and Fromm, 1987	Golden et al., 1987	Olness and Gardner, 1988	Hart and Alden, 1993
Avoidance Distraction: internal and external Age regression Time distortion	Hypnotic relaxation and distraction	Distraction techniques Attention to 'unrelated material' Discussion of details of injury or procedure	Visual Switchbox Change shape/colour Scaling (numbers) Medicinal fluid Regulator Magic pool/mist Imaginative inattention
Alleviation Direct suggestions Numbness Imagined analgesia	Direct and indirect suggestions for analgesia	Direct suggestions for hypnoanaesthesia Numbness Topical anaesthesia Local anaesthesia Glove anaesthesia Switchbox	Sensory Direct/indirect suggestions for analgesia/anaesthesia Glove anaesthesia Substitution Displacement Relaxation Thermal change 'Comfort wool'
Alteration Altered memory, meaning or anticipation Dissociation	Transformation of pain to other body part or other type of sensation Dissociation techniques and cognitive restructuring	Distancing suggestions Moving pain away from self Transferring pain to another body part Paying attention to pain itself: 'Lighted globe'	Cognitive Reinterpretation Distraction Time distortion Amnesia Age regression/progression Dissociation Exploratory methods Inner adviser/counsellor Mystical states Sensory awareness Ego-strengthening

Awareness	Suggestions for feelings	Ericksonian
Focusing on sensations and	antithetical to pain	Truisms
reactions	Comfort	Interspersal
	Laughter	Confusion
	Relaxation	Reminders of comfort
		Future pacing
		Phantom limb pleasure

Note: Modified from Wester and O'Grady (1991)

6.4 TECHNIQUES

There are a number of ways to categorize hypnotic techniques for pain control. Table 6.1 offers four classification systems, including our own which groups techniques into the primary sensory modalities (i.e. visual, sensory and cognitive) called upon to produce the desired effect, plus some of those that appear to be unique to Milton H. Erickson.

Interestingly, most clinicians appear to make use of the same types of hypnotic techniques for pain control, but those with a non-state orientation put less emphasis on the induction and more on contextual factors (e.g. Chaves, 1992). Brief descriptions are offered below for each of the techniques listed by us in Table 6.1, with case examples to demonstrate some applications. All techniques can be used with acute, episodic and chronic pain, unless otherwise specified. Therapist and client will be referred to as T and C, respectively, except when a number follows the letter (e.g. T12 or C5), which indicates either a thoracic or cervical vertebra.

6.4.1 Visual

Switchbox: Olness and Gardner (1988) suggest that T explains to C that pain is transmitted by nerves from the body to the brain which then sends a 'pain message' back to the body. (Coloured drawings can be used to facilitate this.) C is asked to choose a switch that can turn off or modulate incoming nerve signals (e.g. a flip, dimmer or pull) situated wherever C wants (e.g. in the brain or near the site of the pain). C is asked to practise turning off the switches for defined periods of time, starting with only 10–15 seconds and working towards longer periods. Success is judged by touching C with a sharp object and asking for a comparison with feelings on the other side where the nerve signals are unchanged. Vividness of imagery and the degree of control and mastery experienced by C affect the success of this technique.

A variation of this method is to describe the gate control theory of pain perception, with the suggestion that C can imagine 'closing the gate' to modulate pain sensation. This can also be combined with substituting a more acceptable sensation (e.g. warm tingling) for pain.

Change shape or colour: Cs with episodic or chronic pain are asked to picture the shape and colour that best represent the pain, followed by suggestions that it change to a more desirable shape and colour.

Scaling: Barber (1990) describes a method of scaling chronic pain that the present authors have both found to be very useful. C is asked to rate the severity of pain, prior to hypnosis, from 0–10, with 0 representing no pain and 10 the worst pain C has ever experienced. Following a hypnotic induction, C is asked to re-rate the pain and to see the number representing it in his/her mind. T then suggests that as C watches the number, it changes shape into the next lower number, with a commensurate decrease in pain.

A variation of this technique is to raise the numbers first, with a commensurate increase in pain, followed by the suggestion that 'Whatever goes up can come down.' With either approach, T continues by suggesting that the number gets smaller and smaller with consequent decreases in pain, until an agreed level is reached, such as 1 or 2. The post-hypnotic suggestion is then given that C can keep this number (and the associated comfort) in his/her mind after the hypnosis session is over and that he/she can use this technique (of decreasing numbers) when alone whenever needed. This technique can also be modified to reduce anxiety.

Medicinal fluid: Cs with episodic or chronic pain are asked to imagine drinking a special nice-tasting drink that fills their body like an empty vessel and attaches itself to the pain. As it does so, it turns into a dark colour and becomes thick in consistency. The more pain it attaches to the darker and thicker it becomes. When it has gone black and sludgy, C is asked to imagine opening taps at the fingers and toes and to let this dark fluid drain away, taking most if not all the pain with it. The taps are then shut and T suggests that C is now filled with a lovely comfortable feeling inside. Cs with chronic pain are told to use this imagery on a regular basis.

Soskis (1986) describes his 'flowing and discarding' technique, asking C to experience his/her pain as a fluid, to move the fluid through the body to a hand, and then to discard it. This appears to be a variation on Stein's (1963) clenched fist technique for anchoring positive and negative feelings and discarding the latter.

Regulator: In this variation on the switchbox and scaling techniques, C is asked to visualize a dial with numbers or high/low marks, representing the pain. As C rotates it in the direction of lower numbers or marks, suggestions are given for a decrease in pain.

Case 6.1

A 14-year-old boy with a burning pain in paralysed legs chose to imagine a volume control at waist level which he could 'turn down' whenever he needed to. He also needed to retain some of the sensation in his legs, but as a 'warm tingling.' For a spinally injured patient, learning to cope with paralysis requires considerable adjustment. For this teenager, sensation in his legs, even if it was not functional, had significance. Symbolically it indicated that 'something was still alive'.

Magic pool: Alden (1992) asks C to imagine travelling down a path from a garden or beach and to discover a secluded and private pool with special properties to soothe and calm. C is asked to imagine entering the water while T emphasizes its healing properties and suggests it can wash away pain and anxiety, leaving an invisible healing film on the skin. This technique can also be used for skin disorders by suggesting that the water has a medicinal effect.

Magic mist: Wall (1990) invites a child to imagine the chair he/she is relaxing in has become a 'cloud car' that can fly under his/her control. T asks C to imagine flying to a special place and then walking into some healing mist or fog that is suggested will make C feel comfortable, numb, happy and in control. C is told he/she can use this imagery at any time it's necessary to become more comfortable.

Imaginative inattention: T engages C's imagination to conjure up a scene that is incompatible with pain, such as lying on a beach feeling relaxed.

Case 6.2

13-year-old Ryan had suffered with frequent tension headaches for three years and had not responded to analgesic medication. History taking revealed that he enjoyed flying when on holiday and that coolness applied to his head usually eased the pain. Following an eye-roll induction, he was asked to imagine enjoying being on a plane. After he indicated that he was there, Ryan was reminded of no smoking seats on the plane, and he confirmed he knew about these. He was then asked to walk around the plane to find the *no headache* seats, and to ask the stewardess for help if necessary. Once Ryan indicated he was sitting in a no headache seat, T asked him to reach above his head and to turn on the air conditioning by twisting the appropriate knob. T suggested that as Ryan did this, cool air would come out of it and blow across Ryan's forehead and remove any discomfort. These suggestions had an immediately beneficial effect on Ryan, and he was asked to practise this technique daily until next seen. When seen one week later, Ryan was pleased to report that the imagery had been successful in aborting these headaches. He was instructed to use the imagery in a preventative way, and when seen at one and three month follow-up was pleased to report that he had suffered with significantly fewer headaches and felt more able to control a headache if one arose.

6.4.2　Sensory

Direct/indirect suggestions for analgesia/anaesthesia: T simply suggests that the pain will lessen and gradually go away, although probably not completely. Direct suggestions can be used: 'You know what a numb feeling is. Just let that part of your body get numb now' . . . or indirect suggestions can be given: 'I wonder if you'll be surprised or curious to notice how easily you can remember how your (arm, leg, etc.) feels when it falls asleep, either just before or just after your next breath.'

Glove anaesthesia: T asks C to pay attention to his/her hand and to notice tingling feelings develop there. 'When your hand is very numb, touch that hand to your (leg, arm, etc.) and let the numb feelings transfer from your hand to the (leg, arm, etc.). Kuttner (1986) describes the magic glove technique with a child with cancer who had a strong dislike of intravenous (IV) chemotherapy, making her treatment very stressful for her. The suggestion was given for the child to imagine putting a magic glove over her hand to cover, protect and numb the hand. Once the glove was on, the IV needle was inserted into a vein without difficulty or the upset that had plagued previous treatments. Kuttner (1986) claims that part of the success of this technique depends on the child and parent(s) believing in the process.

Substitution: Substituting another sensation (e.g. itching, pressure or warmth) for pain can assist in a re-interpretation of unpleasant sensation. Success is more likely if the substituted sensation is not totally pleasant as this would be somewhat implausible to the client. Like displacement, once a successful substitution is achieved, this demonstrates that change is possible in other aspects of the pain as well. Barber (1986) points out that cancer patients in particular may need some sensation for reassurance that they and the medical team will be aware of any change in their physical condition in order to treat it appropriately.

Displacement: In suggesting that pain can move from one part of the body to another (usually healthy) site, the goal is to make the unpleasant sensations more tolerable and to imply that change in other dimensions (e.g. intensity) is possible. Pain in the extremities is usually less frightening than pain in the abdomen (Karle and Boys, 1987). Humour can also be introduced by displacing pain into a finger or ear lobe. An example of a permissive suggestion for displacement is:

> 'You may have already noticed that the pain moves, ever so slightly, as you can begin to notice that the movement seems to be in an outwardly spiralling circular direction. As you continue to attend to that movement, you may not notice until later that the pain has somehow moved out of your abdomen and seems to be staying in your left hand'.

> *(Barber, 1986, p. 157)*

Relaxation: To the extent that physiological changes associated with tension and anxiety can increase pain, relaxation methods can play a part in pain management. Various types of hypnotic suggestions for relaxation can be administered, such as the following:

Case 6.3

A man of 21 years injured at C5 had very limited hand function. His ability to feed himself was being disrupted by severe spasms which were accompanied by a 'burning electric shock type' pain. Hypnosis was induced and he developed a relaxing image of driving along in a car and becoming more and more comfortable with every mile. Then the following suggestions were given:

'As you relax your eyelids and all the muscles of your face and neck . . . deeper and deeper relaxed . . . you might be surprised to learn that every cell in your body . . . knows how to relax . . . How to tell every other cell in your body to relax . . . And as you experience that comfortable relaxation in your face and neck . . . all the cells in the skin and muscles of your face . . . can tell all the cells of your body . . . right down to your toes . . . to relax . . . deeply . . . and they can send chemical and electrical messages . . . cell to cell . . .' The patient easily learned to induce a deeply relaxed state in himself and both he and the staff on the spinal unit reported a decrease in spasm and improvement in function.

Thermal change: Part of the assessment will be to discover whether coolness or warmth helps to alleviate pain. Suggestions will therefore follow to capitalize upon whichever has been helpful in the past. Suggestions for hand warmth and head cooling are typically used for migraine (Alladin, 1988), and hand warmth to the stomach for irritable bowel syndrome (Whorwell, Prior and Faragher, 1984). Chaves (in press) reports that suggestions for cooling are also often used for causalgias, sympathetic reflex dystrophy and some types of central pain.

Comfort wool: Suggestions are given that C imagine cotton wool being wrapped around his/her body in order to produce comfort as in the following case:

Case 6.4

A female patient with a complete injury at T12 was experiencing severe and constant back pain. Medication was ineffective and her sleep and appetite were affected by her discomfort. She responded well to an eye closure induction and demonstrated the ability to visualize. She had made it clear that any further loss of sensation would be unacceptable, as this was equated in her mind with loss of function. However, she was able to imagine 'comfort so powerful that it could be taken like cotton wool and wrapped around your back' as follows:

'As you enjoy being so comfortable . . . that nothing need bother you . . . nothing need disturb you . . . just imagine you have a very powerful magnifying glass . . . that can magnify comfort . . . just let me know when it is as strong and comfortable as it needs to be . . .' (finger signal given) . . . 'Now . . . it's interesting how feelings can become solid . . . tangible . . . maybe like cotton wool . . . I wonder what that comfort can look like . . . can feel like . . . just let me know when you can see and feel it . . . (A

description of it being like 'pink soft cotton wool' was given) . . .
Now just take that pink soft cotton wool and wrap it around your
back where you need it and just notice how it feels . . . how
comfortable . . . and soft . . . and warm . . .'

She soon learned how to hypnotize herself, produce the 'comfort
wool' and come out of her hypnotic state leaving the 'wool' in
place.

6.4.3 Cognitive

Reinterpretation: T asks C to imagine the painful sensations occurring in
a different, more acceptable context in order to alter their meaning (e.g.
asking a child to imagine that he/she is a spy and the pain in his/her
arm is from getting shot by an enemy spy; or that the pain is due to a
sports injury or important life event).

Distraction: Distraction techniques leave less of C's attention to focus
on pain. Internal distraction methods absorb C in either a pattern of
thought such as mental arithmetic, reciting a poem or pleasurable fantasy or story (e.g. magic carpet ride), or another body part (e.g. breathing), with accompanying suggestions for enhanced comfort. External
distraction shifts attention on to innocuous environmental objects and
stimuli such as watching a favourite television programme or describing
the scenery around oneself (e.g. counting ceiling tiles in a clinic setting).

Kuttner (1984) describes the successful application of her favourite-
story technique used to minimize pain, distress and anxiety in preschool
children undergoing bone marrow aspirations. After the child's favourite story is identified, it is adapted and interwoven with procedural and
sensory information about the ongoing painful treatment. Ross and
Ross (1988) claim that the use of a favourite story can have 'considerable
distraction potentional and a number of positive and reassuring associations for the child' (p. 235).

Greene and Reyher (1972) found that with adults, imagery that was
not body-oriented (e.g. looking at scenery or skiing) was more effective
than body-oriented imagery (e.g. feeling the warmth of the sun) for
pain control. Interestingly, Dane and Brown (1992) similarly find that
Cs initially prefer avoidance and alleviation strategies (see Table 6.1)
that focus attention away from the pain, but advocate gradually shifting
Cs on to alteration and awareness ones.

Time distortion: Suggestions for time distortion capitalize on naturally
occurring experiences of time passing quickly (e.g. when bumping into
an old friend) or slowly (e.g. when waiting for a taxi in the rain). Once
C is hypnotized, the suggestion is given that when pain occurs, time
will pass quickly; during pain-free intervals, however, time will go very
slowly and seem to last forever, in order to produce a subjective sense
of being comfortable for longer periods.

Amnesia: Suggestions that C will forget painful memories can help to decrease anticipatory anxiety and pain associated with medical and dental procedures. Similarly, T can suggest that C can forget current pain immediately after it occurs, in order to prevent it from having a negative emotional effect.

Barber (1977) capitalizes on naturally occurring remembering and forgetting by suggesting it can happen again, as in his permissive and indirect Rapid Induction Analgesia suggestions for dental procedures.

Age regression/progression: T can offer suggestions that promote absoroption in thoughts, ideas and feelings that were enjoyable prior to pain onset or that will be enjoyable in the future (Chaves, in press). These feelings can be anchored to C rubbing fingertips together on one hand, with the posthypnotic suggestion that C can bring back 'most if not all of these feelings of well-being' simply by again rubbing together the fingertips.

Dissociation: Suggestions are given for the separation of either body parts or the whole body from pain by thinking about the body in a detached way. This technique works on the premise that 'If the body isn't here . . . it can't feel pain.' Following Brown and Fromm's (1987) advice to start with either induced or neutral sensation, T can facilitate the experience of dissociation by suggesting that C's hand (or foot, etc.) can float away and be 'somewhere else' prior to focusing on the painful site.

An out-of-body experience can be achieved by suggesting that C experience himself/herself in another time, place or state, as in a vivid daydream (Barber, 1982). This can be useful if C is immobilized by a medical or dental procedure, if the condition renders C immobile, or if there are multiple painful sites. For instance, T can suggest that '. . . While part of you is sitting in that chair, the rest of you can step or float out of your body, walk over to the window and describe for me what you see outside . . . Later on today, when you want to feel more comfortable, you can simply close your eyes and take yourself off in your mind's eye to somewhere you would rather be, such as that favourite museum you told me about.'

Olness and Gardner (1988) claim that every hypnoanalgesic technique they use involves dissociation either directly or indirectly (e.g. in refering to 'that arm' rather than 'your arm').

Ewin (1986) claims that seriously burned patients in an emergency-room setting are already in an altered state due to their focus on the burn and dissociation from external reality. After applying wet towels to the burn, thus producing some instant pain relief, Ewin distracts the patient by asking . . . 'Do you know how to treat this kind of burn?' Upon receiving a negative reply, Ewin reassures the patient that he knows how to treat the burn and the patient did what was necessary in getting to the hospital. Thus, '. . . there is nothing more for you to do and you can hand over the burn to me and then quite happily go to your laughing place . . .' This rapid utilization of the patient's existing focused state of mind followed by strong reassurance facilitates further dissociation and pain control. Suggestions of 'cool, wet grass' are given to lower the temperature of the injury and to keep the site moist. Ewin (1986 and 1992) provides impressive results from this approach.

Exploratory methods: Various uncovering techniques can be used to explore the psychological meaning of chronic pain, or for unconscious co-operation in the control or alleviation of either acute or chronic pain. Age regression, Wolberg's theatre technique and Redlich's jigsaw method are described by Hartland (1971). Rossi and Cheek (1988) provide a very useful review of how unconscious factors related to pain can be explored by ideomotor finger signalling.

Exploratory methods are advised if the pain is associated with past trauma (e.g. incest) or serve unconscious purposes (e.g. self-punishment). This is especially true if the cause of the pain is unknown and cannot be causally related to any organic process, where the pain is more intense than expected, and/or when it lasts longer than expected (Hammond, 1990). For example, Ewin (1980) describes how fear of death can produce 'constant pain syndrome'.

Inner adviser/counsellor: This technique rests on the assumption that at an unconscious level C knows how to control his/her pain. T either suggests a scene with '. . . someone who knows all about you and how to help who you can talk with . . .' or one in which C watches someone similar to himself/herself successfully coping with pain in a new and different way. C thus is being given an opportunity to generate new pain-control techniques that are ego-syntonic.

In an interesting variation of this approach, Dane and Brown (1992) use a hypnoprojective technique for C to discover new pain coping strategies. C is asked to imagine sitting either in a theatre or in front of a television. T suggests that at the count of five C will observe someone on stage or TV who has a very similar pain problem to C. C is asked to simply observe and discover how the person copes with and manages pain, in order to access 'preconscious' coping styles. This is repeated two or three times until C has a clear sense of how to manage pain in a new way. C is then asked to imagine practising the new strategy until a sense of mastery over the pain develops. If a television is being watched, T suggests that C can read subtitles at the bottom of the screen describing the (coping) thoughts going through the mind of the person in the picture. C is told that in time the full meaning of what was observed will become clear.

Mystical states: Sacerdote (1990) offers suggestions for 'introvertive' and 'extrovertive' mystical experiences in order to induce either a state of serenity or to expand C's perception of time and space, respectively. Both are meant to distance C from the reality of pain, illness and death.

In the former, a deep sense of psychological calm, with suggestions for sensory and emotional isolation from pain, is symbolized by C relaxing in the centre of transparent concentric spheres that restrict sensory input. Conversely, an extrovertive state frees C from the limits of time and activities by suggesting multisensory imagery (e.g. climbing a mountain).

Sensory awareness: Instead of giving distancing suggestions from pain, this technique provides C with sensory information about pain either before it occurs (to produce an accurate mental set) or while it is happening. Providing full awareness of the pain experience prompts insight into the nature of pain perception and C's reactivity to it (Brown and Fromm, 1987). T helps C to analyse pain sensations into their more benign components, such as pressure, heat, cold or tingling.

Olness and Gardner (1988) suggest that focusing on a painful medical procedure or injury is useful with children for whom cognitive mastery is a major coping mechanism. T asks C to describe the injury in detail, or with painful procedures, T describes various instruments and asks C to assist by holding them or bandages, counting sutures or checking the time at various points. They also advise on focusing on the 'lesser of two evils' with sensations, such as directing C's attention to cold as opposed to pain.

Ego-strengthening: Chronic pain patients typically develop feelings of low self-esteem or self-worth that can respond to ego enhancing type suggestions. Although Hartland's (1971) ego-strengthening suggestions are well known, refinements of these have been discussed by Heap (1985). Hammond (1990) makes the useful point that teaching self-hypnosis also provides patients with an active self-management strategy that can return some sense of control and mastery to their lives.

6.4.4 Ericksonian

Truisms: Erickson (1990) reminded Cs of their lifelong experiences in developing anaesthesia in all parts of the body, such as limbs going numb ('to sleep') and not noticing objects attached to the body (e.g. shoes on the feet, a watch on the wrist, and glasses on the nose) until attention is drawn to them.

Interspersal: Erickson (1990) 'seeded' ideas by interspersing words or phrases within the context of an apparently neutral story or discussion. Such embedded suggestions were highlighted by using an altered voice pitch or tone or a brief pause (Hammond, 1990). To an elderly florist with facial cancer and intolerable pain, Erickson (1966) said: (suggestions in bold) '. . . Now as I talk, and I can do so comfortably, I wish that you will **listen to me comfortably** as I talk about a tomato plant. . . . One can **feel hope** that a seed will grow into a tomato plant that **will bring satisfaction** by the fruit it has. The seed soaks up water, **not**

much difficulty in doing that because of the rains that **bring peace and comfort** and the joy of growing to flowers and tomatoes . . .'

Confusion and disorientation: Erickson (1990) would attempt to confuse C about the site and direction of pain in order to facilitate displacing it to a more 'healthy' area. This reorientation to a less threatening site produced anaesthesia at the painful site. Erickson would begin by discussing rightness, leftness, centrality and dextrality (Hammond, 1990).

Reminders of comfort: Asking C to recall times of great comfort and relaxation from the past can produce rapid inductions and relaxed states in the here and now. This is especially useful with Cs who are having difficulty responding to more traditional suggestions to relax. Or, after an initial successful relaxing hypnotic experience, in future sessions T can simply remind C of the previous session and ask for the comfortable feelings associated with it to be brought back to the here and now.

Future pace: An interesting variation of age progression is called future pacing or pseudo-orientation in time (Rossi, 1980) where C is asked to imagine going forward in time some weeks or months and see himself/ herself as they want to be (e.g. being pain free). After C has acknowledged that this is visualized, he/she is asked to come back to the present time, keeping eyes closed, and to then slowly review the process of how he/she got from how he/she is now to how he/she wants to be in the future. This can generate new strategies for pain-control.

Phantom pleasure: Erickson and Rossi (1979) ingeniously suggest to a C with a phantom limb pain that he can also have phantom limb pleasure. Erickson did so by telling his patient a story of a double amputee whose itch was relieved by a nurse scratching where his foot used to be. Erickson's patient was in a receptive frame of reference as he had already accepted other anecdotes about learning to change sensory-perceptual experiences.

6.5 CONCLUSION

This chapter has suggested that clinicians will be more effective in treating pain after considering a number of assessment and strategic issues. Ascertaining the 'meaning' and emotional significance of pain is thought to be critical to successful outcome. The focus on hypnotic techniques for pain control may be more relevant for those working within a 'pain perception model' but hopefully others will also be encouraged to apply some of the more innovative and practical ideas presented here.

Interestingly, clinicians differ on the importance they place on unconscious factors in the understanding and treatment of pain. Some advise on starting with an examination of unconscious factors (e.g. Rossi and Cheek, 1990) while others advocate applying a symptomatic approach first (e.g. Brown and Fromm, 1987). Regardless of differences in clinical orientation, there is now an emphasis on enhancing self-efficacy and adopting a 'mastery model' in hypnosis and psychotherapy (Baker, 1987). There is also an acknowledgement that clients have both conscious and unconscious solutions to their problems. This Ericksonian notion of the unconscious having therapeutic resources has influenced a generation of hypnotherapists. The therapist's task thus becomes one of accessing Cs' pre-existing pain coping strategies, generating new ones with C's help, and matching interventions to Cs' unique characteristics.

REFERENCES

Alden, P. A. (1992) The use of hypnosis in the management of pain on a spinal injuries unit. *Paper presented at the 12th International Congress of Hypnosis*, Jerusalem.

Alladin, A. (1988) Hypnosis in the treatment of severe chronic migraine, in *Hypnosis: Current Clinical, Experimental and Forensic Practices*, (ed. M. Heap), Croom Helm, London, pp. 159–66.

Axelrad, A. D. (1990) The role of hypnosis in multiple convergent management of chronic pain. *Houston Medicine*, **6**, 111–19.

Axelrad, A. D. (1992) The role of hypnosis in multiple convergent management of chronic pain. *Paper presented at the 12th International Congress of Hypnosis*, Jerusalem.

Baker, E. L. (1987) The state of the art of clinical hypnosis. *The International Journal of Clinical and Experimental Hypnosis*, **35**(4), 203–14.

Bandura, A. (1977) Self efficacy: Toward a unifying theory of behavior change. *Psychological Review*, **84**, 191–215.

Barber, J. (1977) Rapid induction analgesia: A clinical report. *American Journal of Clinical Hypnosis*, **19**, 138–47.

Barber, J. (1980) Hypnosis and the unhypnotizable. *American Journal of Clinical Hypnosis*, **23**, 4–9.

Barber, J. (1982) Managing acute pain, in *Psychological Approaches to the Management of Pain*, (eds J. Barber and C. Adrian), Brunner Mazel, New York.

Barber, J. (1986) Hypnotic analgesia, in *A Handbook of Psychological Treatment Approaches*, (eds A. Holzman and D. C. Turk), Academic Press, New York, pp. 151–67.

Barber, J. (1990) Techniques of hypnotic pain management, in *Hypnotic Suggestions and Metaphors*, (ed. D. C. Hammond), W. W. Norton & Co, London, pp. 50–2.

Beck, A. T. (1967) *Depression: Clinical, Experimental and Theoretical Aspects*, Holber, New York.

Beck, A. T., Epstein, N., Brown, G. *et al.* (1988) An inventory for measuring clinical anxiety: psychometric properties. *Journal of Consulting and Clinical Psychology*, **56**, 893–7.

Brown, D. P. (1984) A questionnaire study of pain coping strategies. Unpublished manuscript.

Brown, D. P. and Fromm, E. (1987) *Hypnosis and Behavioral Medicine*, Lawrence Erlbaum Associates Publishers, London.

Chaves, J. F. (1992) Hypnotic analgesia: The social-psychological perspective, in *Hypnosis: 175 Years after Mesmer-Recent Developments in Theory and Application*, (eds W. Bongartz, B. Bongartz and V. A. Gheorghiu), Universitats-verlag Konstanz: Konstanz, pp. 109–17.

Chaves, J. F. (in press) Hypnosis in pain management, in *Handbook of Clinical Hypnosis*, (eds J. Rhue, S. Lynn and I. Kirsch), American Psychological Association: Washington, D.C.

Chaves, J. F. and Brown, J. M. (1987) Spontaneous cognitive strategies for the control of clinical pain and stress. *Journal of Behavioral Medicine*, **10**(3), 263–75.

Copp, L. A. (1993) Pain assessment, management and research: The nurse's role, in *Psychology, Pain and Anesthesia*, (ed. H. B. Gibson), Chapman and Hall Ltd., London.

Dane, J. R. and Brown, D. P. (1992) Hypnosis and pain. *Society of Clinical and Experimental Hypnosis Annual Workshop*, Washington D.C.

Dolgin, M. and Jay, S. M. (1989) Pain management in children, in *Treatment of Childhood Disorders*, (eds E. Mash and R. Barkley), The Guilford Press, New York, pp. 383–404.

Erickson, M. (1966) The interspersal hypnotic technique for symptom correction and pain control. *American Journal of Clinical Hypnosis*, **8**, 189–209.

Erickson, M. H. and Rossi, E. L. (1979) *Hypnotherapy: An Exploratory Casebook*, Irvington Publishers, Inc. New York.

Erickson, M. H. (1990) Erickson's suggestions for pain control, in *Handbook of Hypnotic Suggestions and Metaphors*, (ed. D. C. Hammond), W. W. Norton, London, pp. 54; 68–70.

Ewin, D. M. (1980) Constant pain syndrome: Its psychological meaning and cure using hypnoanalysis, in *Clinical Hypnosis in Medicine*, (ed. H. J. Wain), Year Book Medical Publishers, Chicago, pp. 41–50.

Ewin, D. M. (1986) Emergency room hypnosis for the burned patient. *American Journal of Clinical Hypnosis*, **29**(1), 29–37.

Ewin, D. M. (1992) Hypnosis for pain. *Paper presented at the 12th International Congress of Hypnosis*, Jerusalem.

Finer, B. and Melander, B. (1985) Living in Chronic Pain, in *Persistent Pain*, Vol. 5, (ed. S. Lipton), Grune & Stratton, London.

Finer, B. (1987) A multi-disciplinary approach to the hypnotherapy of chronic pain patients. *Hypnosis*, **14**(1), 22–7.

Golden, W. L., Dowd, E. I. and Friedberg, F., (1987) *Hypnotherapy: A Modern Approach*, Pergamon, New York.

Gorassini, D. R. and Spanos, N. P. (1986) A social-cognitive skills training program for the successful modification of hypnotic susceptibility. *Journal of Personality and Social Psychology*, **50**, 1004–12.

Greene, R. J. and Reyher, J. (1972) Pain tolerance in hypnotic analgesic and imagination states. *Journal of Abnormal Psychology*, **79**, 29–38.

Hammond, D. C. (ed) (1990) *Handbook of Hypnotic Suggestions and Metaphors*, W. W. Norton & Co., London.

Hartland, J. (1971) *Medical and Dental Hypnosis*, Bailliere Tindall, London.

Heap, M. (1985) Ego-strengthening: further considerations. *Proceedings of the Second Annual Conference of the British Society of Experimental and Clinical Hypnosis*, London.

Hilgard, E. R. and Hilgard, J. R. (1985) *Hypnosis in the Relief of Pain*, William Kaufmann, Los Altos, California.

Karle, H. W. A. and Boys, J. H. (1987) *Hypnotherapy: A Practical Handbook*, Free Association Books, London.

Kuttner, L. (1984) Favorite stories: A hypnotic pain reduction technique for children in acute pain. *Paper presented at the American Society for Clinical Hypnosis Conference*, San Francisco.

Kuttner, L. (1986) *No Fears . . . No Tears: Children with Cancer Coping with Pain.* A Video/Guide Production, Vancouver: Canadian Cancer Society.

Margolis, C., Byrne, B. and Holst-Goltra, P. (1992) Hypnosis for pain control. *Workshop at the 12th International Congress of Hypnosis*, Jerusalem.

McGrath, P. A. (1990) *Pain in Children: Nature, Assessment and Treatment*, The Guilford Press, London.

Melander, B. and Finer, B. (1986) Co-therapist – hypnotherapist in group hypnotherapy. *Hypnos*, **13**(2), 74–6.

Melzack, R. (1975) The McGill Pain Questionnaire: Major properties and scoring methods. *Pain*, **1**, 277–99.

Mills, J. C. and Crowley, R. J. (1986) *Therapeutic Metaphors for Children and the Child Within*, Brunner Mazel, New York.

O'Grady, D. J. (1991) Hypnosis and pain management in children, in *Clinical Hypnosis with Children*, (eds W. C. Wester and D. J. O'Grady), Brunner Mazel, New York, pp. 213–29.

Olness, K. N. and Gardner, G. G. (1988) *Hypnosis and Hypnotherapy with Children*, 2nd edn, Grune and Stratton, London.

Price, D. D. and Barber, J. (1987) An analysis of factors that contribute to the efficacy of hypnotic analgesia. *Journal of Abnormal Psychology*, **96**(1), 1–6.

Ross, D. M. and Ross, S. A. (1988) *Childhood Pain: Current Issues, Research, and Management*, Urban and Schwarzenberg, Baltimore.

Rossi, E. L. (1980) *The Collected Papers of Milton H. Erickson on Hypnosis, vol. IV*, Irvington Publishers, Inc., New York.

Rossi, E. L. and Cheek, D. B. (1988) *Mind-Body Therapy: Methods of Ideodynamic Healing in Hypnosis*. W. W. Norton & Co., New York.

Rossi, E. L. and Cheek, D. B. (1990) General principles for alleviating persistent pain, in *Handbook of Hypnotic Suggestions and Metaphors*, (ed. D. C. Hammond), W. W. Norton and Co., London, pp. 56–8.

Sacerdote, P. (1990) Hypnotically elicited mystical states in treating physical and emotional pain, in *Handbook of Hypnotic Suggestions and Metaphors*, (ed. D. C. Hammond), W. W. Norton and Co., London, pp. 63–6.

Siegel, L. J. (1983) Hospitalization and medical care of children, in *Handbook of Clinical Child Psychology*, (eds E. Walker and M. Roberts), J. Wiley & Sons: New York, pp. 1089–108.

Siegel, L. J. and Smith, K. E. (1989) Children's strategies for coping with pain. *Pediatrician*, *16*, 110–18.

Soskis, D. A. (1986) *Teaching Self-Hypnosis: An Introductory Guide for Clinicians*, W. W. Norton, London.

Spiegel, H. and Spiegel, D. (1978) *Trance and treatment: Clinical Uses of Hypnosis*, Basic Books, New York.

Spiegel, D. and Spiegel, H. (1990) Pain strategies by hypnotizability level, in *Handbook of Hypnotic Suggestions and Metaphors*, (ed. D. C. Hammond), W. W. Norton and Co., London. pp. 67–8.

Stein, C. (1963) The clenched fist technique as a hypnotic procedure in clinical psychotherapy. *American Journal of Clinical Hypnosis*, **6**, 113–19.

Varni, J. W., Thompson, K. L. and Hanson, V. (1987) The Varni/Thompson Pediatric Pain Questionnaire: I. Chronic musculoskeletal pain in juvenile rheumatoid arthritis. *Pain*, *28*, 27–38.

Vingoe, F. J. (1993) Anxiety and pain, in *Psychology, Pain and Anesthesia*, (ed H. B. Gibson), Chapman & Hall Ltd., London.

Wall, V. J. (1990) Hypnotic procedure for pain control, in *Handbook of Hypnotic*

Suggestions and Metaphors, (ed. D. C. Hammond), W. W. Norton & Co., London, pp. 481–4.

Wester, W. C. and O'Grady, D. J. (eds) (1991) *Clinical Hypnosis with Children*, Brunner Mazel, New York.

Whorwell, P. J., Prior, A. and Faragher, E. B. (1984) Controlled trial of hypnotherapy in the treatment of severe refractory irritable bowel syndrome. *Lancet*, **2**, 1232–4.

CHAPTER 7

Cognitive effects of anaesthesia

Steven P. Mewaldt, M. M. Ghoneim and
Robert I. Block

7.1 INTRODUCTION

This chapter provides an overview of cognitive effects of pharmacological agents commonly used in anaesthesia and of cognitive deficits associated with the post-operative period. As one might expect, drugs which are intended to alter consciousness or influence tranquillity and mood have other effects on cognitive processes. Certain of these effects are desirable. For example, anaesthesiologists often administer drugs with the objective of abolishing memory during surgery. However, at other times the effects of these treatments are undesirable, as with cognitive deficits that may occur as a complication of anaesthesia and surgery. The risk of post-operative cognitive deficits may be a source of anxiety to patients and their families, and may in some cases be life-threatening by interfering with the patient's compliance with therapeutic regimens. Such deficits may also prolong recovery, and reduce the patient's quality of life.

Because of the range of drugs and topics to be covered and limitations in space, this review is not intended to be a complete catalogue of reported results. Rather it should provide the reader with a general understanding of the nature of known cognitive deficits and illustrate how additional research in this area might be conducted. Three major topics are addressed:

- cognitive effects of pre-anaesthetic medications, specifically the benzodiazepines anticholinergics, barbiturates, and opiods;
- cognitive changes caused by subanaesthetic doses of anaesthetic drugs;
- post-anaesthetic and post-surgical cognitive changes. A related

topic: recall of events occurring during anaesthesia is covered in the next chapter of this book.

While other cognitive effects will be discussed, we focus most heavily on memory research for several reasons. First, memory is emphasized in the literature, probably reflecting an appreciation for the central role learning and memory play in cognition. Second, the most consistent finding in the literature is that the treatments reviewed in this chapter produce memory deficits. Third, findings about other cognitive functions are often inconsistent, and typically provide little theoretical insight.

7.2 EFFECTS OF PRE-ANAESTHETIC MEDICATIONS

7.2.1 Benzodiazepines

While there is need for additional research to compare various drugs and modalities of treatment, at this time the similarities among the cognitive effects of different benzodiazepines are much more notable than any observed differences. Reported discrepancies may be the result of variations in dose, timing of tests, subject population, and task selection.

Although the benzodiazepines appear to influence cognitive behaviour similarly, they differ in terms of their times of onset, peak action, and the rate of recovery after administration. The benzodiazepines are classified into 'long-acting', half-life exceeding 10 hours (e.g., diazepam, clorazepate, and prazepam), and 'short-acting', rapidly cleared compounds (e.g., alprazolam, lorazepam, midazolam, oxazepam, and triazolam). Johnson and Chernik (1982) concluded that there are no consistent differences in effects between long-acting and short-acting treatments.

Benzodiazepines also differ in their rate of absorption after oral administration; with diazepam being rapidly absorbed and oxazepam and prazepam being more slowly absorbed. Classifications based on the elimination half-life are misleading when it comes to assumptions about duration of action of the drugs, particularly after single doses. The rate of distribution into the tissues, for which lipophilicity is important, is the determining factor. For example, lorazepam and oxazepam produce effects of longer duration than diazepam (Aranko *et al.*, 1983; Mewaldt et al., 1986). However, even after repeated administration with resultant accumulation of drugs with long half-lives, the development of tolerance obscures the differences between the drugs (Ghoneim *et al.*, 1986).

(a) Memory

It has been well documented that the benzodiazepines have profound and specific effects upon memory. Most notably the drugs greatly impair ability to learn new information, anterograde amnesia (e.g., Brown *et al.*, 1982, 1983; Ghoneim and Mewaldt, 1975, 1977; Hinrichs *et al.*, 1982; Lister, 1985; Mewaldt *et al.*, 1983, 1986). In order to understand the effects of benzodiazepines on memory it is useful to discuss several important distinctions concerning memory. For example, it is important to distinguish among processes involved in forming new memories, i.e., acquisition, maintaining memories, storage, and the processes needed to access memories, i.e. retrieval. In addition, it has been proposed that memories should be classified into two broad categories, declarative and nondeclarative (Graf and Schacter, 1985). Declarative memories are those that can be explicitly and consciously recalled, e.g. memories for facts and personal experiences. Nondeclarative memories, also called procedural or implicit memories, on the other hand, cannot be directly recalled but must be demonstrated through performance. Examples include knowledge of skills like playing a piano or dancing, conditioning phenomena such as classical conditioning, and a phenomenon called priming which is described below. Furthermore, Tulving (1972) has proposed that declarative memory should be further divided into episodic and semantic components. According to Tulving episodic memory involves memory for events that are associated with a particular context, e.g., biographical experience, the learning of a list of words or a story. Semantic memory, on the other hand, concerns representation of knowledge dissociated from the context in which it was learned, such as memory for meaning, rules, and language. Your knowledge that apples are a type of fruit is an example of semantic memory, while a memory that yesterday you ate an apple would be an example of an episodic memory. While much of the support for the usefulness of these distinctions comes from evidence involving patients with various forms of amnesia, the fact that benzodiazepines appear to affect only certain aspects of memory further support their usefulness.

A review of the studies listed above clearly indicates that the benzodiazepines impair acquisition or storage of new declarative episodic information in memory, while having no disruptive effect upon maintenance or retrieval of previously stored episodic memories. For example, if subjects are required to learn one or more lists of words prior to drug administration and then are asked to recall the material after receiving the drug, their recall will not be impaired relative to that of placebo subjects (e.g., Brown *et al.*, 1982, 1983; Ghoneim and Mewaldt, 1975, 1977). In contrast, as cited above, recall of episodic material learned following drug administration is greatly impaired. That recall of predrug material is not impaired while recall of postdrug material is significantly reduced, suggests that differences in postdrug recall are the result of lowered levels of learning in the drugged subjects.

Consistent with this notion, Brown, Brown and Bowes (1983) have shown that when post-treatment acquisition is equated for drug and placebo subjects (by giving drugged subjects extra learning trials) there are no differences in delayed recall between the two groups. One problem with theories which rigidly restrict the drugs' effects to acquisition has been raised by experiments which have shown deficits in retrieval when using a selective reminding task (Block and Berchou, 1984). However, while one aspect of Block and Berchou's data suggest that lorazepam may influence long-term retrieval, they conclude that the effect is probably best attributed to a specific characteristic of the reminding task. Therefore their results do not strongly challenge the hypothesis that drug action in episodic memory is restricted to an impairment of acquisition.

Whether the benzodiazepines also impede the acquisition of information in semantic memory is less certain. Lister and File (1984) found that even though lorazepam prevented some subjects from remembering that they had done the task previously (episodic memory), the drug did not impair their learning of a backwards reading task (semantic memory). However, because tests of semantic memory are comparatively rare in the benzodiazepine literature more firm conclusions must await further research.

Retrieval from semantic memory is most often tested by giving subjects a limited time period to generate words which represent a particular semantic category, e.g. four footed animals, types of music, etc. or which start with a particular letter. Performance on these tasks in general has not been impeded by benzodiazepines (Mewaldt, Ghoneim and Hinrichs, 1986; Weingartner *et al.*, 1992). However, evidence from Brown, Brown and Bowes (1983) and Ghoneim, Hinrichs and Mewaldt (1984a) suggests that speed of retrieval of semantic information may be slowed by the drug.

While tests of the effects of benzodiazepines on declarative episodic memory are now numerous, there is little evidence concerning their influence on nondeclarative memories. Most tasks which might be classified as containing a skill component relevant for assessing implicit memory also contain an episodic memory component. For example, digit symbol substitution and sorting tasks which have a motor skill component and have been found to be disrupted by benzodiazepines (e.g. Ellinwood *et al.*, 1984; Ghoneim, Mewaldt and Hinrichs 1984b) also require learning of the rules governing substitutions or sorting, a matter which requires episodic memory. In addition, in evaluating such tasks care must be taken to separate the drug's effects on learning from its effects on motivation and performance.

Fang, Hinrichs and Ghoneim (1987) conducted a study which directly compared one aspect of declarative and nondeclarative or explicit memory. To test declarative memory subjects learned a list of words which they were asked to recall in any order, an episodic memory task. Nondeclarative memory was evaluated with a priming task. In this task, subjects were presented with a list of words. Then rather than being asked to recall the words they were given the first three letters of each word and were asked to complete it with the first word that came to mind. Priming is said to have occurred if subjects show a greater likelihood of writing words which were previously presented than words which were not. For example, subjects who saw the word 'pension' should be more likely to complete 'pen___' as 'pension' than as pencil, penguin, or others. Fang *et al.* found that diazepam significantly impaired the recall task, but did not affect the priming task.

The results of Fang, Hinrichs and Ghoneim (1987) were confirmed by Danion *et al.* (1989) and with a different implicit memory task by Weingartner *et al.* (1992). However, Brown, Brown and Bowes (1989), who also used the word-stem completion task described above, found that lorazepam impaired implicit memory. The possibility that different benzodiazepines may vary in their effects on implicit memory is intriguing and is currently being investigated by our group.

Another theoretically useful memory distinction is often made between short-term and long-term memory. According to a popular model of memory (Atkinson and Shiffrin, 1968), information coming into memory first enters a short-term store which can only retain a small amount of information for a brief period of time, e.g., a telephone number until dialled. In order to form a more permanent memory it is presumed that the information must be attended to and rehearsed, thereby transferring it into the long-term store. To recall items in long-term storage they must be brought back (retrieved) into the short-term store. A few investigators have suggested that benzodiazepines impair short-term memory (e.g., Angus and Romney, 1984; Jones, Lewis and Spriggs, 1978), however, most studies have failed to find any influence on short-term memory (Curran, Schifano and Lader, 1991; Ghoneim *et al.*, 1975, 1977, 1981a; Lister, 1985; Mewaldt, Hinrichs and Ghoneim, 1983; Rusted, Eaton-Williams and Warburton, 1991). Many tasks generally classified as tests of short-term memory require a contribution from long-term memory in order to achieve accurate performance, i.e. according to the model, information exceeding the capacity of the short-term store must be transferred to long-term memory. We, therefore, suggest that inconsistencies in the literature may be a result of long-term memory processes. That is, by impeding formation of permanent new memories, recall errors may inappropriately be attributed to a disruption of short-term memory for tasks which are near the subject's memory span (see Mewaldt, Hinrichs and Ghoneim, 1983).

It might appear reasonable to suggest that sedative-hypnotics interfere with the transfer of information from short- to long-term memory by reducing subjects' motivation or attention and therefore reducing rehearsal. Consistent with this view, Rich and Brown (1992) found that diazepam reduced overt rehearsals and that number of rehearsals was significantly correlated with recall within the drug and placebo group. Other studies suggest the influence of the benzodiazepines on memory formation is more direct. Mewaldt, Hinrichs and Ghoneim (in press) found that the rehearsal patterns of drugged subjects did not differ from those of their placebo counterparts in either frequency or degree of elaboration. Yet, delayed recall of drugged subjects averaged less than 40% of that of control subjects. Furthermore, when drug and placebo subjects were forced to use the same rehearsal pattern, drug subjects still recalled significantly less than placebo subjects. Similarly, Brown *et al*. (1982) found that recall was impaired in drugged subjects even in an incidental learning task where rehearsal and elaboration would be unlikely, and File and Lister (1982) found that when rehearsal was prevented for both drug and placebo subjects, lorazepam still impaired performance. For further dicussion of evidence supporting a direct impairment of memory by benzodiazepines, see reviews by Curran (1986) and Ghoneim and Mewaldt (1990).

Some investigators have found that when retention of material learned prior to drug administration is tested, drugged subjects not only show no retrograde amnesia for the material, but they may display enhanced recall compared to placebo subjects (Ghoneim, Hinrichs and Mewaldt, 1984a; Mewaldt, Hinrichs and Ghoneim, 1983). Hinrichs, Ghoneim and Mewaldt (1984) have shown that this phenomenon is really just another reflection of the poor learning which occurs while subjects are under the influence of the drug. To demonstrate enhanced recall of material learned prior to drug administration, it is essential that subjects learn interfering material following drug administration. Because this latter material is so poorly learned by the drug subjects, they experience considerably less interference than placebo subjects. As a result drugged subjects recall the predrug material relatively easily.

Some investigators have asked whether benzodiazepines can produce state-dependent memory. State-dependent memory occurs when memories formed in one drug state (e.g. while sedated) are better recalled in the same drug state (e.g. when resedated) than when in a different drug state. The fact that drug subjects recall material learned before drug administration as well as, if not better than, placebo subjects makes it unlikely that benzodiazepines produce symmetrical state-dependency. (When both directions of change in drug state, i.e. placebo to drug or drug to placebo, are equally disruptive to memory, state-dependency is termed symmetrical. When one direction of change in drug states produces recall deficits but the other direction does not, state-dependency is called asymmetric.) Evidence from Petersen and

Ghoneim (1980) and Liljequist, Linnoila and Mattila (1978) suggests that material learned after receiving diazepam may be recalled better while under the influence of the drug than of placebo.

Most results reported above come from tests of normal young adult volunteers who received a single administration of drug in a dosage which would be considered within the therapeutic range for that drug (e.g. 10–20 mg for diazepam). While some investigators have suggested that lower doses may be effective for older subjects, (e.g. Meyer, 1982; Pomara *et al.*, 1985), evidence from Hinrichs and Ghoneim (1987) suggest that memory impairment in older subjects is not greater *per se*. It may only appear greater because lower baseline performance in older subjects makes decrements which are comparable to those in younger subjects more noticeable. In addition, we have observed great individual variability in subjects' response to drugs, perhaps related in part to frequency of prior exposure to these or other CNS active drugs, making it difficult to predict individual reactions. Multiple dose studies suggest that subjects quickly develop some tolerance to the cognitive effects of benzodiazepines, reducing but not eliminating their effects (Ghoneim *et al.*, 1981a, 1986; Liljequist, Linnoila and Mattila, 1978).

(b)   Other cognitive side-effects

In reviewing the literature on anti-anxiety drugs in 1973 McNair found the results contained a 'litany of conflicting, inconclusive, and ambiguous findings'. While the literature on benzodiazepines and memory has obviously advanced past that stage, there is only minor progress concerning other cognitive functions. A major problem is the lack of a theoretical theme with which to tie together the wide variety of tasks which have been tested. Unfortunately, task selection has often been directed by convenience rather than theoretical considerations. In addition, many of the tasks reported below have both a cognitive and motor component, making it uncertain whether an observed effect is the result of impairment in cognitive or motor processes.

Tinklenberg and Taylor (1984) suggested that benzodiazepines influence cognition by reducing attention. If true, vigilance tasks should be particularly sensitive to drug influence. However, while Weingartner *et al.* (1992) found that triazolam impaired vigilance in a task which required simultaneous memory processing, and Clarke *et al.* (1970) found some reduction in vigilance with diazepam, performance in the task was still quite good, and Jones, Lewis and Spriggs (1978) found no effect on vigilance for 5 mg of diazepam. Reduced attention should have an adverse effect on both simple and choice reaction time. (Simple reaction time involves making a decision about when a stimulus is presented, while choice reaction time adds the complexity of choosing the correct response associated with a particular stimulus.) Consistent with this notion some investigators have found that benzodiazepines increased reaction time (e.g. Block and Berchou, 1984; Seppala *et al.*, 1976). However, Ghoneim *et al.* (1981a) and Palva and Linnoila (1978) found no effect. While Ghoneim, Mewaldt and Thatcher (1975) found that 20 mg of diazepam had no effect on median simple or choice reaction time, they found it did increase the variability in response times consistent with the notion that drugged subjects had lapses in attention.

A number of somewhat unrelated tasks are sensitive to the presence of benzodiazepines. For example, ability to distinguish a flashing from a steady light (critical flicker fusion frequency) generally declines under drug (Block and Berchou, 1984; Haffner *et al.*, 1973). Benzodiazepines have also been found to decrease speed but not accuracy in digit-symbol substitution (Ellinwood *et al.*, 1984; Lister and File, 1984; Rich and Brown, 1992), sorting tasks (Haffner *et al.*, 1973; Ghoneim, Mewaldt and Hinrichs, 1984b; Mewaldt, Ghoneim and Hinrichs, 1986), visual search tasks, such as drawing a line through certain target letters in a long series of letters (Jones, Lewis and Spriggs, 1978; Haffner *et al.*, 1973), mental arithmetic (Mewaldt, Ghoneim and Hinrichs, 1986), and a complex logic task (Curran, Schifano and Lader, 1991; Rusted, Eaton-Williams and Warburton, 1991). In addition, studies on driving simultors, tracking tasks, and actual driving tests indicate that moderate doses of benzodiazepines (e.g. 10–15 mg diazepam) impair decision ability and other skills related to safe driving (de Gier *et al.*, 1981; Seppala *et al.*, 1976; van Laar, Volkerts and van Willigenburg, 1992).

Finally, Ghoneim, Mewaldt and Hinrichs (1984b) suggested that some inconsistencies in the literature may be related to the number of times a task is repeated. While benzodiazepines can impair tasks like those described above, Ghoneim *et al.* found that the most obvious way performance was impaired was that drug subjects failed to benefit from practice on the tasks. For example, performance of drug subjects did not decline from predrug levels on mental arithmetic or letter cancellation, but unlike the results for placebo subjects, performance of drug subjects did not improve with practice. Ghoneim *et al.* suggested that the larger the role learning plays in a task, the more sensitive it might be to the presence of a benzodiazepine.

(c) Flumazenil

Flumazenil is used to antagonize the effects of benzodiazepines. The drug effectively reverses their sedative-hypnotic and psychomotor effects but there is limited information on the reversal of amnesia. Review of the literature (Ghoneim, in press) indicates that available studies, due to flaws in their methodologies, have not been able to determine unequivocally whether flumazenil can reverse completely or partially the memory effects of benzodiazepines. This should be explored in future studies.

7.2.2 Anticholinergic drugs

Another class of widely studied pre-operative medications is the anticholinergic drugs. Since the early 1900s it has been thought that hyoscine or scopolamine interfered with memory for events surrounding surgery. However, little concrete data supported that contention until the last twenty years when research on the cholinergic system and memory began in earnest.

(a) Memory

The cholinergic system is intimately involved in memory processes (e.g., Deutsch, 1971; Drachman, 1977; Drachman and Leavitt, 1974). Drugs which disrupt cholinergic pathways interfere with memory (see below), while treatments with cholinergic agonists (e.g., physostigmine, arecoline) have at least small beneficial effects on memory in both normal young subjects and elderly patients with memory disorders (Davis *et al.*, 1978; Sitaram, Weingartner and Gillen, 1978; Weingartner, Sitaram and Gillen, 1979).

The effects of anticholinergic drugs on episodic memory have often been compared to the memory deficits associated with normal ageing and dementia (i.e. Alzheimer's disease) and they also generally resemble those of the benzodiazepines described above. For example, scopolamine impairs the formation or consolidation of permanent new memories while normally leaving retrieval of episodic memories formed prior to drug administration intact (Ghoneim and Mewaldt, 1975, 1977; Mewaldt and Ghoneim, 1979; Rusted and Warburton, 1989). However, scopolamine may disrupt retrieval of episodic memories formed after drug administration. For example, Rusted and Warburton (1989) found that while scopolamine impaired recall of material learned following drug administration it did not influence recognition of the same material. In addition, Caine *et al.* (1981) found a retrieval deficit when a selective reminding task or cued recall task was employed. Retrieval deficits for material learned following drug administration may result from an impaired ability to organize information and use mnemonics. Consistent with this notion, Ghoneim and Mewaldt (1975) found that subjects receiving scopolamine were less capable of using categorical information to organize their recall. In addition, Weingartner, Sitaram and Gillian (1979) found that arecoline improved recall primarily by facilitating the formation of more organized memory structures.

Further parallels with the benzodiazepines are less certain. While several studies suggest that, like the benzodiazepines, neither scopolamine nor atropine impair short-term memory (Broks *et al.*, 1988; Crow, 1979; Crow and Grove-White, 1973; Ghoneim and Mewaldt, 1975; Mewaldt and Ghoneim, 1979), a number of studies reveal at least small deficits (Caine *et al.*, 1981; Molchan *et al.*, 1990; Troster *et al.*, 1989). In addition, some investigators have found that, unlike the benzodiazepines, scopolamine impaired retrieval from semantic memory (e.g., Caine *et al.*, 1981; Drachman and Leavitt, 1974; Molchan *et al.*, 1990). Troster *et al.* (1989) suggests this effect may be a by-product of a drug-induced decrement in sustained and rapid responding. However, as with the benzodiazepines, the drug's effects on learning do not appear to be due to its effects on attention or drowsiness (Drachman, 1977).

Drachman (1977) and Mewaldt and Ghoneim (1979) attempted to reverse the effects of scopolamine with either physostigmine or amphetamine. Both found that physostigmine, an anticholinesterase drug, ameliorated much of the memory deficit caused by scopolamine. However, while Drachman found d-amphetamine had no effect on the memory deficit, Mewaldt and Ghoneim found some improvement with methamphetamine, a more potent stimulant. More recently Molchan *et al.* (1990) demonstrated that thyrotropin-releasing hormone, through its enhancing effect on the cholinergic system, also can reverse memory impairment caused by scopolamine.

Studies which have included methscopolamine (a drug which does not cross the blood–brain barrier) as a control indicate that scopolamine's influence on memory is due to its central effects (e.g., Caine *et al.*, 1981; Drachman and Leavitt, 1974). A study comparing scopolamine and atropine indicates that atropine has little or no effect on memory at the 0.6 mg dose tested (Crow and Grove-White, 1973). Meyers and Abreu (1952) suggested that in order to get degrees of central nervous system depression equal to scopolamine, 8.6 times as much atropine must be used.

(b)   Other cognitive functions

Scopolamine's effects on cognition are not limited to memory. Drachman (1977) and Drachman and Leavitt (1974) demonstrated that 1 mg of scopolamine significantly reduced scores on the performance portion of the Wechsler Adult Intelligence Scale and Wesnes and Revell (1984) found that scopolamine greatly increased confusion in the Stroop color naming task. Subjects receiving scopolamine also performed more poorly on two vigilance tasks (Wesnes and Warburton 1983, 1984). More recent evidence (Broks *et al.*, 1988) suggests that the effect of the drug is primarily on sustained or continuous attention rather than selective attention. Nuotto (1983) found that scopolamine drugged subjects performed poorly on three cognitive-motor tasks involving speed of information processing, simple and choice reaction time and tracking.

However, results from Frith *et al*. (1989) suggest that reaction time and other perceptual motor tasks are relatively insensitive to the drug unless they contain an element of sustained concentration or require acquisition of new skills. Taken together these studies demonstrate that some general cognitive deficits are produced by scopolamine and that tasks involving sustained continuous attention and vigilance may be particularly sensitive to the drug.

7.2.3 Barbiturates

(a) Memory

Research on the cognitive effects of barbiturates has neither been as extensive nor as systematic as on the two previously described drug classes. Although there are a number of studies which found little or no effect of various barbiturates on memory, (e.g. 125 mg amylobarbitone, Crow, 1979; 400 mg heptobarbitone, Wilson and Ellis, 1973; 50 mg pentobarbitone, Heisterkamp and Cohen, 1975; 6.0 mg/kg thiopentone sodium or 4.0 mg/kg methohexitone sodium, Dundee and Pandit, 1972), there is sufficient evidence to indicate that barbiturates do impair memory. For example, Adams (1974) and Evans and Davis (1969) found that secobarbital impaired verbal learning, and Rundell, Williams and Lester (1977) found that 1.5 mg/kg and 2.9 mg/kg of secobarbital reduced both recall and recognition. In a particularly analytical study, Osborn *et al*. (1967) found no effect of continuously infused 0.3% thiopentone, on recall of a six-item list of paired-associates which had been learned before drug administration. However, while this easy list was learned in an average of 1.2 trials before treatment, a similar list took an average of 10 trials to learn following drug administration.

The effects of barbiturates on memory appear to be similar to those of the benzodiazepines and anticholinergics, i.e. they interfere primarily with long-term memory acquisition. However, benzodiazepines produce greater amnesic effects than barbiturates (Bixler *et al*., 1979; Roache and Griffiths, 1985). Talland and Quarton (1965) found that 100 mg of pentobarbitone interfered with a running memory span task at a slow rate of presentation (1 item/4 sec), but not a fast rate (1 item/sec). They interpreted their results as indicating that the drug impaired subjects' ability to select and use appropriate strategies to organize and encode information, a deficit in acquisition. Short-term memory should have played a more important role in performance at the 1 sec than the 4 sec presentation rate. The lack of an effect on recall at the faster rate suggests that as with the benzodiazepines and anticholinergics, barbiturates have little effect on this aspect of memory. That barbiturates impair long-term memory formation is further supported by results from Mohs *et al*. (1980) and Williams and Rundell (1983). Results of these two studies and those of Osborn *et al.* (1967) suggest a possible related impairment in retrieval. This deficit may be a byproduct of the inefficient encoding which occurs when subjects learn under the influence of barbiturates (cf. Tulving and Thompson, 1973).

(b)   Other effects

Barbiturates also influence other cognitive and psychomotor tasks. For example, they have been found to slow reaction time or decision speed (Griffiths, Bigelow and Leibson, 1983; Williams, Rundell and Smith, 1981), alter time perception (Rutschman and Rubinstein, 1966), and impair performance on a scanning task (Crow, 1979). In addition, barbiturates impaired pilots' performance in both simulated and actual aircraft flights (Billings, Gerke and Wick, 1975).

7.2.4   Opioids

In the literature on animal experimentation there is evidence that morphine can either improve or impair memory depending upon the dose and task. However, in this literature drugs are generally used as reinforcement or punishment for behaviour and it is therefore not very instructive when it comes to understanding human cognitive behaviour. In the comparatively sparse literature on human performance, most results suggest that subanaesthetic doses of opioids have little or no effect on memory and cognition. For example, Liljequist, Mattila and Linnoila (1981) found no effect of 50 mg of codeine on learning or retention and Pandit *et al.* (1971) found that opiates produced little anterograde amnesia in either the pre- or post-operative period (see also, Lowenstein and Philbin, 1981). Ghoneim, Mewaldt and Thatcher (1975) found that while 0.2 mg of fentanyl was sufficient to impair performance on a coordination task, it had little influence on memory or reaction time. Similarly, despite the fact that subjects reported feeling a decrease in mental ability, Scamman, Ghoneim and Korttila (1984) found no evidence of memory or cognitive impairment with either fentanyl (1.5 or 3 µg/kg) or alfentanil (7.5 or 15 µg/kg). Even after very large doses administered for pure opioid 'anaesthesia', patients may be aware of certain events during the operation and may recall them post-operatively (Hilgenberg, 1981).

A somewhat contradictory set of results was reported by Kerr *et al.* (1991) who found impairment on a series of motor tasks during intravenous administration of morphine, an effect which was most noticeable when integration of proprioceptive feedback was required. They also found that morphine decreased reading speed. However, while it did not impair comprehension and retention when memory was tested

2 minutes after reading, it did have a small effect when memory was tested 3 hours later.

Patients with advanced malignant diseases may suffer from impaired cognitive performance while being treated with relatively large doses of opioids. The change in their mental state may appear as confusion, hallucinations, delusions, or simply over-sedation. This complicates the care of these patients and impairs their interpersonal relationships. As a result the opioid dose is often reduced resulting in exacerbation of the pain. However, factors other than the opioids may be responsible for the mental impairment, e.g. concurrent treatment with other CNS-depressant drugs, the presence of fever, etc. Correcting these factors may be more effective in improving the patient's mental status while maintaining adequate pain control (Leipzig *et al.*, 1987).

7.3   SUBANAESTHETIC CONCENTRATIONS OF INHALATIONAL ANAESTHETICS

Research on the cognitive effects of anaesthetic drugs has generally involved patients undergoing surgery. While this approach is useful, interpretation of the data concerning various anaesthetics is complicated by use of premedicants, varying age and health of the patients, and the length, type, and stress of surgery. As a consequence, research on the effects of anaesthetics has often been conducted with subanaesthetic doses in normal healthy volunteers. This research is also clinically relevant because nitrous oxide in subanaesthetic concentrations is commonly used in dental, obstetric, and outpatient surgery. Trichloroethylene is also used in the British Isles in similar concentrations for obstetric cases. In addition, nitrous oxide in subanaesthetic concentrations is illegally abused.

7.3.1   Nitrous oxide

(a)   Memory

Substantial impairment of memory is observed when subjects learn and recall information during inhalation of nitrous oxide. When the information (e.g. a list of words) is presented several times, with memory being assessed after each presentation, the memory deficits become greater over successive tests (Ghoneim, Mewaldt and Petersen, 1981b).

The memory impairments produced by nitrous oxide do not vary greatly for different types of stimuli and testing procedures (Block *et al.*, 1988a). They occur with many stimuli including words, nonsense words, numbers, sentences, brief stories, common environmental noises, music, visual designs, and mazes (Biersner, 1972; Block *et al.*, 1988a, b; Edwards, Harris and Biersner 1976; Ghoneim *et al.*, 1981b; Henrie, Parkhouse and Bickford, 1961; Korttila *et al.*, 1981; Mewaldt *et al.*, 1988; Parkhouse *et al.*, 1960; Russell and Steinberg, 1955). Digit span (the longest sequence of digits that can be repeated immediately without error) is also impaired (Cook *et al.*, 1978b; Steinberg, 1954).

Unlike the drug treatments discussed above which apparently affect memory by disrupting learning of new information, nitrous oxide may actually enhance encoding processes in acquisition (Ramsay *et al.*, 1992). Instead the drug's deleterious effects on memory might best be attributed to its ability to impair retrieval. Even material which has been well learned may be difficult to recall if memory is tested while receiving nitrous oxide (Ghoneim, Mewaldt and Petersen, 1981b; Mewaldt *et al.*, 1988; Ramsay *et al.*, 1992).

Do any stimuli resist the drug's effect on memory? Possibilities that have been suggested include personally salient stimuli such as names of relatives (Block *et al.*, 1988a) and visual information (Biersner, 1972). However, some studies have found impairments for visual information (Henrie, Parkhouse and Bickford, 1961; Parkhouse *et al.*, 1960). Ghoneim, Mewaldt and Petersen (1981b) found that nitrous oxide eliminated the recall difference between words whose meaning is easy to visualize (e.g. chair) and words whose meaning is hard to visualize (e.g. law), suggesting that nitrous oxide might reduce effortful processing at a meaningful, semantic level. Compatible with this interpretation, Block *et al.*, (1988a) found that nitrous oxide selectively impaired recognition of nonsense words which were presented once, but did not impair performance on others which were presented multiple times. Therefore, memory disruption may be minimal for information (e.g. frequency of presentation) that is stored automatically in memory, independently of processing that involves intention and cognitive effort (Zacks, Hasher and Sanft, 1982).

These studies involved explicit memory tests in which subjects knew their memory was being assessed. Studies of amnesic patients (Graf, Squire and Mandler, 1984) suggest that tests for nondeclarative or implicit memory, which indirectly assess retention, may be more sensitive to low levels of learning than explicit memory tests. Block *et al.* (1988b) administered three implicit memory tests and corresponding explicit tests to determine if the implicit tests resisted the memory-impairing effects of nitrous oxide. The implicit tests differed in details but each was designed so that words previously presented to the subject provided answers for some of the test items. The test which most resisted impairment by nitrous oxide was the one in which subjects had the most difficulty thinking of answers of their own. This test, in which subjects had to give examples of a specified category like 'metal', might be particularly useful in detecting low levels of learning during anaesthesia.

The decline in subjects' ability to give examples of a specified category on their own suggests that retrieval of simple, pre-experimentally learned semantic memories may be impaired. Other results discussed so far pertain to memory impairment for new episodic information learned under the influence of nitrous oxide.

Some investigators have asked whether nitrous oxide produces 'state-dependent memory'. Mewaldt *et al.* (1988) and Ramsay *et al.* (1992) found no evidence for state-dependent effects when memory was tested with a paired-associate task. In addition, Ghoneim, Mewaldt and Petersen (1981b) using a multi-trial free recall task did not observe the symmetrical form of state-dependent memory described above. However, they did observe a somewhat unusual form of asymmetrical state-dependent memory also obtained in a subsequent study (Mewaldt *et al.*, 1988), in which material learned while receiving placebo was poorly recalled on nitrous oxide, but material learned while receiving nitrous oxide could be recalled in either the placebo or drug state.

(b)   Other effects on performance

Some studies suggest that analgesia produced by subanaesthetic concentrations of nitrous oxide is not purely a sensory effect, rather cognitive, emotional, or motivational factors must contribute to the effect. For example, Chapman, Murphy and Butler (1973) found that nitrous oxide not only reduced sensitivity to pain, but it also decreased subjects' willingness to report pain. Dworkin *et al.* (1986) found that giving subjects preparatory information about the analgesic and sedative effects of nitrous oxide increased its analgesic effect, while instructing subjects that the drug would heighten awareness of body sensations eliminated its analgesic effect.

Other effects of nitrous oxide on cognition have received less attention. The drug impaired performance in solving arithmetic problems and analogies (Ghoneim, Mewaldt and Petersen, 1981b; Russell and Steinberg; 1955; Steinberg, 1954), slowed reaction time (Cook *et al.*, 1978b), but improved subject's ability to discriminate a flickering from a steady light (Korttila *et al.*, 1981; Wernberg, Nielson and Hommelgaard, 1980). It also altered free associations to stimulus words (Block *et al.*, 1988b), but did not affect objective estimates of the passage of time, orientation to time and place, or access to simple information like the name of the President (Biersner, 1972; Parkhouse *et al.*, 1960).

(c) Subjective effects

Steinberg (1956) described the common subjective effects of nitrous oxide as including numbness, tingling, dizziness, dreaminess, euphoria, changes in time perception, auditory and visual changes, and impairments of concentration, memory, and motor abilities. Atkinson *et al.* (1977), using a lengthy questionnaire, observed similar subjective effects. They suggested that nitrous oxide produces a moderate, incomplete psychedelic experience which lacks some effects characteristic of psychedelic drugs, such as special visual and other sensory effects. Such psychedelic experience is consistent with the abuse of nitrous oxide for its subjective effects (Rosenberg, Orkin and Springstead, 1979) and with the descriptions of early investigators such as William James (1882, 1898). Subjects' ratings indicate that nitrous oxide produces sedation (Korttila *et al.*, 1981), but these effects seem less reliable than with other drugs such as benzodiazepines (Ghoneim, Mewaldt and Petersen, 1981b).

A few studies have examined tranquillizing effects of nitrous oxide on behaviour. Under normal conditions, working on an unsolvable task impairs subsequent performance on a solvable task. Nitrous oxide attenuates this effect, i.e., performance on a solvable task under non-drug conditions was better when prior experience with an unsolvable task occurred while breathing nitrous oxide rather than air (Russell and Steinberg, 1955). Nitrous oxide may have attenuated the stress of working on the unsolvable task.

(d) Dose-response effects

Nitrous oxide concentrations of 30% or 33% were used in many of the studies cited above. Several studies have used two or more subanaesthetic concentrations of nitrous oxide, ranging from 5% to 45% (Atkinson *et al.*, 1977; Cook *et al.*, 1978b; Garfield, Garfield and Sampson, 1975; Mewaldt *et al.*, 1988; Wernberg, Nielson and Hommelgaard, 1980). These studies indicate that effects are greater with higher concentrations and suggest that the dose-response curve had a relatively steep slope. Unfortunately, most studies do not indicate the threshold concentration at which significant effects occur. One notable exception is Cook *et al.* (1978b), who found that the two tasks they used (digit span and choice reaction time) were impaired by nitrous oxide concentrations of 20% and 30% but not by concentrations of 10% or less. While effects at 30% concentrations are robust, effects at 20% concentrations appear to be slight, being detected in some individuals but not others (Mewaldt *et al.*, 1988).

In sharp contrast to the preceding results, are reports from one laboratory (Bruce and Bach, 1975, 1976) that nitrous oxide concentrations of

0.005% impaired choice reaction time and 0.05% impaired digit span and other cognitive functions. Cook *et al.* (1978b) were unable to replicate these findings and Bruce and Stanley (1983) and Bruce (1991) have subsequently attributed them to a sampling artifact.

(e)   Time course and tolerance

Korttila *et al.* (1981) administered tasks repeatedly from 2 to 32 minutes after subjects attained a 30% end-tidal concentration of nitrous oxide and during a recovery period after gas inhalation had ceased. Impairments in performance were uniform throughout gas inhalation and in a second gas inhalation phase following recovery, i.e. neither increasing effects nor tolerance was observed. Recovery was rapid, occurring, depending upon the task, within 2 to 22 min after gas inhalation had ceased. Acute tolerance to the analgesic effect of nitrous oxide has been reported with higher concentrations (60%–80%) (Rupreht *et al.*, 1985).

7.3.2   Isoflurance, enflurane, and halothane

Subanaesthetic concentrations of isoflurane, enflurance, and halothane have received less attention than nitrous oxide. The laboratory that reported impairments of digit span and reaction time from trace concentrations of nitrous oxide also reported similar impairments from concentrations as low as 0.0001% halothane plus 0.005% nitrous oxide and 0.0015% enflurane plus 0.05% nitrous oxide (Bruce and Bach, 1975, 1976), but these results are also considered unrepresentative (Bruce, 1991) and others have been unable to replicate them (see Rice, 1983, for a review).

Cook *et al.* (1978b) found 0.2% halothane impaired choice reaction time but not digit span, while 0.02% halothane affected neither task. Cook *et al.* (1978a) examined effects of three concentrations of halothane (0.1, 0.2, and 0.4%) and enflurane (0.2, 0.42, and 0.53%). Performance on digit span, choice reaction time, and pegboard (psychomotor) tests were impaired in a dose-related fashion by both drugs; memory functions also seemed to be impaired. At the lowest concentrations used, the results indicated that neither drug impaired digit span, both impaired choice reaction time, and only halothane impaired the pegboard test.

A recent well done study by Newton *et al.* (1990) examined responding and memory with 0.1, 0.2, and 0.4 MAC concentrations of isoflurane. (MAC is the minimum alveolar concentration of anaesthetic at 1 atmosphere that produces immobility in 50% of patients exposed to a noxious stimulus.) Subjects were asked to follow a number of commands and learn two lists of words while breathing isoflurane. Memory was tested one hour after gas administration ceased. The results indicated that even at the 0.1 concentration there was some impairment of memory for commands. At 0.2 and 0.4 concentrations memory for normal words was absent. At 0.2 concentration some shock words (surprising or humorous words) were still recalled but at the 0.4 concentration even these could not be remembered. No responses to commands were present at the 0.4 concentration. Memory for commands followed performance, i.e., if a subject did not respond to a command, it was not recalled.

More work is needed to determine whether different anaesthetic agents have qualitatively similar or different effects on memory and cognition. If the effects of different agents are similar, it would be useful to determine their dose-response curves in the sub-MAC range to see whether these curves are parallel and whether equal fractions of MAC of different agents produce equal effects on memory and cognition.

7.4 POST-ANAESTHETIC AND POST-SURGICAL COGNITIVE CHANGES

Cognitive changes in the post-operative period may manifest themselves acutely in the recovery period as delirium or as a more gradual mental deterioration. Both syndromes may occur in the same patient, however for convenience, they will be discussed separately.

7.4.1 Post-operative delirium

(a) Incidence

Estimates of the incidence of post-operative delirium vary. Titchener *et al.* (1956) found 7.8 cases per 100, while Tufo, Ostfeld and Schekelle (1970) found an incidence of 24% following open heart surgery.

(b) Causes

Several risk factors have been identified as causative agents for delirium. Pre-operative factors include ageing (over 50 years), pre-operative cognitive deficits, anxiety and personality disorders, and addiction to alcohol or other CNS active drugs. Certain types of operations including open heart surgery, cataract surgery (Weisman and Hackett, 1958), and total joint replacement (Sheppeard *et al.* (1980) seem to make the patients particularly vulnerable. Other factors during the operation include duration of anaesthesia (8+ hours), duration of the extracorporeal circulation (4+ hours), choice of anaesthesia (general versus regional anaesthesia) and operative hypotension, hypoxia, and hypercapnia. Post-operative factors include medications, particularly anticholinergics (which may have been administered pre- or intra-operatively), sleep deprivation, sensory deprivation, cerebrovascular accidents, electrolyte and metabolic abnormalities, hypoxia, fever, and infection (Tune and Folstein, 1986).

(c) Clinical picture

Disturbances of attention are the most prominent feature of post-operative delirium. The patient's attention may either wander aimlessly or be suddenly focused with inappropriate intensity, on an irrelevant stimulus (Mesulam and Geschwind, 1976). Other signs of cognitive impairment include disorientation, memory loss, difficulty with concentration, and difficulty with complex learned motor movements like handwriting. Abnormal mental phenomena, such as hallucinations (especially visual) and delusions, may occur, and abnormal mood states, including depression and anxiety, may also co-exist. The patient may be awake and even hypervigilant or the opposite, drowsy and obtunded.

Depending on the nature of the aetiologic factors, this distressing picture may begin any time within the post-operative period. It may be continuous with the 'emergence delirium' of anaesthesia and be apparent immediately or may appear many days later. Most commonly it is noticed three days after surgery (Mesulam and Geschwind, 1976). Although the symptoms are reversible with treatment, delirium is an important cause of morbidity and mortality in the post-operative period. Among the causes of lethality are failure to take adequate nourishment, hypovolemia or electrolyte imbalance from tearing out of intravenous lines, pulmonary aspiration of gastric material after pulling out a nasogastric tube, pulmonary embolus or pneumonia from lack of early mobility, and trauma due to falls from bed.

(d) Treatment

Proper therapy for delirium requires identification and rectification of the causative factors, e.g. correction of abnormalities of blood gases, electrolytes, etc. as well as symptomatic treatment and nursing care. Easy access to eye glasses and hearing aids helps to prevent sensory deprivation. Use of clocks, calendars, and frequent visits from family members should speed re-orientation. In some cases treatment with drugs is beneficial. For example, haloperidol is beneficial for agitated patients with delirium of non-specific cause, benzodiazepines are the drugs of choice for delirium tremens, and physostigmine is specific for anticholinergically-induced delirium.

7.4.2   Postoperative mental deterioration

(a)   Prevalence and severity

After a major surgical operation many patients complain of mental changes, tiredness, lack of concentration, difficulty with learning and recall, deterioration in verbal capabilities, and the like. For example, Bedford (1955) described 18 cases of gross dementia occurring after anaesthesia and surgery in elderly patients and several cases which showed lesser degrees of dementia. Blundell (1967) studied 86 elderly surgical patients. Patients suffered deterioration of their mental functions, particularly their memory and cognitive abilities which continued to a significant extent for at least several weeks. Hole, Terjesen and Breivik (1980) studied 31 patients who had general anaesthesia for total hip arthroplasty; five displayed mental changes which reduced the quality of their lives for several months post-operatively.

In a study of younger patients (23 to 50 years old) who had gynaecological surgery (Klausen *et al.*, 1983), 30% complained of impairment of intellectual functions three months after surgery and in seven patients (17%) this was severe enough to interfere with their ability to work.

(b)   Type of surgery

The surgical procedure may be an important factor in determining incidence of cognitive deficits. For example high incidence, 23 to 53% of cases, has been reported after cardiac surgery (Sotaniemi, 1983). This may be due to cerebral embolization and/or decreased cerebral perfusion. There is usually a positive relationship between duration of bypass surgery and incidence of complications. The administration of thiopentone during the operation may provide some protection to the brain (Nussmeier, Arlund and Slogoff, 1986). On the other hand, it has been claimed that carotid endarterectomy and cerebral vascular procedures that bypass occluded vessels may improve the cognitive abilities of patients after surgery by restoring the blood supply to ischaemic areas of the brain. Support for this contention is, however, lacking.

(c)   Type of anaesthesia

Effects of general anaesthesia alone have been examined in healthy young volunteers (Davison *et al.*, 1975; Storms *et al.*, 1980). Subjects showed mental impairment for about one week; memory and cognition appeared to be the functions most impaired. A study of patients who had total hip arthroplasty (Hole, Terjesen and Breivik, 1980) showed that none of the 29 patients who received regional anaesthesia, but seven of the 31 patients who received general anaesthesia, had significant post-operative mental changes. However, more recent studies (Asbjorn *et al.*, 1989; Ghoneim *et al.*, 1988; Nielson *et al.*, 1990) showed similar mental performance post-operatively in patients who had surgery performed under either local or general anaesthesia.

(d)   Age

Smith *et al.* (1986) found greater cognitive deficits for older patients than for younger ones following surgery. Elderly patients may stand an increased risk of developing mental sequelae following surgery for several reasons. Some clinicians suggest that the vitality of the brain starts to deteriorate around the age of 60. For example, persons over 60 are more susceptible to delirium when exposed to stressful influences such as trauma, fever, and environmental changes (Carlsson, 1981). Increase in monoamine oxidase activity in the ageing brain (Adolfsson *et al.*, 1980) may provide a basis for increased risk of depression in the elderly, in addition to the many psychosocial factors that increase the risk.

(e)   Type of patient

Some patients suffer from depression post-operatively, particularly after certain types of surgery (Romm, Hutzler and Berggren, 1981). Complaints about poor cognitive function are characteristic of depressed individuals. Kahn *et al.* (1975) found that depression was more highly correlated with complaints about memory than with performance on two mental status tests. However, patients with significant depression also show evidence of cognitive impairment on tasks that demand effort and considerable cognitive capacity. On the other hand, tasks that require little cognitive capacity and that can be accomplished without 'intention' (automatic tasks) are relatively unimpaired in depression (Roy-Byrne *et al.*, 1986). The degree to which effort-demanding cognitive functions are impaired is related to the intensity of disturbed mood (Cohen *et al.*, 1982). Depressive symptomatology should, therefore, be included in any assessment of the cognitive function in patients before and after surgery.

7.5   SUMMARY AND CONCLUSIONS

As is apparent in the above discussion, both drugs associated with anaesthesia and the stress of anaesthesia and surgery may have profound detrimental effects on human cognitive functions. As stated at the outset, the most consistent findings involve disruption of memory. With the exception of the opioids which have not been adequately investigated, the pre-anaesthetic medications reviewed, i.e. the benzo-diazepines, anticholinergics, and barbiturates, have basically similar effects on memory. They impair the formation of new long-term memories, with relatively little influence on other aspects of memory. While disruption of retrieval has not been ruled out in all cases, it would appear that any impairment of this aspect of memory is minor compared to the drugs' effects on acquisition. Because these drugs do not all operate through the same neural transmitter mechanisms, it is appealing to suggest that they act through a general reduction in arousal or motivation. While this proposal has not been conclusively rejected, current evidence suggests that this is not a likely explanation and more direct impairment is implied.

In contrast to the pre-medicant drugs which seem to produce fairly specific effects on memory, nitrous oxide, in subanaesthetic concentrations, produces more general effects. Not only does it disrupt acquisition of new material, but it also interferes with retrieval from long-term episodic and semantic memory. In addition, there is evidence of disruption of short-term memory and a wide variety of other cognitive functions. Although there is little information about other anaesthetics, the scant evidence available suggests it is unlikely that their effects will differ greatly from those of nitrous oxide.

While the cognitive effects of pre-anaesthetic and anaesthetic drugs are profound, in general they are fairly short lived, usually lasting from a few hours to a few days. On the other hand, the combined effects of drug treatments and surgery, while perhaps more subtle, can be considerably more disturbing. Depending on variables such as the length and type of surgery, and the age and health of the patient, disruptions of memory and other cognitive capabilities following surgery may last for several months and may even be indirectly lethal. It is apparent that future research must be directed at identifying the causative factors and remedies for this important problem.

In concluding we would like to point out that while much has been learned about the cognitive effects of anaesthesia it is also clear that there is a need for additional research in the general area of human psychopharmacology. We have mentioned some areas of particular concern, e.g. studies designed to compare various treatments or to resolve particular questions where the existing data is scarce or ambiguous. We have also made some methodological suggestions for specific research areas. As a final point we would like to convey a few general comments which admittedly reflect our biases.

Anyone who has attempted to review the literature in the area of cognitive psychopharmacology is likely to have become frustrated at the melange of data. The array of drugs, dosages, tasks, and timing of tests which have been employed is so broad that one might wonder whether any result has ever been replicated. Some confusion occurs because authors may fail to recognize or convey the precise implications of their results. For example, one paper may report that the particular drug did not affect memory when what was found was that the drug did not impair recall of material learned before drug administration. In contrast, another paper may report that the same drug did impair memory, but memory was tested by examining acquisition of new material learned after drug administration. Apparent contradictions such as these may be resolved when the researcher understands that memory should not be viewed as a unitary process but as a collection of processes, e.g. acquisition or encoding, storage, and retrieval.

In addition, theoretical distinctions between declarative and non-declarative, episodic and semantic memory, short- and long-term memory, and various levels-of-processing (Craik and Lockhart, 1972) should prove useful in understanding the effect of particular treatments on memory. It is certainly not the case that the treatments reviewed influence all stages and processes of memory uniformly. Rather it appears that most drugs have more limited and specific effects upon particular stages or processes of memory. Understanding these distinctions should guild researchers to design experiments aimed at determining in more detail how a treatment influences memory. For example, a drug which impairs memory formation should be expected to interfere with both recall and recognition of material learned after drug administration. However, a drug which interferes with retrieval might impair recall but leave recognition untouched.

While differences in subjects and procedures will exist across studies, when research is aimed at answering particular theoretical questions, consistencies are likely to emerge. We believe that for psychopharmacological research to add significantly to an understanding of human cognitive processes or for the effects of particular pharmacological agents to be clearly understood, the research must be integrated into meaningful models of behaviour.

REFERENCES

Adams, R. G. (1974) Pre-sleep ingestion of two hypnotic drugs and subsequent performance. *Psychopharmacologia* **40**, 185–90.

Adolfsson, R., Gottfries, C. G., Oreland, L. *et al.* (1980) Increased activity of brain and platelet monoamine oxidase in dementia of Alzheimer type. *Life Sciences*, **27**, 1029–34.

Angus, W. R., and Romney, D. M. (1984) The effect of diazepam on patients' memory. *Journal of Clinical Pharmacology*, **4**, 203–6.

Aranko, K., Mattila, M. J. and Seppala, T. (1983) Development of tolerance and cross-tolerence to the psychomotor actions of lorazepam and diazepam in man. *British Journal of Clinical Pharmacology*, **15**, 545–52.

Asbjorn, J., Jakobsen, B. W., Pilegaard, H. K., *et al.* (1989) Mental function in elderly men after surgery during epidural analgesia. *Acta Anaesthesiologica Scandinavica*, **33**, 369–73.

Atkinson, R. C., and Shiffrin, R. M. (1968) Human memory: A proposed system and its control processes, in *The Psychology of Learning and Motivation*, (eds K. W. Spence and J. T. Spence), Academic Press, New York, pp. 89–105.

Atkinson, R. M., Morozumi, P., Green, J. D. *et al.* (1977) Nitrous oxide intoxication: Subjective effects in healthy young men. *Journal of Phychedelic Drugs*, **9**, 317–28.

Bedford, P. D. (1955) Adverse effects of anaesthesia in the elderly. *Lancet*, **II** 259–73.

Biersner, R. J. (1972) Selective performance effects of nitrous oxide. *Human Factors*, **14**, 187–94.

Billings, C. E., Gerke, R. J., and Wick, R. L. (1975) Comparisons of pilot performances in simulated and actual flights. *Aviation Space and Environmental Medicine*, **46**, 304–8.

Bixler, E. O., Scharf, M. B., Soldatos, C. R. *et al.* (1979) Effects of hypnotic drugs on memory. *Life Sciences*, **25**, 1379–88.

Block, R. I., and Berchou, R. (1984) Alprazolam and lorazepam effects on memory acquisition and retrieval processes. *Pharmacology, Biochemistry and Behavior*, **20**, 233–41.

Block, R. I., Ghoneim, M. M., Hinrichs, J. V. *et al.* (1988a) Effects of a subanesthetic concentration of nitrous oxide on memory and subjective experience: Influence of assessment procedures and types of auditory stimuli. *Human Psychopharmacology*, **3**, 257–65.

Block, R. I., Ghoneim, M. M., Pathak, D. *et al.* (1988b) Effects of a subanesthetic concentration of nitrous oxide on overt and covert assessments of memory and associative processes. *Psychopharmacology*, **96**, 324–31.

Blundell, E. (1967) A psychological study of the effects of surgery on eighty-six elderly patients. *British Journal of Social and Clinical Psychology*, **6**, 297–303.

Broks, P., Preston, G. C., Traub, M. *et al.* (1988) Modelling dementia: Effects of scopolamine on memory and attention. *Neuropsychologia*, **26**, 685–700.

Brown, J., Brown, M. W. and Bowes, J. B. (1983) Effects of lorazepam on rate of forgetting, on retrieval from semantic memory and on manual dexterity. *Neuropsychologia*, **21**, 501–12.

Brown, J., Lewis, V., Brown, M. *et al.* (1982) A comparison between transient amnesias induced by two drugs (diazepam and lorazepam) and amnesia of organic origin. *Neuropsychologia*, **20**, 55–77.

Brown, M. W., Brown, J. and Bowes, J. (1989) Absence of priming coupled with substantially preserved recognition in lorazepam induced amnesia. *Quarterly Journal of Experimental Psychology*, **41A**, 599–617.

Bruce, D. L. (1991) Recantation Revisited. *Anesthesiology*, **74**, 1160–1.

Bruce, D. L., and Bach, M. J. (1975) Psychological studies of human performance as affected by traces of enflurane and nitrous oxide. *Anesthesiology*, **42**, 194–6.

Bruce, D. L., and Bach M. J. (1976) Effects of trace anaesthetic gases on behavioural performance of volunteers. *British Journal of Anaesthesia*, **48**, 871–6.

Bruce, D. L., and Stanley, T. H. (1983) Research replication may be subject specific. *Anesthesia and Analgesia*, **62**, 617.

Caine, E. D., Weingartner, H., Ludlow, C. L. *et al.* (1981) Qualitative analysis of scopolamine-induced amnesia. *Psychopharmacology*, **74**, 74–80.

Carlsson, A. (1981) Aging and brain neurotransmitters, in *Strategies for the development of an effective treatment for senile dementia*, (eds. T. Crook and S. Gershon), Mark Powely Associates, New Canaan, C.T., pp. 93–104.

Chapman, C. R., Murphy, T. M. and Butler, S. H. (1973) Analgesic strength of 33 percent nitrous oxide: A signal detection theory evaluation. *Science*, **179**, 1246–8.

Clarke, P. R. F., Eccersley, P. S., Frisby, J. P. and Thornton, J. A. (1970) The amnesic effect of diazepam (Valium). *British Journal of Anaesthesia*, **42**, 690–7.

Cohen, R. M., Weingartner, H., Smallberg, S. and Murphy, D. L., (1982) Effort in cognitive processes in depression. *Archives of General Psychiatry*, **39**, 593–7.

Cook, T. L., Smith, M., Starkweather, J. A., and Eger II, E. I. (1978a) Effect of subanesthetic concentrations of enflurane and halothane on human behavior. *Anesthesia and Analgesia*, **57**, 434–40.

Cook, T. L., Smith, M., Starkweather, J. A. *et al.* (1978b) Behavioral effects of trace and subanesthetic halothane and nitrous oxide in man. *Anesthesiology*, **49**, 419–24.

Craik, F. I. M. and Lockhart, R. S. (1972) Levels of processing: A framework for memory research. *Journal of Verbal Learning and Verbal Behavior*, **11**, 671–84.

Crow, T. J. (1979) Action of hyoscine on verbal learning in man: Evidence for a cholinergic link in the transition from primary to secondary memory, in *Brain Mechanisms in Memory and Learning: From the Single Neuron to Man*, (ed. M. A. B. Brazier), Raven Press, New York, pp. 269–75.

Crow, T. J. and Grove-White, I. G. (1973) An analysis of the learning deficit following hyoscine administration to man. *British Journal of Pharmacology*, **49**, 322–7.

Curran, H. V. (1986) Tranquillizing memories: A review of the effects of benzodiazepines on human memory. *Biological Psychology*, **23**, 179–213.

Curran, H. V., Schifano, F. and Lader, M. (1991) Models of memory dysfunction? A comparison of the effects of scopolamine and lorazepam on memory, psychomotor performance and mood. *Psychopharmacology*, **103**, 83–90.

Danion, J. M. Zimmmermann, M. A., Willard-Schroeder, D. *et al.* (1989) Diazepam induces a dissociation between explicit and implicit memory. *Psychopharmacology*, **99**, 238–43.

Davis, K. L., Mohs, R. C., Tinklenberg, J. R. *et al.* (1978) Physostigmine improvements of long-term memory processes in normal humans. *Science*, **201**, 272–4.

Davison, L. A., Steinhelber, J. C., Eger, E. I., *et al.* (1975) Psychological effects of halothane and isoflurane anesthesia. *Anesthesiology*, **43**, 313–24.

de Gier, J. J., Hart, B. J., Nebmans, F. A. *et al.* (1981) Psychomotor performance and real driving performance of out-patients receiving diazepam. *Psychopharmacology*, **73**, 340–4.

Deutsch, J. A. (1971) The cholinergic synapse and the site of memory. *Science*, **174**, 788–94.

Drachman, D. A. (1977) Memory and cognitive function in man: Does the cholinergic system have a specific role? *Neurology*, **27**, 783–90.

Drachman, D. A. and Leavitt, J. (1974) Human memory and the cholingeric system. *Archives of Neurology*, **30**, 113–21.

Dundee, J. W. and Pandit, S. K. (1972) Studies on drug-induced amnesia with intravenous anaesthetic agents in man. *British Journal of Clinical Practice*, **26**, 164–6.

Dworkin, S. F., Schubert, M. M., Chen, A. C. N. and Clark, D. W. (1986) Psychological preparation influences nitrous oxide analgesia: Replication of laboratory findings in a clinical setting. *Oral Surgery, Oral Medicine, Oral Pathology*, **61**, 108–12.

Edwards, D., Harris, J. A. and Biersner, R. (1976) Encoding and decoding of connected discourse during altered states of consciousness. *Journal of Psychology*, **92**, 97–102.

Ellinwood, E. H., Easler, M, E., Linnoila, M., *et al.* (1984) Effects of oral contraceptives on diazepam-induced psychomotor impairment. *Clinical Pharmacology and Therapeutics*, **35**, 360–6.

Evans, W. O., and Davis, K. E. (1969) Dose-response effects of secobarbital on human memory. *Psychopharmacology*, **14**, 46–61.

Fang, J. C., Hinrichs, J. V. and Ghoneim, M. M. (1987) Diazepam and memory: Evidence for spared memory function. *Pharmacology, Biochemistry and Behavior*, **28**, 347–52.

File, S. E. and Lister, R. G. (1982) Do lorazepam-induced deficits in learning result from impaired rehearsal, reduced motivation or increased sedation? *British Journal of Clinical Pharmacology*, **14**, 545–50.

Frith, C. D., McGinty, M. A., Gergel, I. and Crow, T. J. (1989) The effects of scopolamine and clonidine upon the performance and learning of a motor skill. *Psychopharmacology*, **98**, 120–5.

Garfield, J. M., Garfield, F. B. and Sampson, J. (1975) Effects of nitrous oxide on decision-strategy and sustained attention. *Psychopharmacologia*, **42**, 5–10.

Ghoneim, M. M. The reversal of benzodiazepine-induced amnesia by flumazenil: A review. *Anesthesiology Review* (in press).

Ghoneim, M. M., and Mewaldt, S. P. (1975) Effects of diazepam and scopolamine on storage, retrieval, and organizational processes in memory. *Psychopharmacologia*, **44**, 257–62.

Ghoneim, M. M., and Mewaldt, S. P. (1977) Studies on human memory: The interactions of diazepam, scopolamine, and physostigmine. *Psychopharmacology*, **52**, 1–6.

Ghoneim, M. M., and Mewaldt, S. P. (1990) Benzodiazepines and human memory: A review. *Anesthesiology*, **72**, 926–38.

Ghoneim, M. M., and Mewaldt, S. P. and Thatcher, J. W. (1975) The effects of diazepam and fentanyl on mental, psychomotor, and electroencephalographic functions and their rate of recovery. *Psychopharmacologia*, **44**, 61–6.

Ghoneim, M. M., and Mewaldt, S. P., Berie, J. L. and Hinrichs, J. V. (1981a). Memory performance effects of single and 3-week administration of diazepam. *Psychopharmacology*, **73**, 147–51.

Ghoneim, M. M., and Mewaldt, S. P. and Petersen, R. C. (1981b) Subanesthetic concentration of nitrous oxide and human memory. *Progress in Neuro-Psychopharmacology*, **5**, 395–402.

Ghoneim, M. M., Hinrichs, J. V. and Mewaldt, S. P. (1984a) Dose-response analysis of the behavioral effects of diazepam: I. Learning and memory. *Psychopharmacology*, **82**, 291–5.

Ghoneim, M. M., and Mewaldt, S. P., and Hinrichs, J. V. (1984b) Dose-response analysis of the behavioral effects of diazepam: II. Psychomotor performance, cognition and mood. *Psychopharmacology*, **82**, 296–300.

Ghoneim, M. M., Hinrichs, J. V., and Mewaldt, S. P. (1986) Comparison of two benzodiazepines with differing accumulation: Behavioral changes during and after three-week administration. *Clinical Pharmacology and Therapeutics*, **39**, 491–500.

Ghoneim, M. M., Hinrichs, J. V., O'Hara, M. W. *et al.* (1988) Comparison of psychological and cognitive function after general or regional anesthesia. *Anesthesiology*, **69**, 507–15.

Graf, P. and Schacter, D. L. (1985) Implicit and explicit memory for new associations in normal and amnesic patients. *Journal of Experimental Psychology: Learning, Memory, and Cognition*, **11**, 501–18.

Graf, P. Squire, L. R. and Mandler, G. (1984) The information that amnesic patients do not forget. *Journal of Experimental Psychology: Learning, Memory, and Cognition*, **10**, 164–78.

Griffiths, R. R., Bigelow, G. E., Liebson, I. (1983) Differential effects of diazepam and pentobarbital on mood and behavior. *Archives of General Psychiatry*, **40**, 865–73.

Haffner, J. F. W., Moreland, J., Setekleiu, J. *et al.* (1973). Mental and psychomotor effects of diazepam and ethanol. *Acta Pharmacologica et Toxicologica*, **32**, 161–78.

Heisterkamp, D. R. and Cohen, P. J. (1975) The effect of intravenous premedication with lorazepam (Ativan), pentobarbitone or diazapam on recall. *British Journal of Anaesthesia*, **47**, 79–81.

Henrie, J. R., Parkhouse, J. and Bickford, R. G. (1961) Alteration of human consciousness by nitrous oxide as assessed by electroencephalography and psychological tests. *Anesthesiology*, **22**, 247–59.

Hilgenberg, J. C. (1981) Intraoperative awareness during high-dose fentanyl-oxygen anesthesia. *Anesthesiology*, **54**, 341–4.

Hinrichs, J. V and Ghoneim, M. M. (1987) Diazepam, behavior, and aging: Increased sensitivity or lower baseline performance? *Psychopharmacology*, **92**, 100–5.

Hinrichs, J. V., Ghoneim, M. M., Mewaldt, S. P. (1984) Diazepam and memory: Retrograde facilitation produced by interference reduction. *Psychopharmacology*, **84**, 158–62.

Hinrichs, J. V., Mewaldt, S. P., Ghoneim, M. M. and Berie, J. L. (1982) Diazepam and learning: Assessment of acquisition deficits. *Pharmacology, Biochemistry, and Behavior*, **17**, 165–70.

Hole, A., Terjesen, T. and Breivik, H. (1980) Epidural versus general anaesthesia for total hip arthroplasty in elderly patients. *Acta Anaesthesiologica Scandinavica*, **24**, 279–87.

James, W. (1882) II On some Hegelisms. *Mind*, **7**, 186–208.

James, W. (1898) Consciousness under nitrous oxide. *Psychological Review*, **5**, 194–6.

Johnson, L. C. and Chernik, D. A. (1982) Sedative-hypnotics and human performance. *Psychopharmacology*, **76**, 101–13.

Jones, D. M., Lewis, M. J. and Spriggs, T. L. B. (1978) The effects of low doses of diazepam on human performance in group administered tasks. *British Journal of Clinical Pharmacology*, **6**, 333–7.

Kahn, R. L., Zarit, S. H., Hilbert, N. M., and Niederehe, G. (1975) Memory complaint and impairment in the aged. *Archives of General Psychiatry*, **32**, 1569–73.

Kerr, B., Hill, H., Coda, B. *et al.* (1991) Concentration-related effects of morphine on cognition and motor control in human subjects. *Neuropsychopharmacology*, **5**, 157–66.

Klausen, N-O., Wiberg-Jorgensen, F., and Chraemmer-Jorgensen, B. (1983) Psychomimetic reactions after low-dose ketamine infusion. *British Journal of Anaesthesia*, **55**, 297–301.

Korttila, K., Ghoneim, M. M., Jacobs, L. *et al.* (1981) Time course of mental and psychomotor effects of 30 per cent nitrous oxide during inhalation and recovery. *Anesthesiology*, **54**, 220–6.

Leipzig, R. M., Goodman, H., Gray, G. *et al.* (1987) Reversible, narcotic-associated mental status impairment in patients with metastatic cancer. *Pharmacology*, **35**, 47–54.

Liljequist, R., Linnoila, M., Mattila, M. J. (1978) Effect of diazepam and chlorpromazine on memory functions in man. *European Journal of Clinical Pharmacology*, **13**, 339–43.

Liljequist, R., Mattila, M. J. and Linnoila, M. (1981) Alterations in human memory following acute maprotiline, diazepam and codeine administration. *Acta Pharmacologica et Toxicologica*, **48**, 190–2.

Lister, R. G. (1985) The amnesic action of benzodiazepines in man. *Neuroscience and Biobehavioral Reviews*, **9**, 87–94.

Lister, R. G., and File, S. E. (1984) The nature of lorazepam-induced amnesia. *Psychopharmacology*, **83**, 183–7.

Lowenstein E., and Philbin D. M. (1981) Narcotic 'anesthesia' in the eighties. *Anesthesiology*, **55**, 195–7.

McNair, D. M. (1973). Antianxiety drugs and human performance. *Archives of General Psychiatry*, **29**, 611–17.

Mesulam, M. M. and Geschwind, N. (1976) Disordered mental states in the post-operative period. *Urologic Clinics of North America*, **3**, 199–215.

Mewaldt, S. P. and Ghoneim, M. M. (1979) The effects and interactions of scopolamine, physostigmine and methamphetamine on human memory. *Pharmacology, Biochemistry, and Behavior*, **10**, 205–10.

Mewaldt, S. P., Hinrichs, J. V. and Ghoneim, M. M. (1983) Diazepam and memory: Support for a duplex model of memory. *Memory and Cognition*, **11**, 557–64.

Mewaldt, S. P., Ghoneim, M. M. and Hinrichs, J. V. (1986) The behavioral profiles of diazepam and oxazepam are similar. *Psychopharmacology*, **88**, 165–71.

Mewaldt, S. P., Ghoneim, M. M. Choi, W. W. *et al.* (1988) Nitrous oxide and human state-dependent memory. *Pharmacology, Biochemistry and Behavior*, **30**, 83–7.

Mewaldt, S. P., Hinrichs, J. V. and Ghoneim, M. M. Memory impairment with diazepam is not the result of a rehearsal deficit. *Psychopharmacology* (in press).

Meyer, B. R. (1982). Benzodiazepines in the elderly. *Medical Clinics of North America*, **66**, 1017–35.

Meyers, F. H. and Abreu, B. E. (1952) A comparison of the central and peripheral effects of atropine, scopolamine and some synthetic atropine-like compounds. *Journal of Pharmacology and Experimental Therapeutics*, **104**, 387–94.

Mohs, R. C., Tinklenberg, J. R., Roth, W. T. *et al.* (1980) Sensitivity of some human cognitive functions to effects of methamphetamine and secobarbital. *Drug and Alcohol Dependence*, **5**, 145–50.

Molchan, S. E., Mellow, A. M., Lawlor, B. A. *et al.* (1990) TRH attenuates scopolamine-induced memory impairment in humans. *Psychopharmacology*, **100**, 84–9.

Newton, D. E. F., Thornton, C., Konieczko, K. *et al.* (1990) Levels of consciousness in volunteers breathing sub-mac concentrations of isoflurane. *British Journal of Anaesthesia*, **65**, 609–15.

Nielson, W. R., Gelb, A. W., Casey, J. E. *et al.* (1990) Long-term cognitive and social sequelae of general versus regional anesthesia during arthroplasty in the elderly. *Anesthesiology*, **73**, 1103–9.

Nuotto, E. (1983) Psychomotor, physiological and cognitive effects of scopolamine and ephedrine in healthy man. *European Journal of Clinical Pharmacology*, **24**, 603–9.

Nussmeiser, N. A., Arlund, C., and Slogoff, S. (1986) Neuropsychiatric complications after cardioplumonary bypass: Cerebral protection by a barbiturate. *Anesthesiology*, **64**, 165–70.

Osborn, A. G., Bunker, J. P., Cooper, L. M. *et al.* (1967) Effects of thiopental sedation on learning and memory. *Science*, **157**, 574–6.

Palva, E. S. and Linnoila, M. (1978) Effect of active metabolites of chlordiazepoxide and diazepam, alone or in combination with alcohol, on psychomotor skills related to driving. *European Journal of Clinical Pharmacology*, **13**, 345–50.

Pandit, S. K., Dundee, J. W. and Keilty, S. R. (1971) Amnesia studies with intravenous premedication. *Anaesthesia*, **26**, 421.

Parkhouse, J. D., Henrie, J. R., Duncan, G. M., *et al.* (1960) Nitrous oxide analgesia in relation to mental performance. *Journal of Pharmacology and Experimental Therapeutics*, **128**, 44–54.

Petersen, R. C. and Ghoneim, M. M. (1980) Diazepam and human memory: Influence on acquisition, retrieval, and state-dependent learning. *Progress in Neuro-Psychopharmacology*, **4**, 81–9.

Pomara, N., Stanley, B., Block, R. *et al.* (1985) Increased sensitivity of the elderly to the central depressant effects of diazepam. *Journal of Clinical Psychiatry*, **46**, 185–7.

Ramsay, D. S., Leonesio, R. J., Whitney, C. W. *et al.* (1992) Paradoxical effects of nitrous oxide on human memory. *Psychopharmacology*, **106**, 370–4.

Rice, S. A. (1983) Behavioral toxicity of inhalation anaesthetic agents, in *Clinics in Anaesthesiology* (Volume 1, No. 2) (ed. R. I. Mazze), W. B. Saunders, Philadelphia, pp. 507–19.

Rich, J. B. and Brown, G. G. (1992) Selective dissociations of sedation and amnesia following ingestion of diazepam. *Psychopharmacology*, **106**, 346–50.

Roache, J. D. and Griffiths, R. R. (1985) Comparison of triazolam and pentobarbitol: Performance impairment, subjective effects and abuse liability. *Journal of Pharmacology and Experimental Therapeutics*, **234**, 120–33.

Romm. S., Hutzler, J. and Berggren, R. B. (1981) Sexual identity and prophylactic mastectomy. *Annals of Plastic Surgery*, **7**, 35–7.

Rosenberg, H., Orkin, F. K., and Springstead, J. (1979) Abuse of nitrous oxide. *Anesthesia and Analgesia*, **58**, 104–6.

Roy-Byrne, P. P., Weingartner, H., Bierer, L. M. *et al.* (1986) Effortful and automatic cognitive processes in depression. *Archives of General Psychiatry*, **43**, 265–7.

Rundell, O. H., Williams, H. L. and Lester, B. K. (1977) Comparative effects of alcohol, secobarbital, methaqualone and meporbamate on information processing and memory, in *Alcohol Intoxication and Withdrawal*, **85A**, *Biological Aspects of Ethanol*, (ed. M. M. Gross), Plenum, New York, pp. 617–28.

Rupreht, J., Dworacek, B., Bonke, B. *et al.* (1985) Tolerance to nitrous oxide in volunteers. *Acta Anaesthesiologica Scandinavica*, **29**, 635–8.

Russell, R. W. and Steinberg, H. (1955) Effects of nitrous oxide on reactions to 'stress'. *Quarterly Journal of Experimental Psychology*, **7**, 67–73.

Rusted, J. M. and Warburton, D. M. (1989) Effects of scopolamine on verbal memory; a retrieval or acquistion deficit? *Neuropsychobiology*, **21**, 76–83.

Rusted, J. M., Eaton-Williams, P. and Warburton, D. M. (1991) A comparison of the effects of scopolamine and diazepam on working memory. *Psychopharmacology*, **105**, 442–5.

Rutschman, J. and Rubinstein, L. (1966) Time estimation, knowledge of results and drug effects. *Journal of Psychiatric Research*, **4**, 107–14.

Scamman, F. L., Ghoneim, M. M. and Korttila, K. (1984) Ventilatory and mental effects of alfentanil and fentanyl. *Acta Anaesthesiologica Scandinavica*, **28**, 63–7.

Seppala, T., Korttila, K., Hakkinen, S. and Linnoila, M. (1976) Residual effects and skills related to driving after a single oral administration of diazepam, medazepam or lorazepam. *British Journal of Clinical Pharmacology*, **3**, 831–41.

Sheppeard, H., Cleak, D. K., Ward, D. K. and O'Connor, B. T. (1980) A review of early mortality and morbidity in elderly patients following Charnley total hip replacement. *Archives of Orthopaedic and Trauma Surgery*, **97**, 243–8.

Sitaram, N., Weingartner, H. and Gillen, J. C. (1978) Human serial learning: Enhancement with arecholine and choline and impairment with scopolamine. *Science*, **201**, 274–6.

Smith, R. J., Roberts, N. M., Rodgers, R. J. and Bennett, S. (1986) Adverse cognitive effects of general anaesthesia in young and elderly patients. *International Clinical Psychopharmacology*, **1**, 253–9.

Sotaniemi, K. A. (1983) Cerebral outcome after extracorporeal circulation: Comparison between prospective and retrospective evaluations. *Archives of Neurology*, **40**, 75–7.

Steinberg, H. (1954) Selective effects of an anaesthetic drug on cognitive behaviour. *Quarterly Journal of Experimental Psychology*, **6**, 170–80.

Steinberg, H. (1956) 'Abnormal behaviour' induced by nitrous oxide. *British Journal of Psychology*, **47**, 183–94.

Storms, L. H., Stark, A. H., Calverly, R. K. and Smith, N. T. (1980) Psychological functioning after halothane or enflurane anesthesia. *Anesthesia and Analgesia*, **59**, 245–9.

Talland, G. A., and Quarton, G. C. (1965) The effects of methamphetamine and pentobarbital on the running memory span. *Psychopharmacology*, **7**, 379–82.

Tinkleberg, J. R., and Taylor, J. L. (1984) Assessments of drug effects on human memory functions, in *Neuropsychology of Memory* (eds L. Squire and N. Butters) Guilford Press, New York, pp. 213–23.

Titchener, J. L., Zwerling, I., Gottschalk, L. *et al.* (1956) Psychosis in surgical patients. *Surgery, Gynecology and Obstetrics*, **102**, 59–65.

Troster, A. I., Beatty, W. W., Staton, R. D. and Rorabaugh, A. G. (1989) Effects of scopolamine on anterograde and remote memory in humans. *Psychobiology*, **17**, 12–18.

Tufo, H. M., Ostfeld, A. M., and Schkelle, R. (1970) Central nervous system dysfunction following open-heart surgery. *Journal of the American Medical Association*, **212**, 1333–40.

Tulving, E. (1972) Episodic and semantic memory, in *Organization and Memory*, (eds E. Tulving and W. Donaldson) Academic Press, New York.

Tulving, E., and Thompson, D. M. (1973) Encoding specificity and retrieval processes in episodic memory. *Psychological Review*, **80**, 352–73.

Tune, L., and Folstein, M. F. (1986) Post-operative delirium, in *Psychological Aspects of Surgery*, (ed. F. G. Guggenheim), S. Karger, Farmington, CT, pp. 51–68.

van Laar, M. W., Volkerts, E. R. and van Willigenburg, A. P. P. (1992) Therapeutic effects and effects on actual driving performance of chronically administered buspirone and diazepam in anxious outpatients. *Journal of Clinical Psychopharmacology*, **12**, 86–95.

Weingartner, H., Sitaram, N. and Gillin, C. (1979) The role of cholinergic nervous system in memory consolidation. *Bulletin of the Psychonomic Society*, **13**, 9–11.

Weingartner, H. J., Hommer, D., Lister, R. G. *et al.* (1992) Selective effects of triazolam on memory. *Psychopharmacology*, **106**, 341–5.

Weisman, A. D., and Hackett, T. P., (1958) Psychosis after eye surgery: Establishment of specific doctor–patient relationship in prevention and treatment of black patch delirium. *New England Journal of Medicine*, **258**, 1284–9.

Wernberg, M., Nielson, S. F. and Hommelgaard, P. (1980) A comparison between reaction time measurement and critical flicker fusion frequency under rising nitrous oxide inhalation in healthy subjects. *Acta Anaesthesiologica Scandinavica*, **24**, 86–9.

Wesnes, K. and Revell, A. (1984) The separate and combined effects of scopolamine and nicotine on human information processing. *Psychopharmacology*, **84**, 5–11.

Wesnes, K. and Warburton, D. M. (1983) Effects of scopolamine on stimulus sensitivity and response bias in a visual vigilance task. *Neuropsychobiology*, **9**, 154–7.

Wesnes, K. and Warburton, D. M. (1984) Effects of scopolamine and nicotine on human rapid information processing performance. *Psychopharmacology*, **82**, 147–50.

Williams, H. L. and Rundell, O. H. (1983) Secobarbitol effects on recall and recognition in levels-of-processing paradigm. *Psychopharmacology*, **80**, 221–5.

Williams, H. L., Rundell, O. H., and Smith, L. T. (1981) Dose effects of secobarbitol in a Sternberg memory scanning task. *Psychopharmacology*, **72**, 161–5.

Wilson, J. and Ellis, F. R. (1973) Oral premedication with lorazepam (Ativan): A comparison with heptabarbitone (Medomin) and diazepam (Valium). *British Journal of Anaesthesia,***45**, 738–44.

Zacks, R. T., Hasher, L. and Sanft, H. (1982) Automatic encoding of event frequency: Further findings. *Journal of Experimental Psychology: Learning, Memory, and Cognition*, **8**, 106–16.

CHAPTER 8

Awareness and memory for events during anaesthesia

Steven P. Mewaldt, Robert I. Block and

M. M. Ghoneim

8.1 INTRODUCTION

Imagine lying immobilized but cognizant in front of a surgical team which is in the process of cutting into your body. You feel the pain of the incision caused by the surgeon's scalpel and though you hear the conversations of the medical personnel as they work, you are unable to do anything to attract their attention to alert them of your plight. Perhaps few situations could be more feared by a patient facing surgery, nor could few events associated with surgery be more likely to produce psychological or emotional trauma.

Reports of cases dating to the mid–1800s suggest that incidents of awareness during general anaesthesia have been observed since the origin of anaesthetic use (e.g., Calverley, 1989; Crile, 1947; Peirson, 1846). However, the problem became more apparent after the early 1940s when Griffith and Johnson (1942) introduced the use of muscle relaxants into surgery, thereby permitting physicians to employ lighter levels of anaesthesia than previously possible. Subsequently, numerous reports of cases dealing with awareness during anaesthesia have appeared in the literature.

Recently the topic has received a great deal of attention, being the focus of numerous articles in the medical literature, the lay press, and the subject of three recent conferences. There are several reasons for interest in the topic. First, awareness and recall of events from surgery can have powerful effects upon the well-being of the patient. Second, it has been a basis for litigation against physicians (Utting, 1982). Third, the topic is theoretically interesting because general anaesthesia is intended to abolish awareness and subsequent memory for intraoperative events, therefore awareness during general anaesthesia seems almost a contradiction in terms.

8.2 TERMINOLOGY

Before examining this phenomenon in more detail it should be helpful to consider a number of terms used in the ensuing discussion. First, it will be helpful to review some of the memory distinctions referred to in the last chapter. For example, one should be aware of the distinction between declarative or explicit memory and nondeclarative or implicit memory (Graf and Schacter, 1985). Declarative memory refers to situations where the remembered event can be consciously or explicitly brought to mind and recalled. Recall, therefore, can be made in an overt verbal fashion. In contrast, nondeclarative memory must be demonstrated implicitly through its influence on performance. Nondeclarative memory tests are also referred to as implicit or covert memory tests as subjects are typically unaware that their memory is being evaluated. For example, we will later refer to a test situation in which an anaesthetized patient is given a suggestion to perform some act following surgery, e.g., touching his or her ear during a post surgery interview. A patient who later states, 'I recall being told to touch my ear during this interview' would be displaying explicit memory for the event. On the other hand, a patient who touched his or her ear during the interview could be displaying implicit memory for the event. These two forms of memory can be independent. Therefore, a person who recalled the instructions to touch one's ear might not perform the act, and a person who touched his or her ear during the interview might have no recollection of being told to do so.

It is also useful to discuss distinctions among the terms 'awareness', 'memory', and 'recall'. Unfortunately, these terms have been used interchangeably in much of the anaesthesia literature. Awareness refers to whether or not an individual is cognizant or conscious of some event. A person who can respond to commands or reports feeling pain during surgery might be said to be aware during surgery. However, while postoperative recall of events which occurred during anaesthesia can be interpreted as indicating postoperative awareness of the events, it has also sometimes been interpreted as indicating prior awareness of the events, i.e., consciousness or awareness during surgery. Such an interpretation may not be valid; it is possible that some patients may recall events following surgery of which they were unaware during surgery (cf. Bogod *et al.*, 1990). More importantly, the absence of postoperative recall should not be interpreted as indicating that there was no prior awareness of surgical events. For example, Tunstall (1977) tested 12 patients who were receiving Caesarean sections; while 75% responded in some form to commands during surgery no patient showed any recall postoperatively. Normal forgetting could have occurred, or drugs employed in surgery and the shock of surgery itself may have impaired the formation of stable retrievable memories (see the previous chapter of this text). In the following discussion, we will use the term 'awareness' to refer to situations in which the patient displays concurrent signs of consciousness during surgery or explicit recall following surgery of some event which occurred during surgery. 'Recall' shall refer to only explicit or declarative memory performance, and 'memory' will be used to refer to either explicit or implicit memory situations.

8.3 INCIDENCE AND CHARACTERISTICS

8.3.1 Clinical studies

A number of clinical surveys of patients have been conducted to determine the incidence and characteristics of awareness during general anaesthesia. A brief review is reported here; for more detailed information see reviews by Guerra (1986) and Utting (1982). The first systematic study of the problem of awareness during general anaesthesia was conducted by Hutchinson (1960) who carried out an extensive retrospective survey of surgical patients. Interviewing 656 patients following surgery Hutchinson found 8 (1.2%) who could recall some events which had occurred during surgery. Another large clinical study involved interviews with 490 postsurgical patients (Wilson *et al.*, 1975). Almost all patients received premedication, induction with thiopentone, and 50%–70% nitrous oxide supplemented (in varying concentrations) with halothane, enflurane, innovar, ketamine, and opioids. The incidence of awareness was again about 1%. Awareness did not appear meaningfully related to the type of premedication or anaesthetic agents used, the duration or type of surgery, or the age or sex of the patients. However, with such low incidence, relationships of these kinds are difficult to establish. Dreaming during anaesthesia was substantially more common than awareness (8%). Utting (1975, 1982) has suggested that dreaming lies along a continuum between unconsciousness and awareness.

A more recent study (Utting, 1987) examined 500 surgical patients who received 70% nitrous oxide in oxygen as the only anaesthetic. Recall of events during anaesthesia was 2%. When the concentration of nitrous oxide was lower (60–67%) the number of patients displaying recall of surgical events ranged from 2–4% (Agarwal and Sikh, 1977; Brice, Hetherington and Utting, 1970; Scott, 1972). In a study of obstetric cases, Crawford (1971) found explicit recall in up to 4% of the women when a 67% concentration of nitrous oxide was employed, and an incidence as high as 25% when the nitrous oxide concentration was reduced to 50%. One of the lowest positive reports of explicit recall of events during anaesthesia was reported by Liu *et al.* (1991) who found only a 0.2% incidence. This recent lower rate of occurrence may result from changes in anaesthetic use to deeper levels of anaesthesia (cf. Lyons and Macdonald, 1991) perhaps because of increasing awareness of the problem in the medical community.

In these and a number of other clinical studies, patients were asked after surgery whether they remembered anything that happened during anaesthesia and affirmative answers were used to establish the incidence of awareness. This could underestimate the frequency of the problem since patients might be aware during anaesthesia but be unable to remember anything afterward (Tunstall, 1977). On the other hand, it could overestimate the incidence because often patients' reports of awareness have been accepted with little attempt to establish the veracity of their memories. In addition, questioning might itself encourage some patients to 'recall' events when their recollections have little validity.

When explicit recall of events during surgery occurs, it most often involves memory for operating room sounds and conversations. More rarely, pain and other physical sensations are reported. Personally meaningful, stressful, or emotional events are supposedly more likely to be recalled than meaningless events (Bennett and Boyle, 1986; Goldmann, 1990). It is often reported that unfavorable comments are particularly likely to be remembered (e.g., Levinson, 1965; Trustman, Dubovsky and Titley, 1977).

While recall of actual events or comments from surgery is relatively rare, more common is the recall of 'dreams' which appear to be associated with the anaesthetic (Brice, Hetherington and Utting, 1970). In a sample of 500 patients receiving nitrous oxide for surgery, Utting (1987) found dreams were reported by approximately 7% of the patients. Many of the dreams were disturbing and were often considered by the patient as one of the worst features of their postoperative experience. In addition, studies discussed below suggest the existence of nondeclarative or implicit memory for events occurring during anaesthesia.

8.3.2 Factors influencing incidence

Higher incidence of awareness during anaesthesia is likely in surgeries which require lighter levels of anaesthesia. For example, awareness is more frequently reported for Caesarean sections (7–28%) (Barr *et al.*, 1977; Bogod *et al.*, 1990). It is also more common in cardiopulmonary bypass surgery (up to 23%) (Mark and Greenberg, 1983; Kim, 1978; Goldmann, Shah and Helden, 1987), surgery for major trauma (11–43%) (Bogetz and Katz, 1984) and bronchoscopy (8%) (Moore and Seymour, 1987). Similarly, higher incidence rates are likely when anaesthesia involves induction with thiopentone and maintenance with nitrous oxide and muscle relaxants but without supplementary inhalational or intravenous anaesthetics or opioids (Utting, 1975, 1982). The incidence of awareness may then be more than 1% with 66%–70% concentrations of nitrous oxide and may increase substantially with lower concentrations.

The general conclusion that emerges from such clinical studies is a common sense one, i.e. that the incidence of awareness increases as the depth of anaesthesia decreases. Since nitrous oxide is a weak anaesthetic, with a 70% concentration equivalent to only 0.67 MAC, awareness is more likely to occur with unsupplemented nitrous oxide than when adjuvants are given.

One should not infer, however, that awareness occurs only when anaesthesia becomes excessively light. While some cases of awareness undoubtedly result from technical errors that permit emergence from anaesthesia, awareness occasionally occurs without technical errors and with use of potent inhalational agents. Awareness can occur in patients who clinically appear to be adequately anaesthetized (Barr *et al.*, 1977); however, judgments of depth of anaesthesia are neither quantitatively precise nor infallible (Evans and Davies, 1984).

A number of other factors besides situations involving light anaesthesia may influence the occurrence of the phenomenon. For example, it has also been suggested that awareness is more likely towards the beginning or end of anaesthesia (Utting, 1975). Other cases may arise because of equipment malfunction or misuse. For example, cylinders of anaesthetic may become empty, gauges may become inaccurate or be misread, air may leak into a ventilator, or a vaporizer may become empty. In addition, personal characteristics of the patient may make some patients less susceptible to anaesthesia than others. Given the well-documented individual differences in responding to many drugs which affect the central nervous system, it would seem likely that there should be variability in effectiveness of anaesthetics also. While individual characteristics that might decrease responsiveness to anaesthetics have not been established, some factors have been suggested, e.g. heavy use of alcohol (Tammisto and Tigerstedt, 1977; Lemmens *et al.*, 1989; Swerdlow *et al.*, 1990), and previous exposure to anaesthetics (Sia, 1969). In addition, Guerra (1986) has suggested that the incidence of awareness may be higher in obese patients because physicians may use lower concentrations of nitrous oxide and lower doses of other drugs to reduce the risk of respiratory depression following surgery.

8.4 METHODS OF ASSESSMENT

In contrast to clinical studies that simply involve questioning patients about their recollections of surgery, several more specific methods have been used to study awareness of events during general anaesthesia.

Obviously it would be beneficial if physicians had a reliable technique to detect awareness during surgery, and, following sugery, if they had a procedure to detect memory for events which had occurred during anaesthesia. As mentioned above, these are really two different questions which might be labelled as methods focusing on 'awareness' vs. 'memory'. We will first examine methods which have been developed to detect the depth of an anaesthetic state during the course of anaesthesia. If effective, one or more of these techniques might be useful as a means of assuring that a patient is kept at an adequate depth of anaesthesia during surgery, thereby making the undesirable consequences of awareness and recall unlikely.

8.4.1   Methods used during general anaesthesia

(a)   Clinical signs of depth of anaesthesia

The simplest technique for attempting to gauge the depth of anaesthesia during surgery is to monitor physical signs of the patient's condition. For example, during general anaesthesia, the absence of purposeful behaviour or response to surgical stimuli is assumed to indicate an absence of awareness. But this assumption may not be valid, particularly when the commonly administered muscle relaxants prevent the patient from moving. One might also watch for indications of sympathetic nervous system activity such as hypertension, sweating, pupil response, tachycardia, pallor, or tearing. However, there are a number of problems with the use of such clinical signs as an accurate source of information. For example, the signs may be missing or be significantly attenuated because they are interfered with by muscle relaxants or other drugs used during surgery. Signs could be missed or misinterpreted as a somatic reflex response or physical response to something other than light anaesthesia. Finally, the importance of these signs may be unclear because of the frequent experience of physicians who have observed some of them without having the patient complain of any problems following surgery, or they may have received complaints in situations in which none of the signs had been present.

Since physical signs alone are therefore not an adequate indicator of depth of anaesthesia, more sophisticated techniques have been proposed. Each involves the use of some method which might somewhat complicate operating room procedures, but if accurate might be worth the effort.

(b)   Isolated forearm technique

The most important of these methods is Tunstall's (1977, 1979) 'isolated forearm technique'. Prior to administering a muscle relaxant, a blood pressure cuff is inflated to prevent circulation of the muscle relaxant into one arm. The patient, if aware, can then use the unparalysed hand to respond to commands, e.g. to grip the anaesthesiologist's hand. In a recent review, Jessop and Jones (1991) suggested that this technique is the closest currently available to a 'gold standard' for detection of awareness, against which other methods can be evaluated. More recently, Wang *et al.* (1992) tested the procedure in subjects receiving muscle relaxants without anaesthesia. They found that subjects maintained enough fine motor control of the hand on the occluded arm that they could still write intelligibly for 20 minutes following isolation of the forearm. In addition, writing was still possible after removal of the bloodpressure cuff but before neuromuscular recovery. Wang *et al.* argue strongly that the technique should be more widely employed in general anaesthesia. Tests with patients also indicate that the technique may be useful. For example, Tunstall (1979) reported that 72% of patients undergoing Caesarean section and using the technique responded in the early minutes following induction of anaesthesia with thiopentone, and Russell (1986) reported that 44% of patients anaesthetized with nitrous oxide and intravenous fentanyl increments were wakeful at some time during surgery. However, the technique is not without problems. Criticisms include: it is sometimes difficult to distinguish responses to commmands from reflex or involuntary muscle movements (Millar and Watkinson, 1983), the method cannot be used for more than 20 minutes because of the risk of temporary paralysis or injury to the arm (Breckenridge and Aitkenhead, 1983), movement of the isolated arm may interfere with surgery (Breckenridge and Aitkenhead, 1981), and some patients may be unable to communicate with the arm despite being awake (Russell, 1989). In addition, interpretation of the results from the technique must be tempered by the fact that even if subjects show wakefulness during surgery they may later show no awarenes or recall of the events (Tunstall, 1977); and a few patients have displayed the opposite, i.e. they have recalled intraoperative events but did not respond to commands during anaesthesia (Bogod *et al.* 1990).

(c) · *Electroencephalography*

Perhaps because of its usefulness in the study of sleep, many investigators have attempted to use the electroencephalograph (EEG) as an indicator of the depth of anaesthesia. Unfortunately, while some EEG patterns have been identified which always signify unconsciousness, e.g., burst suppression and isoelectricity, there is no pattern which has been identified which always accompanies consciousness (Plourde, 1991). Stanski (1990) in a recent review points out that use of the EEG in surgery is complicated by the unknown effects of drugs or drug combinations used in surgery, and by the need for an independent measure of consciousness with which to compare EEG results.

In contrast to global EEG patterns, which have not been very successful in monitoring depth of anaesthesia, evoked responses (which are EEG changes tied to specific auditory, visual, or somatosensory stimuli) have proved somewhat promising. Anaesthetics at clinical concentrations alter the amplitudes and latencies of evoked responses, but do not completely abolish the responses (e.g., Sebel *et al.*, 1985, 1986; Thornton *et al.*, 1983). Changes in visual (VEP) or somatosensory (SEP) evoked potentials in response to anaesthetics have received some attention (e.g. Chi and Field, 1986; Peterson, Drummond and Todd, 1986). Much more attention has been given to auditory evoked potentials (AEP) such as the middle latency evoked response (MLR) (Houston, McClelland and Fenwick, 1988; Jones, 1990; Thornton *et al.*, 1983, 1986), 40 Hz oscillatory activity (Plourde and Picton, 1990), and the P3 or P300 response which occurs when a subject notices a difference in a series of presented stimuli (Jessop *et al.*, 1991; Plourde, 1991).

(d)   Other suggested responses

Evans *et al.* (1984) suggested that measurement of lower oesophageal contractility (LEC) could be used as an indicator of depth of anaesthesia because the smooth muscles of the lower oesophagus are not affected by the paralysis induced by muscle relaxants. Edmonds *et al.* (1987) and Herregods and Rolly (1987) tested the usefulness of electromyograph (EMG) responses and Jänig and Räth (1980) have shown that anaesthetics dampen the skin conductance response. Unfortunately, with each of these measures there is a wide range of typical responding which makes it unlikely that a single standard can be found to indicate consciousness.

8.4.2   Methods used after recovery from general anaesthesia

Methods used following surgery obviously involve evaluation of memory. The results of memory studies will be more easily understood if they are divided into two categories, those resulting from studies which have attempted to assess explicit or declarative memory and those from studies which tested for implicit or nondeclarative memories. In addition, explicit recall has been tested in either a normal awake state or with the aid of hypnosis.

(a)   Explicit memory tests (awake state)

In the clinical studies discussed earlier, patients were asked after surgery whether they remembered anything that occurred during anaesthesia. It is difficult with this method to distinguish veridical memories from confabulations; only when patients recall specific details during surgery that can be confirmed by others can much confidence be placed in their reports. An obvious way to handle this difficulty is by presenting specific information during anaesthesia and assessing memory for this information afterward. Several studies have presented words, poems, stories, music, or other sounds via tape recordings during anaesthesia. The results of recall and recognition tests administered following surgery have been generally negative, i.e. no recall or recognition has been detected (Brice, Hetherington and Utting, 1970; Dubovsky and Trustman, 1976; Lewis, Jenkinson and Wilson, 1973; Loftus *et al.*, 1985; McIntyre, 1966; Wilson, Lewis and Jenkinson, 1970). Two studies, however, produced positive results (Block *et al.*, 1991b; Millar and Watkinson, 1983). In the earlier of these two studies (Millar and Watkinson) general anaesthesia was induced with thiopentone or althesin and maintained with 66% nitrous oxide supplemented, in some patients, with 0.25%–1.0% halothane. Patients who were played a list of words during anaesthesia performed better on a later recognition test than controls who were played noise. However, the difference was significant only for a measure of sensitivity derived from signal detection theory, not for basic measures of the number of correct responses; and the report does not indicate whether the words played during anaesthesia were later recognized at a level above chance. In the Block *et al.* (1991b) study, patients who heard nonsense words presented sixteen times during anaesthesia recognized them following surgery significantly better than less frequently presented words, while not showing this pattern under control conditions. However, we will argue below that both of these experiments reflect the contribution of implicit rather than explicit memory and therefore that they do not contradict the results of the other studies which show no explicit recall of controlled test materials.

(b) Explicit memory tests under hypnosis

Some investigators have asked whether use of hypnosis might increase explicit memory for intraoperative events. The method involves hypnotizing subjects and regressing them to the time of surgery. This, it has been suggested, might enable patients to recall information which might not otherwise be available. Hypnosis it is argued might improve rapport with the patient, remove barriers of repression from the recall of traumatic events, and aid in memory retrieval, perhaps by increasing concentration. It has also been suggested that the hypnotized state might more closely resemble the anaesthetized state than does normal waking consciousness. Therefore, patients might benefit from a state-dependent memory effect. (As discussed in the previous chapter state-dependent memory refers to the situation where memories formed in one state of consciousness are better recalled later when in the same state of consciousness than when in a different one.) Of course the appropriateness of the analogy between the state of consciousness during anaesthesia and that created during hypnosis is somewhat dubious.

Most research which has investigated the effects of hypnosis on recall of intrasurgical events consists of clinical studies. For example, Cheek (1959) found that when patients who had complaints concerning a previous surgery were hypnotized they were able to recall negative statements made about them by members of their operating team. This recall was following by a remission of their symptoms. In another frequently cited study (Levinson, 1965), a fake surgical crisis was staged during dental surgery on patients anaesthetized with thiopentone, nitrous oxide, and ether. Although no patients recalled this event under normal conditions, four subjects (40%) supposedly recalled it in near verbatim detail under hypnosis. Another four subjects became so anxious while attempting recall that they emerged from hypnosis. Bennett and Davis (1984) reported in an abstract that verbatim recall of intraoperative events was elicited under hypnosis in half of a group of patients anaesthetized with thiopentone, nitrous oxide, and enflurane or halothane. Similar instances of recall under hypnosis of events occurring during anaesthesia have been reported by Bennett (1988), Goldmann, Shah and Helden, (1987), and Howard (1987).

While these clinical case reports of recall under hypnosis of events which occurred during anaesthesia are anecdotally interesting, their importance is difficult to judge. Because they were not true experiments there is no nonhypnosis control condition with which to compare results. Subject assignment and other details were not handled under double-blind conditions, and controls over the test environment were generally not as tight as one would expect in an experiment. For example, few attempted to control the depth of anaesthesia or measure the end-expired concentration of anaesthetics. As a result one cannot be certain that subjects were really under deep anaesthesia. Consistent with this notion, Eger *et al.* (1990) recently have argued that the EEG patterns observed in subjects in the Levinson (1965) study suggest a light level of anaesthesia was present.

A further problem in interpreting the results of studies employing hypnosis is that material recalled under hypnosis is frequently incorrect. In 1985 a special panel established by the Council on Scientific Affairs of the American Medical Association after reviewing the literature on hypnosis and memory stated that 'recollections obtained during hypnosis can involve confabulations and pseudomemories, and not only fail to be more accurate, but actually appear to be less reliable than nonhypnotic recall' (Council on Scientific Affairs, 1985). Without specific stimuli to score, it is therefore hard to separate accurate from bogus recall in many of the above studies.

Studies which have employed controlled stimuli and more objective recall measures suggest that hypnosis is unlikely to contribute much to an understanding of memory for events which occurred during anaesthesia. For example, Terrell *et al.* (1969) tested recall of specific verbal stimuli presented during anaesthesia and found no evidence of recall of these stimuli under hypnosis. Similarly, Bennett, Davis and Giannini (1985), Goldmann (1988), and Goldmann and Levey (1986) tested subjects under hypnosis for recognition of cues or recall of commands given during anaesthesia and found no evidence of enhanced recall.

(c) *Implicit memory tests for verbal material*

The second set of research methods which employ tests done after recovery from anaesthesia address implicit memory. They ask whether it is possible that awareness and learning might occur during anaesthesia but not be consciously accessible afterwards. Eich, Reeves and Katz (1985) distinguished between memory and the awareness of remembering. They suggested that information presented during anaesthesia might be stored in memory but not be available for intentional memory retrieval as is required in a recognition or recall test. Therefore, covert tests, which do not overtly assess memory but in which performance might be influenced by memories of previously presented information, might be more sensitive to memories stored during anaesthesia. Implicit memory tests with amnesic patients have successfully detected memories that were not evident with the more common explicit tests.

Several forms of implicit memory tasks have been employed. Most use some form of priming task in which information is presented during anaesthesia and the effect of the presentation or 'priming' is covertly evaluated following surgery. For example, Eich, Reeves and Katz (1985) chose words which could be spelled in more than one way (e.g. homophones such as EIGHT/ATE) and presented phrases during anaesthesia (e.g. dinner at EIGHT) which were intended to influence patients towards giving a particular spelling on a test administered after recovery. The results were negative, i.e. no effect of the priming exposure was found. At least two factors may have contributed to these negative results: First, the interval between presentation of the material during anaesthesia and its testing was long (4–5 days). Second, it is possible that this priming task required more cognitive processing than subjects could muster during anaesthesia, i.e. subjects had to determine the meaning and the correct spelling of an item from the context in which it was presented.

A more popular priming task is the word completion test. In this task subjects are presented with a list of words during anaesthesia. Then following recovery they are presented with a series of three-letter word stems. The subject's task is to complete the word stems by writing the first word that comes to mind. For example, the subject might receive the stimulus 'For____' during testing, to which he or she could write foreign, fork, forfeit, forgive, etc. Evidence of priming is found when subjects complete the stems by making words they were exposed to during anaesthesia with greater frequency than they make control words to which they were not exposed. In creating this test the experimenter typically attempts to ensure that the target word is not one of the most frequent responses to the test stimulus. Block *et al.* (1991b) tested subjects with this task one day after surgery and found a significant priming effect. Presenting a word during surgery almost doubled the probability of giving that word on the test, relative to control words.

Block *et al.* (1991b) also employed a nonsense word task to test for both implicit and explicit memory. During anaesthesia patients were presented with a series of nonsense words, e.g. 'goral'. Some nonsense words were repeated up to 16 times. Then during testing patients listened to a series of pairs of nonsense words and were asked to identify the item they had heard before. In a separate test they were asked to tell which item they found more pleasant sounding. Patients more accurately selected the nonsense words that had been played most frequently during anaesthesia relative to those played less frequently, but showed no such patterns in additional control test. In the preference task they also displayed a partiality for the most frequently presented items. Presumably the preference task measured implicit memory, while the recognition task tested explicit memory. However, Block *et al.* argued that in this case even the results of the recognition task reflected implicit memory because patients viewed the recognition task as pure guesswork, i.e., they were not aware of having heard the items before. In addition, Block *et al.* suggested that the recognition judgements may have been mediated by information concerning frequency of presentation, which may be encoded automatically and independently of other types of memory (cf. Zacks, Harker and Sanft, 1982).

A similar argument can be made that the results of the Millar and Watkinson (1983) study mentioned above reflect the effects of implicit rather than explicit memory. They tested for recognition of a list of ten low-frequency words presented originally during anaesthesia induced by nitrous oxide and halothane. When recognition was tested by asking patients to select the presented words from a long list of presented and nonpresented words, no evidence of learning was observed. However, when subjects were asked to select (which may have meant 'guess' for subjects who had no explicit memory) the presented item from a pair of items, patients displayed some evidence of having been exposed to the items before.

Another common priming task is a category production test. In this task patients are given the name of a series of semantic categories and are asked to give exemplars of the category. For example, one category could be 'a type of fruit' to which one might respond, 'peach'. In this task it is important that the category exemplars which are provided during anaesthesia not be the most common examples of the category. While Block *et al.* (1991b) found no priming effect with this task, a number of investigators have found significant effects. Millar (1987) presented a list of words during anaesthesia which consisted of moderately common examples of a semantic category. During testing patients were asked to list exemplars from that category and five other categories each of which had been presented to other patients. Patients were significantly more likely to generate words that had been presented during anaesthesia early in their protocols than they were to generate target words from the control categories.

More recently, Jelicic, Bonke and Appleboom (1990) using nitrous oxide supplemented with fentanyl or sufentanil, and Roodra-Hrdlickova *et al.* (1990) using nitrous oxide and isoflurane also found a significant priming effect with this task. Given that the category task is therefore apparently sensitive to priming during anaesthesia, it is puzzling that Block *et al.* did not find a category priming effect when two other tasks in their study did produce significant effects. Possible explanations for the discrepancy may lie in the retention interval which was relatively short in the Jelicic *et al.* study (approximately 80 min) and the Roodra-Hrdlickova *et al.* study (approximately 200 min) compared to 24 h in the Block *et al.* study. In addition, Block *et al.* used categories for which it is more difficult to generate exemplars (e.g. types of male clothing) than the other studies which used relatively easy categories (e.g. colours).

Two other recent studies provide evidence that nondeclarative or implicit memories may be formed during anaesthesia. Before anaesthesia, Goldmann (1988) gave patients a questionnaire consisting of unusual questions such as 'What is the blood pressure of an octopus?' During anaesthesia patients heard the answers. Following recovery subjects did better at selecting the correct answers to questions for which they had been presented the answers during anaesthesia than for other questions. This occurred despite the fact that they did not recall having heard the answers before. In a more recent study, Kihlstrom *et al.* (1990) presented patients receiving isoflurane anaesthesia with a series of stimulus words and the corresponding most frequent response to those stimuli. When asked following surgery to give a response to each stimulus subjects performed better on the pairs which had been presented during surgery than on control pairs.

While there have been failures to detect priming effects following anaesthesia, (e.g. Standen, Hain and Hosker, 1987; Winograd *et al.*, 1990), other studies are consistent in suggesting that implicit memory functions may be partially preserved during anaesthesia. Other approaches to implicit memory are also suggestive of this conclusion.

(d)   Implicit memory for behavioural suggestions

Another method for testing implicit memory involves presenting a suggestion during anaesthesia that the subject engage in a specific behaviour after recovery. During anaesthesia with thiopentone, nitrous oxide, and enflurane or halothane, some patients were given suggestions to touch their ear during a post-anaesthesia interview (Bennett, Davis and Giannini, 1985). Ear-touching was more frequent in patients who were given these suggestions than in others who were not. While there have been a number of criticisms of this initial study (Ghoneim and Block, 1992) its importance lies in suggesting this research approach. In a similar study, Goldmann, Shaha and Helden (1987) also found an effect for behavioural suggestions, however, one should be concerned that the levels of anaesthesia in this study were quite light as explicit recall occurred in 23% of the patients.

Recently Block *et al.* (1991b) employed a design with an additional internal control condition. During surgery half the patients were told to touch their ear during the postsurgery interview and half were told to touch their nose. Therefore, one could determine the effect of the suggestion by determining the difference in ear and nose touching for each patient. They found that patients touched the suggested body part significantly longer than the nonsuggested body part. A similar but nonsignificant trend was observed when number of touches was the dependent variable. As in the Bennett *et al.* study, patients could not correctly guess which body part they had been asked to touch.

(e)   Implicit memory for therapeutic suggestions

The technique of presenting suggestions during anaesthesia has also been used with therapeutic suggestions rather than suggestions to engage in a specific, observable behaviour like ear-touching. Some favourable outcomes for therapeutic suggestions have been obtained providing possible further evidence of implicit memory effects. These studies are reviewed in a later section of this chapter dealing with the consequences of awareness and memory for events occurring during anaesthesia.

(f)   Implicit memory for conditioning

Another form of implicit or nondeclarative memory is represented by classical or Pavlovian conditioning. Animal studies have shown that conditioning can be established and/or elicited during general anaesthesia under favourable conditions (Pirch, Corbus and Ebenezer, 1985;

Weinberger, Gold and Sternberg, 1984). This suggests that conditioning methods might be used to study responsiveness and learning during anaesthesia in humans. Studies of this kind have not been reported, but we have demonstrated the feasibility of using a classical conditioning method to study responsiveness and learning during inhalation of a subanaesthetic (30%) concentration of nitrous oxide (Block *et al.*, 1987). The method used in that study could prove useful in studying the extent to which language is processed during anaesthesia.

8.5 CONSEQUENCES

There can be important consequences for both patients and physicians resulting from awareness or memory for events occurring during anaesthesia. Many of the possible consequences are undesirable. However, we shall discuss a few which may be beneficial.

8.5.1 Adverse physical and psychological effects

As the introduction to this chapter suggests, awareness or recall of events which happened during surgery could have profound psychological effects on the patient. Prior to surgery fear of not being adequately anaesthetized or asleep during the operation had been found to be a source of preoperative anxiety in patients, (McCleane and Cooper, 1990). Some patients whose fears are realized apparently can down-play the event and seem to suffer no long-term effects. For others a traumatic neurotic syndrome characterized by nightmares, irritability, anxiety, and occasionally, preoccupation with death has been reported. Depression and rage have also been frequently observed (Blacher, 1975, 1984; Brahams, 1989; Guerra, 1986). Such psychological responses can obviously have an adverse effect on adjustment and recovery following surgery. In extreme cases there are even claims of stress-induced myocardial infarction (Anonymous, 1986).

Several factors may account for these effects. Acute pain, of course, should be a major factor. Additionally the feeling of being unable to control oneself or to communicate during surgery that one is in distress, may create the impression that things have gone wrong. Patients who discuss the experience after surgery may find that they are not believed by friends, family, or their physicians, thereby increasing their distress and perhaps causing some to question their own sanity.

8.5.2 Beneficial effects

One of the most intriguing notions concerning memory for events during anaesthesia is its possible use to promote recovery and patient well-being following surgery. It is well established that mentally and emotionally preparing a patient before surgery will benefit recovery (Rogers and Reich, 1986). Particularly useful are suggestions which encourage the patient to behave appropriately during recovery. According to Barber (1984) the effect of hypnotic suggestions is more pronounced when subjects are relaxed and feel that they are in a special situation where unusual events might occur. Perhaps the administration of suggestions during anaesthesia contains some of the same desirable conditions as hypnosis which might make those suggestions more effective.

Interpretation of many of the existing studies on therapeutic suggestion is somewhat difficult because often details are missing concerning control procedures, or if reported, the studies lack adequate controls. Ideally subjects should be matched for sex, age, type of surgery, general health prior to surgery, and related complications like extent of malignancy or other disorders. Socioeconomic status of the patients may also be important, as lower socioeconomic status is related to a higher risk of infection (Duff, 1986). While therapeutic suggestions could be effective in uncontrolled studies, one cannot rule out alternative explanations for the observed effects.

While the literature is somewhat inconsistent, probably in part because of failures in control procedures, a number of positive outcomes have been reported. For example, Wolfe and Millett (1960) and Hutchings (1961) in uncontrolled studies claimed that there were significant therapeutic effects from the presentation of positive suggestions to patients under anaesthesia. Similarly, Pearson (1961) found that patients who received therapeutic suggestions during anaesthesia were released from the hospital an average of 2.4 days earlier than control subjects who listened to music or blank tape. However, type of surgery was not controlled, thereby making it difficult to know whether the results were really due to the suggestions. Bonke *et al.* (1986) reported a controlled study in which groups of patients undergoing cholecystectomy or choledochostomy were presented with therapeutic suggestions, noise, or operating room sounds. The groups did not differ in subjectively-rated well-being, pain, or nausea and vomiting after surgery, but they did differ in the length of their post-operative hospital stay. The latter difference appeared to result more from a longer stay for patients in the control group exposed to noise than from a shorter stay for patients exposed to therapeutic suggestions. If receiving noise during anaesthesia was harmful to recovery, the effect of beneficial suggestions may have been attenuated in this study as the experimental group heard the same noise on the tape interspersed with the therapeutic suggestions. Unfortunately, a more tightly controlled follow-up study did not replicate the earlier beneficial effects of suggestions (Boeke *et al.*, 1988). Nor could two other studies (Abramson, Greenfield and Heron, 1966; Woo,

Seltzer and Marr, 1987) although those were based on rather small sample sizes. Evans and Richardson (1988) obtained positive results in a study of 39 hysterectomy patients who were tested in a double blind and randomized design. Patients who heard therapeutic suggestions during anaesthesia had shorter postoperative stays (7.1 vs. 8.4 days), shorter periods of pyrexia (2.2 vs. 3.9 half days), and were rated by nurses as showing better recovery (16 vs. 6 rated as displaying better recovery than expected). In addition, on a 0–100 self-rating scale, subjects receiving positive suggestions gave lower ratings to a question concerning difficulty with their bowels (31.3 vs. 55.7). Pyrexia was affected despite the fact that it was not mentioned on the tape. On the other hand, there were no effects on perceived pain, nausea and vomiting, and urinary problems, even though these conditions were explicitly mentioned on the tape. There were also no differences between groups in anxiety or mood ratings.

Three recent studies provide some evidence that hearing positive suggestions during anaesthesia may reduce pain. Münch and Zug (1990) published a brief report which lacks many details. They tested patients receiving thyroidectomies. The group receiving positive suggestions rated their overall well-being on a visual analogue scale running from 0–10 as better than the non-suggestion group (3.4 vs. 4.5), however, there was no effect on more direct measures of pain or nausea. A small pilot study which also does not report a number of important postoperative details (Furlong, 1990) found that surgical patients who received positive suggestions during anaesthesia required less pain medication during recovery than the control group. Finally, McLintock et al. (1990) tested 63 patients who received abdominal hysterectomies. Patients controlled their own analgesia following surgery. Patients who received positive suggestions during surgery took on average less morphine (51.0 vs. 65.7 mg) than the control group which listened to a blank tape during surgery.

More recently Block *et al.* (1991a) studied 209 patients who had received surgery for a variety of reasons. As in the McLintock *et al.* (1990) study patients in the experimental group listened to positive suggestions during anaesthesia while the control group listened to a blank tape. A large assortment of techniques were used to assess postoperative recovery, but none indicated a meaningful improvement in recovery in the experimental group.

Why a number of discrepant results have been reported is uncertain. Because of differences in patient populations, type of surgery, and other details of patient care it is difficult directly to compare various studies. In addition, subtle differences between studies could be significant. For example, it may not only be important to deliver positive suggestions, but it may matter at what speed they are delivered, what terms are used in the suggestions and how often a suggestion is repeated. It might also matter that the voice delivering the suggestions sounds pleasing, relaxing, or sympathetic. Some researchers have proposed that the suggestions incorporate the patient's name to gain attention, and that the voice delivering the suggestions be one that the patient can recognize, such as the patient's physician. One should also consider what the control group will listen to. The results of Bonke *et al.* (1986) indicate noise might have a detrimental effect. On the other hand,, music could have a relaxing beneficial effect that might mask the effects of suggestions.

In conclusion, while a number of encouraging results have been reported there is certainly need for much more work. Unfortunately, this is not an easy area to control all the factors one should consider and also obtain a reasonable sample size. We suggest that as much as possible researchers attempt to match subjects on as many health and socio-economic variables as possible. We also encourage researchers to give a complete description of their subjects and procedures. Without clear reporting of experimental details, a study may add to the confusion rather than enhance an understanding of the phenomenon.

8.5.3   Potential legal consequences

Significant legal implications may be one of the unintended by-products of awareness and memory for events during anaesthesia. Even without a full understanding of the phenomenon, and a generally accepted medical approach to avoiding awareness under anaesthesia, claims have been made and suits filed by patients. Public interest in the United Kingdom was heightened by two highly publicized and successful lawsuits. These cases, which arose in 1985 and 1989, each involved plaintiffs who asserted that they were awake during a Caesarean section performed under general anaesthesia (Aitkenhead, 1990; Powers, 1987; Puxon, 1987). Similar claims followed. It was reported that the Medical Defence Union, which defends physicians in the United Kingdom, receives four to five cases involving consciousness and recall each year (Hargrove, 1987).

Perhaps because of the lack of similar publicity and therefore public knowledge, a reviewer during the same time period found only one reported lawsuit involving a claim for awareness in the United States (Thompson, 1987). There is no available count of claims which were made and settled before the filing of a lawsuit, or of lawsuits settled before trial. However, the Committee on Professional Liability of the American Society of Anesthesiologists has obtained information from insurance carriers on closed malpractice claims related to anaesthetic care which may provide useful information (Cheney *et al.*, 1989).

8.5.4 Recommendations concerning legal consequences

It is a matter of general agreement in the medical and legal communities that both good medical practice and a desire to avoid being a defendant is furthered by communication with the patient and by evidencing a caring attitude. Before surgery this means that the anaesthesiologist should explain the possibility of consciousness, particularly if the patient is at relatively high risk. If there is a valid reason not to discuss this matter with the patient, that should be documented in the chart, and the anaesthesiologist may instead consider discussing the matter with the patient's family (e.g. when a child is the patient). It may be argued by some that the incidence of awareness under anaesthesia is low enough that raising the issue will cause undue anxiety. Avoiding the subject, however, puts the anaesthesiologist at risk. He or she may later have to explain why the information was withheld in the face of the patient's claim of a right to know.

During surgery, if the anaesthesiologist suspects the patient might be conscious, obviously taking steps to induce unconsciousness is reasonable. At the same time speaking reassuringly to the patient and advising the surgical team of the situation may go far in avoiding a later claim.

Finally, steps can also be taken if a patient complains of surgical awareness during the postoperative visit. The anaesthesiologist can explore through questioning the accuracy of the patient's recall. This can be compared with actual surgical events to determine whether the awareness is real, or whether the patient is confusing reality with dreaming. Dreaming may occur at any time in the perioperative period and pain experienced postoperatively may be confused with pain during surgery.

When the patient's recall is consistent with actual operative events, acknowledging the account and demonstrating compassion and concern for the patient is perhaps the most effective tool to avoid creating the adversarial relationship which is a necessary precursor to litigation. The anaesthesiologist should explain to the patient that consciousness will occasionally and unavoidably occur because of the tradeoffs made in the use of anaesthesia. With the employment of muscle relaxants, the anaesthesiologist must strike a balance, seeking to avoid high and potentially toxic doses of the anaesthetic drugs, yet induce unconsciousness. The anaesthesiologist should also be prepared to refer the patient to a clinical psychologist or a psychiatrist with expertise in the area, should the patient's distress continue.

Defence counsel and insurers would contend that if avoidable error is responsible for consciousness, the anaesthesiologist who admits fault is at great risk. This risk must be weighed against the possibility of preventing a lawsuit by avoiding an adversarial relationship with the patient. Additionally, thought must be given to alleviating the patient's concern about future surgery.

Time spent with the patient at this stage is almost certainly well spent. In contrast to his or her treating physician, the patient is unlikely to have a personal relationship with the anaesthesiologist. This is perhaps the last chance to show the ocncern and care for the patient which may prevent litigation. The literature supports an assertion that claims might be avoided in some cases if the anaesthesiologist listens sympathetically and explains honestly what happened (Aitkenhead, 1990).

8.6   SUMMARY AND CONCLUSIONS

In this chapter we have reviewed five basic categories of research concerning awareness and memory for events during anaesthesia:

1) clinical studies which first indicated the presence and characteristics of the phenomenon and which suggest its incidence is low but not insignificant;
2) studies which have evaluated possible methods for detecting consciousness during the course of surgery;
3) a small group of controlled experiments which tested for explicit recall of selected stimuli presented during surgery and which provide essentially no evidence for explicit memory for events during anaesthesia;
4) a somewhat larger group of controlled experiments which suggest that implicit memories may be formed during anaesthesia and perhaps may influence behaviour and recovery following surgery; and
5) research which describes possible mental, physical, emotional, and legal consequences of the phenomenon.

In the typical surgical situation the consequences of awareness and memory for events during surgery are neutral at best, with most evidence suggesting they are undesirable. (Beneficial effects are uncertain and have only been reported when specific steps were taken during surgery to produce them, i.e. administration of therapeutic suggestions.) Therefore, physicians should be careful to take steps to reduce the risk of awareness and recall. While more specific recommendations can be found elsewhere (e.g., Aldrete and Wright, 1985; Ghoneim and Block, 1992; Hargrove, 1987; Lunn and Rosen, 1990), a number of steps should be apparent from the above discussion. For example, when possible, light levels of anaesthesia should be avoided so as to maintain unconsciousness. Alertness by operating room personnel and routine checking of equipment should reduce incidents due to accident or equipment malfunction. Reducing the use of muscle relaxants when feasible should increase the possibility of detecting physical signs of wakefulness. Of course, those in the field should attend to developments in the literature and employ more explicit methods of monitoring alertness as they become available.

Operating room personnel should be careful about comments made during surgery since some evidence suggests that negative remarks about the patient or his or her condition may be particularly likely to be recalled. Even in the absence of explicit recall of such comments, it seems reasonable that if therapeutic suggestions can benefit recovery, negative comments might also have an implicit memory effect and impede postoperative recovery. Therefore, especially when anaesthesia must be light, it may be worthwhile to provide the patient with earplugs, or earphones over which music is played. Finally, as suggested by discussion in the previous chapter, patients can be premedicated with benzodiazepines or anticholinergic drugs to enhance amnesia.

If despite all efforts awareness and recall still occurs, additional steps are necessary. The first should be to acknowledge to the patient that such events can happen and to provide an explanation. This may allay some fears and help restore the patient's trust. Care should also be taken to provide a sympathetic and supportive environment which encourages discussion of the patient's fears and other feelings. In cases where depression is prominent or other undesirable sequelae are apparent, referral to a mental health professional may be appropriate (Guerra, 1980).

Awareness and memory for events during anaesthesia are legitimate possibilities. While the frequency of reported incidents is low, the possible humanitarian and legal consequences of such events underlines the need for better understanding of the phenomenon. Development of a reliable measure of unconsciousness would greatly facilitate this research. With such a measure effective drug combinations and concentrations for maintaining unconsciousness can be determined. Additionally, recommendations concerning drug treatments might then be adjusted for individual factors, such as age, sex, weight, or other characteristics which are determined to be relevant. Finally, one would hope that the possibility that the phenomenon might be turned to the benefit of patient health and recovery will be explored further.

REFERENCES

Abramson, M., Greenfield, I. and Heron, W. T. (1966) Response to or perception of auditory stimuli under deep surgical anesthesia. *American Journal of Obstetrics and Gynecology,* **96**, 584–5.

Agarwal, G. and Sikh, S. S. (1977) Awareness during anaesthesia: A prospective study. *British Journal of Anaesthesia,* **49**, 835–8.

Aitkenhead, A. R. (1990) Awareness during anaesthesia: What should the patient be told? *Anaesthesia,* **45**, 351–2.

Aldrete, J. A. and Wright, A. J. (1985) Concerning the acceptibility of awareness during surgery (Correspondence). *Anesthesiology,* **63**, 460–1.

Anonymous (1986) The depth of anaesthesia (Editorial). *Lancet,* **II**, 553–4.

Barber, T. X. (1984) Changing 'unchangeable' bodily processes by (hypnotic) suggestions: A new look at hypnosis, cognitions, imagining, and the mind–body problem, in *Imagination and Healing,* (ed A. A. Sheikh), Baywood Publishing Company, Farmingdale, New York, pp. 89–105.

Barr, A. M., Moxon, A., Woollam, C. H. M. and Fryer, M. E. (1977) The effect of diazepam and lorazepam on awareness during anaesthesia for Caesarian section. *Anaesthesia,* **58**, 873–8.

Bennett, H. L. (1988) Perception and memory for events during adequate general anesthesia for surgical operations, in *Hypnosis and Memory,* (ed H. M. Pettinati), Guilford Press, New York, (pp. 193–231).

Bennett, H. L. and Boyle, W. A. (1986) Selective remembering: Anesthesia and memory (Letter). *Anesthesia and Analgesia,* **65**, 988–9.

Bennett, H. L. and Davis, H. S. (1984) Nonverbal response to intraoperative conversation (Abstract). *Anesthesia and Analgesia,* **63**, 185.

Bennett, H. L., Davis, H. S. and Giannini, J. A. (1985) Nonverbal response to intraoperative conversation. *British Journal of Anaesthesia,* **57**, 174–9.

Blacher, R. S. (1975) On awakening paralyzed during surgery: A syndrome of traumatic neurosis. *Journal of the American Medical Association,* **234**, 67–8.

Blacher, R. S. (1984) Awareness during surgery (Editorial). *Anesthesiology,* **61**, 1–2.

Block, R. I., Ghoneim, M. M., Fowles, D. C. *et al.* (1987) Effects of a subanesthetic concentration of nitrous oxide on establishment, elicitation, and semantic and phonemic generalization of classically conditioned skin conductance responses. *Pharmacology, Biochemistry and Behavior,* **28**, 7–14.

Block, R. I., Ghoneim, M. M., Sum Ping, S. T. and Ali, M. A. (1991a) Efficacy of therapeutic suggestions for improved postoperative recovery presented during general anesthesia. *Anesthesiology,* **75**, 746–55.

Block, R. I., Ghoneim, M. M., Sum Ping, S. T. and Ali, M. A. (1991b) Human learning during general anaesthesia and surgery. *British Journal of Anaesthesia,* **66**, 170–8.

Boeke, S., Bonke, B., Bouwhuis-Hoogerwerf, M. L. *et al.* (1988) Effects of sounds presented during general anaesthesia on postoperative course. *British Journal of Anaesthesia,* **60**, 697–702.

Bogetz, M. S. and Katz, J. A. (1984) Recall of surgery for major trauma. *Anesthesiology,* **61**, 6–9.

Bogod, D. G., Orton, J. K., Yau, H. M. and Oh, T. E. (1990) Detecting awareness during general anaesthetic Caesarean section: An evaluation of two methods. *Anaesthesia,* **45**, 279–84.

Bonke, B. and Rupreht, J. (1986) Response to intraoperative conversation (Letter). *British Journal of Anaesthesia,* **58**, 134.

Bonke, B., Schmitz, P. I. M., Verbage, F. and Zwaveling, A. (1986) Clinical study of so-called unconscious perception during general anaesthesia. *British Journal of Anaesthesia,* **58**, 957–64.

Brahams, D. (1989) Anesthesia and the law. Awareness and pain during anaesthesia. *Anaesthesia,* **44**, 352.

Breckenridge, J. L. and Aitkenhead, A. R. (1981) Isolated forearm technique for detection of wakefulness during general anaesthesia. *British Journal of Anaesthesia,* **53**, 665–6.

Breckenridge, J. L. and Aitkenhead, A. R. (1983) Awareness during general anaesthesia: A review. *Annals of the Royal College of Surgeons of England,* **65**, 93–6.

Brice, D. D., Hetherington, R. R. and Utting, J. E. (1970) A simple study of awareness and dreaming during anaesthesia. *British Journal of Anaesthesia*, **42**, 535–42.

Calverley, R. K. (1989) Anesthesia as a speciality: Past, present and future, in *Clinical Anesthesia*, (eds P. G. Barash, B. F. Gullen and R. K. Stoeling), Lippincott, Philadelphia, pp. 3–33.

Cheek, D. B. (1959) Unconscious perception of meaningful sounds during surgical anaesthesia as revealed under hypnosis. *American Journal of Clinical Hypnosis*, **1**, 101–13.

Cheney, F. W., Posner, K., Caplan, R. A. and Ward, R. J. (1989) Standard of care and anesthesia liability. *Journal of the American Medical Association*, **261**, 1599–603.

Chi, O. Z. and Field, C. (1986) Effects of isoflurane on visual evoked potentials in humans. *Anesthesiology*, **65**, 328–30.

Council on Scientific Affairs. (1985) Council report: Scientific status of refreshing recollection by the use of hypnosis. *Journal of the American Medical Association*, **253**, 1918–23.

Crawford, J. S. (1971) Awareness during operative obstetrics under general anaesthesia. *British Journal of Anaesthesia*, **43**, 179–82.

Crile, G. (1947) *George Crile: An Autobiography*. Lippincott, Philadelphia, p. 197.

Dubovsky, S. L. and Trustman, R. (1976) Absence of recall after general anesthesia: Implications for theory and practice. *Anesthesia and Analgesia*, **55**, 696–701.

Duff, P. (1986) Pathophysiology and management of postcesarean endomyometritis. *Obstetrics and Gynecology*, **67**, 269–76.

Edmonds, H. L., Jr., Stolzy, S. L. and Couture, L. J. (1987) Surface electromyography during low vigilance states, in *Consciousness, Awareness and Pain in General Anaesthesia*, (eds M. Rosen and J. N. Lunn), Butterworths, London, pp. 89–98.

Eger, E. I., II, Lampe, G. H., Wauk, L. Z. *et al.* (1990) Clinical pharmacology of nitrous oxide: An argument for its continued use. *Anesthesia and Analgesia*, **71**, 575–85.

Eich, E., Reeves, J. L. and Katz, R. L. (1985) Anesthesia, amnesia, and the memory/awareness distinction. *Anesthesia and Analgesia*, **64**, 1143–8.

Evans, C., and Richardson, P. H. (1988) Improved recovery and reduced postoperative stay after therapeutic suggestions during general anaesthesia. *Lancet*, **II**, 491–3.

Evans, J. M. and Davies, W. L. (1984) Monitoring anaesthesia. *Clinics in Anaesthesiology*, **2**, 243–62.

Evans, J. M., Davies, W. L. and Wise, C. C. (1984) Lower oesophageal contractility: A new monitor of anaesthesia. *Lancet*, **1**, 1151–4.

Furlong, M. (1990) Positive suggestions presented during anaesthesia, in *Memory and Awareness in Anaesthesia*, (eds B. Bonke, W. Fitch, K. Millar and M. A. Rockland), Swets and Zeitlinger, Amsterdam, pp. 170–5.

Ghoneim, M. M. and Block, R. I. (1992) Learning and consciousness during general anaesthesia. *Anaesthesiology*, **76**, 279–305.

Goldmann, L. (1988) Information-processing under general anaesthesia: A review. *Journal of the Royal Society of Medicine*, **81**, 224–7.

Goldmann, L. (1990) Factors determining the probability of recollections of intraoperative events, in *Memory and Awareness in Anaesthesia*, (eds B. Bonke, W. Fitch, K. Millar, and M. A. Rockland), Swets and Zeitlinger, Amsterdam, pp. 45–9.

Goldmann, L. and Levey, A. B. (1986) Orienting responses under general anaesthesia. *Anaesthesia*, **41**, 1056–7.

Goldmann, L., Shah, M. V. and Helden, M. W. (1987) Memory of cardiac anaesthesia: Psychological sequelae in cardiac patients of intraoperative suggestion and operating room conversation. *Anaesthesia,* **42**, 596–603.

Graf, P. and Schacter, D. L. (1985) Implicit and explicit memory for new associations in normal and amnesic patients. *Journal of Experimental Psychology: Learning, Memory, and Cognition,* **11**, 501–18.

Griffith, H. R., and Johnson, G. E. (1942) Use of curare in general anesthesia. *Anesthesiology,* **3**, 418–20.

Guerra, F. (1980) Awareness during anesthesia (Letter). *Canadian Anaesthetists' Society Journal,* **27**, 178.

Guerra, F. (1986) Awareness and recall, in *International Anesthesiology Clinics, Volume 24, Neurological and Psychological Complications of Surgery and Anesthesia,* (ed. B. T. Hindman), Little Brown, Boston, pp. 75–99.

Hargrove, R. L. (1987) Awareness: A medicolegal problem, in *Consciousness, Awareness and Pain in General Anaesthesia,* (eds M. Rosen, and J. N. Lunn), Butterworths, London, pp. 149–54.

Herregods, L. and Rolly, G. (1987) The EMG, the EEG zero crossing frequency and mean integrated voltage analysis during sleep and anaesthesia, in *Consciousness, Awareness and Pain in General Anaesthesia,* (eds M. Rosen, and J. N. Lunn), Butterworths, London, pp. 82–8.

Houston, H. G., McClelland, R. J. and Fenwick, P. B. C. (1988) Effects of nitrous oxide on auditory cortical evoked potentials and subjective thresholds. *British Journal of Anaesthesia,* **61**, 606–10.

Howard, J. F. (1987) Incidents of auditory perception during general anaesthesia with traumatic sequelae. *Medical Journal of Australia,* **146**, 44–6.

Hutchings, D. D. (1961) The value of suggestion given under anesthesia: A report and evaluation of 200 consecutive cases. *American Journal of Clinical Hypnosis,* **4**, 26–9.

Hutchinson, R. (1960) Awareness during surgery: A study of its incidence. *British Journal of Anaesthesia,* **33**, 463–9.

Jänig, W. and Räth, B. (1980) Effects of anaesthetics on reflexes elicited in the sudomotor system by stimulation of pacinian corpuscles and of cutaneous nociceptors. *Journal of the Autonomic Nervous System,* **2**, 1–14.

Jelicic, M., Bonke, B., and Appleboom, D. K. (1990) Indirect memory for words presented during anaesthesia (letter). *Lancet,* **II**, 249.

Jessop, J. and Jones, J. G. (1991) Conscious awareness during general anaesthesia – What are we attempting to monitor (Editorial). *British Journal of Anaesthesia,* **66**, 635–7.

Jessop, J., Griffiths, D. E. and Sapsford, D. J. *et al.* (1991) Changes in amplitude and latency of an event-related potential with depression of consciousness by nitrous oxide (abstract). *British Journal of Anaesthesia,* **66**, 400.

Jones, J. G. (1990) Use of the auditory evoked response to evaluate depth of anaesthesia, in *Memory and Awareness in Anaesthesia,* (eds B. Bonke, W. Fitch, K. Millar and M. A. Rockland), Swets and Zeitlinger, Amsterdam, pp. 303–15.

Kim, C. L. (1978) Awareness during cardiopulmonary bypass. *AANA Journal,* **46**, 373–83.

Kihlstrom, J. F., Schacter, D. L., Cork, R. C. *et al.* (1990) Implicit and explicit memory following surgical anesthesia. *Psychological Science,* **1**, 303–6.

Lemmens, H. J. M., Bovill, J. G., Hennis, P. J. *et al.* (1989) Alcohol consumption alters the pharmacodynamics of alfentanil. *Anesthesiology,* **71**, 669–74.

Levinson, B. W. (1965) States of awareness during general anaesthesia: Preliminary communications. *British Journal of Anaesthesia,* **37**, 544–6.

Lewis, S. A., Jenkinson, J. and Wilson, J. (1973) An EEG investigation of awareness during anaesthesia. *British Journal of Psychology*, **64**, 413–15.

Liu, W. H. D., Thorp, T. A. S., Graham, S. G. and Aitkenhead, A. R. (1991) Incidence of awareness with recall during general anaesthesia. *Anaesthesia*, **46**, 435–7.

Loftus, E. F., Schooler, J. W., Loftus, G. R. and Glauber, D. T. (1985) Memory for events occurring under anesthesia. *Acta Psychologica*, **59**, 123–8.

Lunn, J. N. and Rosen, M. (1990) Anaesthetic awareness (Correspondence). *British Medical Journal*, **300**, 938.

Lyons, G. and Macdonald, R. (1991) Awareness during Caesearean section. *Anaesthesia*, **45**, 62–4.

Mark, J. B. and Greenberg, L. M. (1983) Intraoperative awareness and hypertensive crisis during high-dose fentanyl-diazepam-oxygen anesthesia. *Anesthesia and Analgesia*, **62**, 698–700.

McCleane, G. J. and Cooper, R. (1990) The nature of pre-operative anxiety. *Anaesthesia*, **45**, 153–5.

McIntyre, J. W. R. (1966) Awareness during general anesthesia: Preliminary observations. *Canadian Anaesthetists' Society Journal*, **13**, 495–9.

McLintock, T. T. C., Aitken, H., Downie, C. F. A. and Kenny, G. N. C. (1990) Post-operative analgesic requirements in patients exposed to positive intraoperative suggestions. *British Medical Journal*, **301**, 788–90.

Millar, K. (1987) Assessment of memory for anaesthesia, in *Aspects of Recovery from Anaesthesia*, (eds I. Hindmarch, J. G. Jones, and E. Moss), John Wiley, New York, pp 76–91.

Millar, K. and Watkinson, N. (1983) Recognition of words presented during general anaesthesia. *Ergonomics*, **26**, 585–94.

Moore, J. K. and Seymour, A. H. (1987) Awareness during bronchoscopy. *Annals of the Royal College of Surgeons of England*, **69**, 45–7.

Münch, F. and Zug, H. D. (1990) Do intraoperative suggestions prevent nausea and vomiting in thyroidectomy patients? An experimental study, in *Memory and Awareness in Anaesthesia*, (eds B. Bonke, W. Fitch, K. Millar and M. A. Rockland), Swets and Zeitlinger, Amsterdam, pp. 185–8.

Pearson, R. E. (1961) Response to suggestions given under general anaesthesia. *American Journal of Clinical Hypnosis*, **4**, 106–14.

Peirson, A. L. (1846) Surgical operation with the aid of the 'new gas.' *Boston Medical and Surgical Journal*, **35**, 362–4.

Peterson, D. O., Drummond, J. C. and Todd, M. M. (1986) Effects of halothane, enflurane, isoflurane and nitrous oxide on somatosensory evoked potentials in humans. *Anesthesiology*, **65**, 35–40.

Pirch, J. H., Corbus, M. J. and Ebenezer, I. (1985) Conditioned cortical slow potential responses in urethane anesthesized rats. *International Journal of Neuroscience*, **25**, 207–18.

Plourde, G. (1991) Depth of anaesthesia (Editorial). *Canadian Journal of Anaesthesia*, **38**, 270–4.

Plourde, G. and Picton, T. W. (1990) Human auditory steady-state response during general anesthesia. *Anesthesia and Analgesia*, **71**, 460–8.

Plourde, G. and Picton, T. W. (1991) Long-latency auditory evoked potentials during general anaesthesia: N1 and P3 components. *Anesthesia and Analgesia*, **72**, 342–50.

Powers, M. J. (1987) A lawyer's view of the problem, in *Consciousness, Awareness and Pain in General Anaesthesia*. (eds M. Rosen, and J. N. Lunn), Butterworths, London, pp. 155–64.

Puxon, M. (1987) Awareness under anaesthesia: A QC's view, in *Consciousness,*

Awareness and Pain in General Anaesthesia, (eds M. Rosen, and J. N. Lunn), Butterworths, London, pp. 155–60.

Rogers, M. and Reich, P. (1986) Psychological intervention with surgical patients: Evaluation outcome, in *Psychological Aspects of Surgery*, (ed: F. G. Guggenheim), Karger, Basel, pp. 23–50.

Roodra-Hrdlickova, V., Wolters, G., Bonke, B. and Phaf, R. H. (1990) Unconscious perception during general anesthesia, demonstrated by an implicit memory task, in *Memory and Awareness in Anesthesia*, (eds B. Bonke, W. Fitch, K. Millar, and M. A. Rockland), Swets and Zeitlinger, Amsterdam, pp. 150–5.

Russell, I. F. (1986) Comparison of wakefulness with two anesthetic regimens. *British Journal of Anaesthesia*, **58**, 965–8.

Russell, I. F. (1989) Conscious awareness during general anaesthesia, in *Depth of Anaesthesia*, (ed. J. G. Jones), Bailliere Tindall, London, pp. 511–32.

Scott, D. L. (1972) Awareness during general anaesthesia. *Canadian Anaesthetists' Society Journal*, **19**, 173–83.

Sebel, P. S., Heneghan, C. P. and Ingram, D. A. (1985) Evoked responses: A neurophysiological indicator of depth of anaesthesia? (Editorial), *British Journal of Anaesthesia*, **57**, 840–2.

Sebel, P. S., Ingram, D. A., Flynn, P. H. *et al.* (1986) Evoked potentials during isoflurane anaesthesia. *British Journal of Anaesthesia*, **58**, 580–5.

Sia, R. L. (1969) Consciousness during general anaesthesia. *Anesthesia and Analgesia*, **48**, 363–6.

Standen, P. J., Hain, W. R. and Hosker, K. J. (1987) Retention of auditory information presented during anaesthesia: A study of children who received light general anaesthesia. *Anaesthesia*, **42**, 604–8.

Stanski, D. R. (1990) Monitoring depth of anesthesia, in *Anesthesia*, (3rd edition), (ed R. D. Miller) Churchill Livingstone, New York, pp. 1001–29.

Swerdlow, B. N., Holley, F. O., Maitre, P. O. and Stanski, D. R. (1990) Chronic alcohol intake does not change thiopental anesthetic requirement, pharmacokinetics, or pharmacodynamics. *Anesthesiology*, **72**, 455–61.

Tammisto, T. and Tigerstedt, I. (1977) The need for halothane supplementation of $N_2O–O_2$ relaxant anesthesia in chronic alcoholics. *Acta Anaesthesiologica Scandinavica*, **21**, 17–23.

Terrell, R. K., Sweet, W. O., Gladfelter, J. H. and Stephen, C. R. (1969) Evidence of partial recall during general anesthesia (Abstract). *Anesthesia and Analgesia*, **48**, 86–90.

Thompson, B. H. (1987) An American legal view, in *Consciousness, Awareness and Pain in General Anaesthesia*, (eds M. Rosen and J. N. Lunn), Butterworths, London, pp. 161–4.

Thornton, C., Catley, D. M., Jordan, C. *et al.* (1983) Enflurane anaesthesia causes graded changes in the brainstem and early cortical auditory evoked response in man. *British Journal of Anaesthesia*, **58**, 422–7.

Thornton, C., Heneghan, C. P. H., Navaratnarajah, M. and Jones, J. G. (1986) Selective effect of althesin on the auditory evoked response in man. *British Journal of Anaesthesia*, **58**, 422–7.

Trustman, R., Dubovsky, S. and Titley, R. (1977) Auditory perception during general anesthesia: Myth or fact? *International Journal of Clinical and Experimental Hypnosis*, **25**, 88–105.

Tunstall, M. E. (1977) Detecting wakefulness during general anaesthesia for Caesarean section. *British Medical Journal*, **1**, 1321.

Tunstall, M. E. (1979) The reduction of amnesic wakefulness during Caesarean section. *Anaesthesia*, **34**, 316–19.

Utting, J. E. (1975) Philip Gett memorial lecture: Awareness in anaesthesia. *Anesthesia and Intensive Care,* **3**, 334–40.

Utting, J. E. (1982) Awareness during surgical operations, in *Recent Advances in Anaesthesia and Analgesia,* (eds R. S. Atkinson and C. L. Hewer), Churchill Livingstone, New York, pp. 106–19.

Utting, J. E. (1987) Awareness: Clinical aspects, in *Consciousness, Awareness and Pain in General Anaesthesia,* (eds M. Rosen and J. N. Lunn), Butterworths, London, pp. 171–9.

Wang, M., Russell, I. F., Charlton, P. F. C. and Conlon, J. (1992) An experimental simulation of anaesthetic awareness and validation of the isolated forearm technique. Paper presented at the Second International Symposium on Memory and Awareness in Anaesthesia, Atlanta.

Weinberger, N. M., Gold, P. E. and Sternberg, D. B. (1984) Epineprine enables Pavlovian fear conditioning under anesthesia. *Science,* **223**, 605–7.

Wilson, J., Lewis, S. A. and Jenkinson, J. L. (1970) Electroencephalographic investigation of awareness during anaesthesia. *British Journal of Anaesthesia,* **42**, 804–5.

Wilson, S. L., Vaughan, R. W. and Stephen, C. R. (1975) Awareness, dreams, and hallucinations associated with general anesthesia. *Anesthesia and Analgesia,* **54**, 609–17.

Winograd, W., Sebel, P. S., Goldman, W. P. and Clifton, C. L. (1990) Indirect assessment of memory for music under anaesthesia, in *Memory and Awareness in Anaesthesia,* (eds B. Bonke, W. Fitch, K. Millar, and M. A. Rockland), Swets and Zeitlinger, Amsterdam, pp. 181–4.

Wolfe, L. S. and Millett, J. B. (1960) Control of post-operative pain by suggestion under general anesthesia. *American Journal of Clinical Hypnosis,* **3**, 109–12.

Woo, R., Seltzer, J. L. and Marr, A. (1987) The lack of response to suggestion under controlled surgical anesthesia. *Acta Anaesthesiologica Scandinavica,* **31**, 567–71.

Zacks, R. T., Hasher, L. and Sanft, H. (1982) Automatic encoding of event frequency: Further findings. *Journal of Experimental Psychology: Learning, Memory, and Cognition,* **8**, 106–16.

CHAPTER 9

The management of intractable low back pain

Michael O'Connor and Anne K. Goddard

9.1 EPIDEMIOLOGY AND REFERRAL PATTERNS

. . . and there shall be no more death, neither sorrow, nor crying, neither shall there be any more pain.

The revelation of St John the Divine

Back pain is an important cause of medical, psychological, social and economic problems. In the United Kingdom in any 14 day period 21% of adults experience low back pain (Dunnell and Cartwright, 1972), while over 60% of people can expect to have low back pain at some time in their lives (Walsh *et al.*, 1989). In any year 375 000 people, a proportion approaching 1% of the population, have a period of certified sickness incapacity because of back pain (Working Group on Back Pain, 1979). Although the incidence of low back pain across the country is probably uniform, sufferers in the North are three times more likely to consult their general practitioner than those in the South (Walsh, Cruddas and Coggon, 1992a) for reasons that are not yet explained. In general a one in five rule can be applied to sufferers' contact with doctors (Papageorgiou and Rigby, 1991). At any time one in five of the population have back pain; of these one in five consult their general practitioner and one in five are referred to a specialist. One in five of those seen in the out patient department are admitted to hospital and one in five will have an operation.

Most episodes of back pain are brief and self limiting irrespective of medical intervention; however, a few people will go on to develop chronic (i.e. long lasting) back pain. It is likely that most people with chronic back pain do not have severe symptoms and may simply describe their pain as 'a bad back' or 'backache'. A few will have low back disability with time lost from work, sickness certification, and effects on psychological, social and family life. It has been suggested that although back pain is a common problem in all societies low back disability is a relatively recent phenomenon associated with modern Western medicine (Waddell, 1987). Only a very few sufferers will be referred to a pain clinic (O'Connor and Glynn, 1991), usually by their general practitioner or an orthopaedic surgeon. This chapter is primarily concerned with the small number of patients with low back disability who are seen in pain clinics.

9.2 STRUCTURE AND FUNCTION OF THE SPINE

Today we have naming of parts.

Lessons of the War – Henry Reed

The spine serves a number of functions that put conflicting demands upon it. It has to provide support for the trunk and protect the delicate spinal cord, and yet it must also allow movement. The spine consists of a jointed column of seven cervical, twelve thoracic, five lumbar and five fused sacral vertebrae; this arrangement provides mechanical strength and protection but still permits movement. The sacral bones are fused and the thoracic spine is fairly rigid, so that most movement occurs in the cervical and lumbar areas. Each individual vertebra is essentially a solid bony cylinder, called the body, connected to a bony ring which forms the spinal canal (Figure 9.1). An intervertebral disc lies between adjacent vertebral bodies, and two facet joints connect adjacent rings of the spinal canal (Figure 9.2). Unlike the arrangement of vertebral bodies and intervertebral discs the facet joints are 'typical' joints like the hip and knee, and have a joint capsule lined by a synovial membrane.

The spinal canal contains the spinal cord and nerve roots. The spinal cord ends at the level of the second lumbar vertebra; below this the canal contains only the spinal nerve roots (Figure 9.3). Surrounding the cord and nerve roots are the three covering layers of meninges called, from inside to out, the pia, the arachnoid and the dura. Between the dura and the bony and ligamentous borders of the spinal canal is the epidural space.

9.3 OVERVIEW OF CAUSES OF BACK PAIN

Felix qui potuit rerum cognoscere causas.
(Happy is he who has been able to learn the causes of things.)

Georgics I – Virgil

There is a widespread belief that the human predisposition to back pain is due to an unfortunate decision by our ancestors a few million years

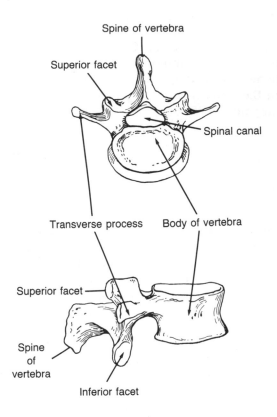

Spine of vertebra

Superior facet

Spinal canal

Transverse process   Body of vertebra

Superior facet

Spine
of
vertebra

Inferior facet

Fig. 9.1 Superior and lateral views of a typical lumbar vertebra.

ago to adopt an upright posture. The evidence for this is scanty and indeed dinosaur skeletons show evidence of back problems (Blumberg and Sokoloff, 1961; Dixon, 1980) while some of our domestic pets have much worse spinal problems than we humans (Dixon, 1980). Nonetheless, one effect of the upright posture is that back pain is commonest in the lower lumbar area (low back pain), probably because this area is subject to the greatest mechanical stresses; it takes the weight of the trunk but is also an area where much of the spinal movement occurs. Many patients with low back pain also complain of pain which goes down into the leg.

9.3.1 Causes of leg pain

Who like a foul and ugly witch doth limp
So tediously away.

Henry V – William Shakespeare

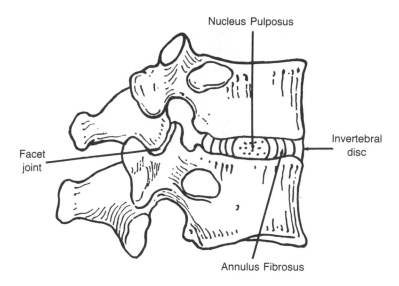

Fig. 9.2 Connections between adjacent vertebrae.

There are two quite distinct causes of leg pain. Pain emanating from any structure in the back can be experienced in the leg due to the way the spinal cord and brain process information. This is called **referred** pain; it seldom goes below the knee and is commonly described as dull or aching. Unfortunately, there is no clear-cut relationship between the distribution of the pain in the leg and the site of the problem in the back. The second type of leg pain is caused by compression and inflammation of a nerve root in the spinal canal. This is called **radicular** pain (Latin radicula = root) and radiates down the leg in the distribution of a branch of the major sensory nerve of the leg, the sciatic nerve (hence sciatica). It goes down the back of the leg beyond the knee and into the foot and is associated with feelings of numbness or tingling.

Radicular pain that persists for more than a few weeks may indicate a need for operative treatment to free the compressed nerve; however, even in orthopaedic clinics referred pain is twice as common as radicular pain (Waddell, 1980) and in pain clinics it is quite rare to see radicular pain.

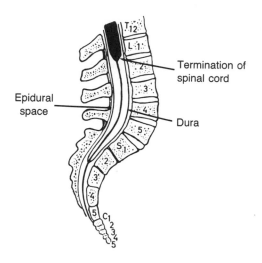

Fig. 9.3   Contents of the spinal canal in the lumbar region.

9.3.2   A classification of back pain

Although he is slightly odd I think his pain is genuine.

Pain Clinic referral letter

Before attempting to classify back pain it is worth discussing a few frequently used and misused terms. **Arthritis** (Greek arthron = joint) means inflammation of joints; the two most common forms are osteoarthritis and rheumatoid arthritis. **Osteoarthritis** is a common disorder of ageing synovial joints such as the hip and knee; it can be thought of as 'wear and tear arthritis' although this is rather an over-simplification. Because it is a disease of synovial joints it does not occur between the bodies of the vertebrae or in the discs, but it can occur in the facet joints. **Rheumatoid arthritis** is a relatively common disease caused by a malfunction of the immune system which produces chronic joint inflammation. Although back pain is not a major feature of rheumatoid arthritis, some back pain sufferers have a mental picture of the crippling deformity and disability occasionally seen in this disease if they are told they have 'arthritis'.

Most textbooks give long lists of causes of back pain. Sadly their half-remembered features are of frustratingly little use when confronted with a patient rather than an end of term examination. Nonetheless some form of classification does seem to be necessary to structure

Table 9.1 Waddell's classification of back pain

		Examples
Mechanical		
	Disc	
	Facet joint	
	Instability	
Spinal pathology		
	Tumour	
	Infections	
	Inflammatory	Ankylosing spondylitis, Polyarthritis, Paget's disease, Primary neurological disease
Nerve root pain		
	Prolapsed intervertebral disc	
	Spinal stenosis	

one's ideas; that suggested by Waddell (1982) (Table 9.1) is appealingly practical. The conditions discussed here are based on this classification.

(a)   Mechanical back pain

This is predominantly a problem of the middle years of life, and is thought to arise from a predisposition to back pain coupled with external factors. Some of the factors involved are: smoking (Frymoyer *et al.*, 1980; Battié *et al.*, 1989), height (in men) (Walsh, Cruddas and Coggon, 1991), occupational driving (Walsh *et al.*, 1989), regular heavy lifting (Walsh *et al.*, 1989), and admission to hospital following a traffic accident or fall (Walsh, Cruddas and Coggon, 1992b). The possible sources of pain lie in the connections between adjacent vertebrae and in the soft tissues.

The intervertebral disc is a complex structure with a rich nerve supply and may be a source of pain. The centre is a viscous gel called the nucleus pulposus which is surrounded by a tough ring of collagen called the annulus fibrosus. The concept of a soft deformable centre surrounded by a tough outer casing is that used in the car tyre; such a structure provides exactly the properties of mechanical strength and mobility required by the spine. With age, discs degenerate and shrink producing X-ray appearances of loss of disc space and bony overgrowth, a condition known as spondylosis (Greek spondulos = vertebra). Although this is a common finding on spinal X-rays its relationship to chronic back pain is obscure, particularly since the X-ray changes of spondylosis become more common with advancing years whereas mechanical back pain is predominantly a problem of middle age.

The facet joints can have new stresses imposed on them as the intervertebral discs degenerate and lose height; abnormal movements can occur leading to osteoarthritis. Facet joint pain is said to radiate typically to the front of the thighs or the buttocks and to be provoked by extension of the back from the flexed position.

Spondylolisthesis (Greek lusis = loosening) is the slippage forward of one vertebra on another. It is common and usually asymptomatic. When it does cause problems it tends to present in adolescence with symptoms of nerve root entrapment (Meyerding, 1941; Scoville and Corkill, 1974). If it is found on an X-ray of an adult with mechanical low back pain there is a natural tendency to assume that the pain and X-ray appearances are connected. It is important to remember however that both pain and spondylolisthesis are common and can occur independently in the same patient.

Soft tissue pain can arise from most of the structures in the back, and indeed ligamentous strain is probably the cause of the common 'bad back' which occurs after unusual exercise and subsides over a few days. **Fibromyalgia**, formerly known as fibrositis, is a syndrome of generalized musculo-skeletal aching, stiffness, fatigue, poor sleep, and tenderness at trigger points. It is associated with headache, irritable bowel syndrome, a subjective sense of swelling in articular and periarticular areas, paraesthesiae and anxiety. Most sufferers are women aged between 20 and 55. The mechanisms are not understood but it shares features of other functional disorders such as irritable bowel syndrome and tension headache (Yunnus, 1989).

(b) Spinal pathology

Waddell uses this term to include tumours, infections and miscellaneous 'inflammatory' conditions. It is not intended to imply that no identifiable disease process is present in other sorts of back pain. Suspicion of spinal pathology should be higher in the young, the elderly, and those with pain in the upper back.

Tumours can involve the lumbar spine and cause pain. The history is usually short and they present as acute, not chronic, back pain.

Ankylosing spondylitis (Greek agkulosis = crooked) is characterized by inflammation where ligaments join bones. It used to be thought to be a rare disease almost exclusively confined to men (West, 1949) but more recent studies suggest that most sufferers are undiagnosed and there is a prevalence of about 1% of the general population with an equal male to female ratio (Calin and Fries, 1975), although women tend to have a milder disease with less spinal involvement. The condition usually has an insidious onset and presents as chronic low back pain associated with stiffness which is at its worst in the morning and tends to improve with exercise (Calin *et al.*, 1977). Interestingly 98% of sufferers have the HLA-B27 blood type as compared with only 8% of the general population. Diagnosis is by the typical clinical picture and characteristic changes on the X-ray of the sacro-iliac joints between sacrum and pelvis. The vertebrae eventually fuse and the pain diminishes.

(c)   Nerve root pain

Prolapsed intervertebral disc (pid) or 'slipped disc' is a diagnosis that has taken a peculiarly firm hold on the public and medical imaginations when one considers its fairly recent description (Mixter and Barr, 1934) and its relative rarity as a cause of back pain. Contrary to popular belief the disc does not actually 'slip', nor can it be manipulated back into place. What actually happens is that as the disc degenerates with age cracks appear in the annulus fibrosus. Sudden stress can then lead to herniation of part of the nucleus pulposus through the weakest part of the annulus into the side of the spinal canal; this causes nerve root compression and sciatica. Most cases improve spontaneously over a few weeks. Those that do not are further investigated using myelography (injection of radio opaque dye around the spinal cord) or high resolution imaging techniques such as computed tomography (CT scan) or magnetic resonance imaging (MRI); if a prolapsed disc is demonstrated a decompression operation is performed. It is, however, becoming clear from improved radiological techniques that not all cases of acute sciatica are due to pid, nor do all episodes of pid cause sciatica (Jinkins, Whittemore and Bradley, 1989).

Spinal stenosis (Greek stenosis = narrowing): **Central canal stenosis** is caused by a spinal canal which is either congenitally narrow or which has become narrow following degenerative change, spondylolisthesis, or interventions such as trauma or operation (Nelson, 1973). Patients complain of radicular pain, sensory and motor symptoms; these come on after walking a certain distance and are relieved by stopping or by manoeuvres which increase the volume of the canal such as flexing the spine. Treatment is by operative decompression. **Lateral canal stenosis** occurs when lumbar spondylosis and bony overgrowth compress single nerves as they leave the spinal canal giving rise to radicular pain. Treatment is by operative decompression. In contrast to pid the nerve may not recover function after decompression and patients can have persistent radicular pain.

Chronic spinal arachnoiditis is a relatively rare condition in which there is scar tissue within and between the meninges affecting the spinal nerve roots. Most cases seen in the United Kingdom have lumbar arachnoiditis following myelography and/or surgery. Patients present with low back pain or leg pain aggravated by movement and may have neurological signs involving several nerve roots. Diagnosis is based on myelographic appearances (Shaw, Russell and Grossart, 1978) although there is a poor correlation between myelography, clinical signs and operative findings. There is no specific treatment.

9.3.3 Problems of classifications

When *I* use a word, Humpty Dumpty said, in rather a scornful tone, it means just what I choose it to mean – neither more nor less.

Alice Through the Looking Glass – Lewis Carroll

In our present state of knowledge no classification can hope to be comprehensive or universally accepted; however, the problem is even greater than it might first seem. There is no agreement as to how frequently a precise anatomical diagnosis can be made, nor how important it is to do so (O'Brien, 1984; Kirwan, 1989). Conventional doctors, such as general practitioners, orthopaedic surgeons, orthopaedic physicians, neurosurgeons and pain clinic doctors, often have differing views on the causes of back pain. Even when they do agree, the terminology used for the same condition can vary between specialties and also between countries; Macnab (1977) lists ten different synonyms for prolapsed intervertebral disc (without in fact including the precise term 'prolapsed intervertebral disc'). Furthermore, different sorts of back pain are seen by different specialists, for example patients with ankylosing spondylitis are more likely to be seen in a rheumatology clinic than an orthopaedic or pain clinic (Jajić, 1979; Grahame *et al.*, 1974; Sandström, Andersson and Rydberg, 1984; O'Connor and Glynn, 1991). Many chronic pain sufferers also see alternative or complementary therapists such as osteopaths, chiropractors, acupuncturists or faith healers, some of whom would have no sympathy at all with anatomically based classifications. Their terminology and explanations reflect their different outlooks.

Perhaps the most serious problem with the classification used above is that it is based on the medical model, which presupposes that illness is due to an identifiable underlying disorder and that symptoms, signs and disability are directly related and proportionate to that underlying disorder. The case for a biopsychosocial model incorporating distress, illness behaviour and social interaction has subsequently been cogently argued by the same author (Waddell, 1987) and in our view is a more accurate reflection of the reality of the situation. Like the classification based on the medical model this has been bedevilled by a lack of agreed terminology; although a comprehensive taxonomy has recently been proposed (Harper *et al.*, 1992), it is probably too complex for routine use by harassed doctors. This is less of a criticism of the taxonomy and more of a demonstration that **full** assessment needs to be multidisciplinary.

9.3.4 Chronic back pain

I've got this terrible pain in all the diodes down my left hand
side. . . . I've asked for them to be replaced but no one ever listens.
Marvin the Android in The Hitch Hikers Guide to the Galaxy
Douglas Adams

A review of the literature by Humphrey (1980) suggests that pain persisting for more than six months, in the absence of a remediable cause,
is usually regarded as chronic. The reasons why chronicity becomes
established in some sufferers and not others are still poorly understood.
Financial or psychosocial factors such as outstanding compensation
claims, or secondary gains for the patient and his family may contribute
in some cases. The availability of support from family members and the
form this support takes may also be important; an over-solicitous spouse
may reinforce and ensure the continuance of overt pain behaviour
(Block, Kremer and Gaylor, 1980). We have also observed in our own
clinic the disruptive effects of chronic back pain on some marital
relationships. Lack of understanding and support from spouses are
frequently identified as causes of tension, and may lead to exaggerated
pain behaviour in order to establish the authenticity of the pain.

9.4 PAIN CLINIC ASSESSMENT

I learned of the vital necessity to know as much about the patient
who has the backache as about the backache the patient has.
I Macnab

In our clinic, as in most others in the UK, the initial assessment is by a
doctor only. Psychologists, physiotherapists and occupational therapists
are involved only when a patient is individually referred or has reached
the stage of entering the pain management programme (see below and
Chapter 2). This approach reflects the manner in which pain clinics
have evolved in this country and also arises from the necessity to
husband scarce resources. In a few clinics a psychologist is present at
the patient's initial assessment and management is thereafter integrated
between the physical and psychological. We believe that this approach
has a lot to commend it; early involvement of a psychologist and advice
on managing the consequences of back pain is then seen as a routine
part of treatment. Referral after medical treatment has failed can make
the patient feel that the doctor does not believe in the reality of the
pain and has lost interest.

Medical assessment follows the usual format of history and examination. It has specific aims: to identify patients who have a surgically
remediable condition, to identify patients with inappropriate symptoms

and signs, and to formulate a treatment plan. The vast majority of patients will have some form of mechanical back pain which in our experience seldom has an identifiable anatomical source. Unlike obtaining the usual medical history which is purely an information gathering exercise, the taking of a pain history is also the start of treatment.

9.4.1 History

Pain is an unpleasant sensory and emotional experience associated with actual or potential tissue damage or described in terms of such damage.

International Association for the Study of Pain (IASP)

Although the IASP definition of pain is comprehensive and emphasizes the subjective nature of pain it is of necessity long. We find a more useful *aide-mémoire* is the definition of McCaffrey (1983), 'Pain is what the patient says it is'. Both patient and doctor will find that application of this definition makes life much easier.

Many patients feel that no doctor has ever had the time to listen and understand their problem properly; they usually have long, complicated histories and it is important not to rush the first consultation. We allot about an hour for the first meeting which is far more than general practitioners or surgeons are usually able to give. We start with an open question such as, 'Tell me about your pain'. This gives the patient an opportunity to express his concerns and helps us to start to gain an understanding of the patient's beliefs, preoccupations and anxieties.

We ask direct questions about the site, character, daily pattern and severity of the pain, and about sleep disturbance and limitation of activity. We make a detailed record of the history of the back pain and in particular how it has changed with time. Going through the story with the patient, with the aid of the old medical notes, can be very enlightening and often reveals surprising discrepancies between the patient's ideas and expectations and those of his medical attendants.

We ask about drugs the patient takes and those that have been tried in the past. The fact that an analgesic is currently being consumed does not mean that it is useful; it is commonplace for patients to be on high doses of drugs for long periods of time which they say are of no benefit. Continued consumption of analgesics despite lack of benefit reflects desperation rather than addiction.

9.4.2 Examination

For every ill beneath the sun
There is some remedy or none;

If there be one, resolve to find it;
If not, submit, and never mind it.

Maxims and Morals – Anon

Examination of the patient begins in the waiting room. Escorting the
patient from the waiting room to the office offers several benefits: it
gives the doctor a little exercise, it provides the opportunity to see the
patient sitting, standing and walking naturally, and last but not least it
is courteous. The more formal part of the examination occurs after the
history has been taken. The back is examined taking note of previous
scars, range of movement and tenderness. Range of movement is
notoriously difficult to assess, describe and interpret; in contrast to
many of his patients who are incapacitated by back pain the present
medical author has never been able to touch his toes! This is partly
because the ability to touch one's toes depends not only on movement
in the lumbar spine but also on movement in the hips and laxity of the
ham strings; however it also illustrates the poor correlation between
symptoms and physical signs in chronic pain patients.

The legs are examined to detect evidence of nerve root compression
or irritation which produce numbness, weakness and loss of tendon
reflexes in the part of the leg supplied by the affected nerve. Longstand-
ing compression of any nerve also gives muscle wasting in the calf
which can be easily detected with a tape measure. Straight leg raising
is a non-specific test for nerve irritation; with the patient lying supine
the examiner raises each leg in turn keeping it straight. It should normally be possible to raise the leg to 80° or more without pain. The test
is positive if the range is diminished to 30° or less because of pain down
the back of the leg.

The abdomen and peripheral pulses are examined to exclude the very
rare but important extra spinal causes of back pain such as pelvic cancer
or abdominal aortic aneurysm.

9.4.3 Surgically remediable conditions

Is this a knife I see before me?
Minimally misquoted from Macbeth – apologies to William Shakespeare

Patients who have symptoms and signs of nerve root compression and
those with extra spinal causes of pain may require an operation; they are
best investigated by the surgeon who might have to undertake treatment.

9.4.4 Inappropriate symptoms and signs

Except ye see signs and warders ye will not believe.

Gospel of St John

Waddell (1980, 1984) has described a set of inappropriate physical symptoms and signs. It cannot be emphasized too strongly that these tests are neither designed to pick up malingerers nor to separate out 'real' and 'unreal' pains, whatever these terms might be thought to mean. Their function is to allow accurate assessment. The inappropriate symptoms are: never being free of pain, being intolerant of treatments, having emergency admissions to hospital, and having pain, numbness, or giving way of the whole leg. The inappropriate signs are: superficial or non-anatomical tenderness, pain on simulated movement of the spine such as axial loading or passively rotating the shoulders and pelvis in the same plane, reduced straight leg raising which markedly improves on distraction, pain affecting a widespread part of the body which cannot be explained by accepted neuroanatomy, 'cogwheel' weakness, stocking sensory disorder, or over-reaction during examination such as collapsing or sweating.

Patients with these symptoms and signs are almost never indulging in a conscious effort to deceive and indeed some of the inappropriate signs such as sweating are completely outside voluntary control. These patients frequently have a long history of failed interventions; their inappropriate signs are a largely unconscious attempt to impress upon the examiner the reality and severity of the pain. In practice of course they tend to have the effect of convincing a naive examiner of the non-existence of the pain and so provoking even greater efforts by the patient to be believed. Such patients require particularly careful assessment; a galaxy of inappropriate signs does not exclude a remediable condition.

Some of these tests require careful interpretation. For example rotating the shoulders and pelvis in the same plane while the patient stands with feet together is somewhat similar to straight leg raising and may provoke completely appropriate radicular leg pain in a patient with nerve root compression; however since the spine moves as a whole a complaint of back pain is inappropriate. Other tests such as 'over-reaction' during examination can show wide cultural variation. We therefore use only two of the tests routinely; axial loading and distracted straight leg raising. In axial loading we press on the standing patient's head; an inappropriate response is to complain of low back pain. For distracted straight leg raising we sit the patient up from the supine position with the legs still outstretched. This is functionally exactly the same manoeuvre as leaving the trunk supine and raising the legs, and it is therefore inappropriate if the patient can achieve a substantially greater degree of leg raising in this position than in the conventional test.

9.5 TREATMENT

Desperate diseases require desperate remedies.

Guy Fawkes

9.5.1 Aims

It is part of the cure to wish to be cured.

Lucius Annaeus Seneca

There is a conflict between what most patients request from a pain clinic and what the clinic can provide. Patients state two aims, 'To find out what is really wrong with my back' and 'To take the pain away'. Although these are eminently reasonable desires and reflect the usual expectations of both doctor and patient of the outcome of a medical consultation, we believe that they are seldom achievable in patients with low back disability. The primary aim should be rehabilitation and any period of temporary pain relief that we can provide is an aid to this end, rather than an end in itself.

As explained above, the first stage of treatment is a careful and detailed medical assessment which has therapeutic as well as information gathering aspects. The next stage is explanation. Patients expect a diagnostic label and will be disappointed if they do not receive one. In some cases this may be more important than relief of the pain itself. A precise diagnosis serves a number of functions for the patient: it reassures him that the doctor understands what is wrong; it tells him that he does not have a feared condition such as cancer; and it provides an acceptable explanation for others as to why he is in pain. The problem is that there is seldom an identifiable source of pain. Textbooks usually include an exhortation such as, 'The patient should be given a sympathetic and firm explanation'. In our experience this is easier said than done. Patients seen in pain clinics have usually already seen a considerable number of conventional and complementary therapists. Therapists of whatever persuasion are as keen to diagnose and explain as patients are to grasp at straws of hope. It has been suggested that the label 'non-specific back pain' is of little use to patients or their doctors (Lancet editorial, 1989). While this may be true, it is more honest and causes fewer problems than the numerous, different, incompatible explanations for their pain that patients actually receive.

Terminology is a further problem. Even when different practitioners have tried to explain similar concepts it is likely that different words will have been used. Patients also bring their own preconceptions as to causes of pain and the meaning of medical terms. To a doctor the terms wear and tear, lumbar spondylosis and arthritis carry similar meanings but different degrees of accuracy. To most sufferers wear and tear is a normal part of ageing, lumbar spondylosis is incomprehensible but encouragingly scientific, while arthritis is a sentence to progressive disability and eventual condemnation to a wheelchair.

9.5.2 Specific treatments

When a lot of remedies are suggested for a disease, that means it can't be cured.

The Cherry Orchard – Anton Chekhov

There are many treatments for chronic back pain, each of which may produce a period of relief in some patients; all have their enthusiastic advocates but permanent cure from any of them is extremely rare. Where conventional methods have been subjected to clinical trials reviewers tend to be despairing (Waddell, 1987). The results attributed to complementary medicine are more often anecdotal and eulogistic (Greenhalgh, 1992). To what extent the direct financial connection between patient and private practitioner affects satisfaction with treatment is not known.

It may be that the lack of widespread success of any one treatment is due to the variety of different disorders underlying the common symptom of back pain. The heterogeneous nature of back pain, the existence of powerful placebo effects and uncertainty as to appropriate criteria for success make evaluation of any treatment extremely difficult. Achieving symptomatic relief by a placebo effect may be reasonable but it must be remembered that all treatments have costs, not only in financial terms but also in terms of time, risk to health, and further confirmation of the sick role.

(a) Acupuncture

Acupuncture was developed in China and has been in use for several thousand years. Although few western doctors subscribe to the theoretical basis of Chinese medicine there is a strong view that acupuncture can have an important analgesic effect. Unfortunately it is not easily amenable to standard methods of investigation such as double blind trials. Acupuncture analgesia for low back pain has been reviewed (Richardson and Vincent, 1986); short term benefits are common, longer term benefits are uncertain. It is commonly stated that acupuncture releases the body's 'natural pain killers', however the mechanism of any analgesic effect is in fact not known.

(b) Analgesics

Analgesics can be classified as conventional or unconventional (Table 9.2). The conventional analgesics can be further subdivided into periph-

Table 9.2 A classification of analgesics

			Examples
Conventional			
	Peripherally acting		Aspirin
		NSAIDs	Ibuprofen Naproxen
	Centrally acting	Weak	Codeine Dextropropoxyphene
		Strong	Morphine Pethidine
Unconventional			
	Antidepressants		Amitryptiline Lofepramine
	Anticonvulsants		Sodium valproate Carbamazepine

erally acting drugs which are relatively weak, and centrally acting drugs which have a range of efficacy.

Peripherally acting drugs include aspirin and the non-steroidal anti-inflammatory drugs (NSAIDs). These drugs probably act by a number of mechanisms; the best understood is the inhibition of production of pain promoting prostaglandins in the tissues. Prostaglandins have a range of actions: as well as mediating pain they inhibit gastric acid secretion, stimulate the production of mucus, and help to maintain renal blood flow. This explains some of the side-effects of these drugs such as gastritis, peptic ulceration and depres sion of renal function, all of which are particularly likely to occur in the elderly. It is relatively unusual for us to prescribe any of these drugs because failure to respond to them, or intolerance of their side-effects is one of the factors that leads to patients being referred to a pain clinic.

Centrally acting analgesics act by binding to receptors in the brain and spinal cord. The archetypal drug is morphine which is derived from the opium poppy; although morphine is a powerful analgesic many other opioids are quite weak. Weak opioids are commonly prescribed as compound preparations with other drugs such as aspirin and paracetamol, for example co-proxamol is a mixture of paracetamol and the weak opioid dextropropoxyphene. As with the NSAIDs, patients have usually worked their way through an impressive number of these drugs before referral and we seldom prescribe them. There is controversy over whether it is ever reasonable to prescribe strong opioids to patients with chronic non-malignant pain; fears of addiction and tolerance seem to have been overstated in the past but still cause concern. Other arguments are based on a belief in the lack of efficacy of opioids in chronic non-malignant pain; this belief is at odds with the huge popularity of the compound drugs mentioned above. Perhaps the most serious objection is the undeniable and important problem of constipation. We believe that powerful opioids do have an occasional role to play but with a number of important caveats: one must be sure that the pain is opioid responsive, treatment should only be started after discussion with the patient's general practitioner, and one should follow the principles already established for the use of these drugs in malignant pain. On the very rare occasions that we use them we prescribe long-acting drugs given at fixed intervals; slow release morphine sulphate is probably ideal. However, buprenorphine is perceived to cause less dependence and it may therefore be better tolerated by the patient's medical attendants, if not by the patient. Short-acting drugs such as pethidine prescribed to be taken as required have a number of disadvantages: they focus the patient's attention on their pain and on the clock, and they tend to have a higher incidence of side-effects such as dysphoria.

Unconventional analgesics such as tricyclic antidepressants can be effective in relieving chronic pain in conditions such as post-herpetic neuralgia where the nervous system has obviously been damaged. They have also been used with apparent success in other conditions such as chronic low back pain, both with (Hameroff *et al.*, 1982; Ward *et al.*, 1984; Ward, 1986) and without (Alcoff *et al.*, 1982) depression. The mechanism of action is unknown but they are effective at lower doses and with a shorter latency of action than when they are used to treat depression. At these low doses they do not have a significant effect on mood (McQuay, Carroll and Glynn, 1992).

Depression is three to four times commoner in patients with low back pain than in the general population and may respond to higher doses of antidepressants (Sullivan *et al.*, 1992). Unfortunately even the small dose of an antidepressant required for analgesia can have significant side-effects; many patients experience unacceptable day time drowsiness and an uncomfortably dry mouth. The most commonly used drug is amitryptiline but the risks of confusion, cardiovascular and urinary side effects make it unsuitable for use in the elderly. Lofepramine has fewer side-effects but also a less convincing track record as an analgesic.

Anticonvulsants are also established as effective analgesics in some conditions of obvious nervous system damage such as trigeminal neuralgia; their effectiveness in other conditions is less certain. The most commonly used drugs are sodium valproate and carbamazepine, both of which can have serious side-effects.

Drug withdrawal is one of the most useful treatments for many patients. As discussed above, it is commonplace for patients to be taking drugs which do not help their pain but which do have significant side-effects and reduce quality of life. Since these drugs are taken in desperation it can be difficult to convince the patient to abandon them and even more difficult to stop the quest for the Holy Grail of the completely effective analgesic with no side-effects. Clear information about the function and limitations of analgesics may help as may the discovery that without analgesics the pain is no worse and troublesome side-effects disappear.

(c) Epidurals

Drugs can be injected into the epidural space either at the base of the spine through a gap in the sacrum (the caudal hiatus) or in the lumbar region using a rather more difficult loss of resistance technique. Both local anaesthetics and steroids may have beneficial effects. Local anaesthetics interrupt activity in the nervous system which may be a cause of pain; they also relax paraspinal muscle spasm, which in turn may allow disarticulated surfaces of the facet joints to move back into alignment (Kirkaldy-Willis, 1983). The beneficial effect of steroids may be due to an anti-inflammatory action on nerve roots. The outcome of epidural steroid injections has been reviewed (Kepes and Duncalf, 1985; Benzon, 1986). Patients particularly likely to benefit are those with radicular pain of relatively brief duration; those who respond do so within six days. The steroid depresses natural cortisol production for about three weeks but this is not thought to have any clinical importance.

(d) Facet joint injections

There is little agreement on the clinical features of pain arising from the facet joints and even less agreement as to the mechanism of analgesia produced by injections into or close to the joints. Published studies report 6% (Ogsbury, Simon and Lehman, 1977) to 20% (Mooney and Robertson, 1976) long-term relief after facet joint injection and most pain clinics perform these injections. Under X-ray image intensifier control a mixture of local anaesthetic and steroid is injected into or close to the joints. A dilemma arises in those patients who respond briefly but whose pain returns after a short time. A variety of 'denervation' techniques have been described but, with the elucidation of the complex nerve supply to these joints (Bogduk and Long, 1979), it has been realized that few of the techniques achieved their purpose. Some clinics use a radio-frequency lesion generator to perform a destructive lesion of the posterior primary ramus of the nerve as it runs over the transverse process; this is claimed to produce good results but controlled trials are lacking.

(e) Manipulation

Manipulation for chronic back pain is carried out by doctors, physiotherapists, osteopaths, and chiropractors, each working within a different theoretical framework. Anecdotal reports are often enthusiastic (Greenhalgh, 1992); considered reviews less so (Jayson, 1986). A recent study which has shown significant long-term benefits in patients treated with chiropractic rather than conventional hospital out-patient treatment (Meade *et al.*, 1990) demonstrates the difficulties inherent in conducting trials in low back pain. Although the result seems unequivocal the trial design meant that no specific component of treatment could be identified as being responsible for improvement. The chiropractic patients received on average 44% more treatments, and placebo, educational or counselling effects of this alone could be invoked to explain the difference in outcome.

How manipulation might work is not known. It may break down adhesions or mobilize stiff joints, or the barrage of nerve impulses entering the spinal cord might suppress pain sensation in a manner similar to transcutaneous electrical nerve stimulation (see below). Any mode of treatment requiring direct physical contact between therapist and patient has the potential for powerful placebo effects.

(f) Occupational therapy

The occupational therapist is involved in the assessment and management of functional disabilities, most commonly as part of a rehabilitation or pain management programme (Chapter 2).

(g) Physiotherapy

The physiotherapist can use a series of sessions to encourage mobility, and educate the patient. This can be done either individually, or with groups of patients in a 'back school', or as part of a rehabilitation or pain management programme (see below and Chapter 2).

(h) Psychological intervention

The clinical psychologist's role is to enhance the patient's perception of control over his pain, to provide training in a range of coping strategies, and to facilitate improvements in quality of life. Psychological interventions are intended to interrupt the vicious cycles which become established in chronic back pain sufferers; pain increases muscle tension which intensifies the pain, the conscious fear of injuring the painful area leads to avoidance of movement and disuse which in turn produces more pain. Reduced mobility and fear of injury curtail activities and social contacts outside the family and increase problems within the family. Negative mood states increase awareness of pain and vice versa. These aspects are addressed in individual sessions or in group pain management programmes.

(i)   *Rehabilitation and pain management programmes*

These are discussed in detail in Chapter 2. Rehabilitation and pain management programmes differ in emphasis; rehabilitation programmes focus more on physical than psychological aspects. The contributions of physiotherapists and occupational therapists to both types of programme have been briefly mentioned above.

Our own pain management programme is fairly typical; it includes formal education about medical aspects of pain and its treatment, and about pain perception and the psychological factors affecting it. We teach the use of relaxation techniques and cognitive methods involving re-labelling and de-catastrophizing the pain experience to interrupt the vicious cycle of pain and tension and to increase perceived control. Chronic back pain sufferers tend to vacillate between immobility and strenuous bursts of activity. We use the concept of 'pacing' in which the patient plans intervals of activity and rest, and becomes more aware of signs of fatigue. Patients are encouraged to set realistic goals to enhance their quality of life, including taking up new activities compatible with their mobility levels. Group-based programmes are particularly useful in allowing sufferers to exchange coping strategies and reduce feelings of isolation and hopelessness. Although there is widespread belief in the importance of family relationship factors in chronic pain (Humphrey, 1989), there is less certainty about whether and how these should be tackled as part of the pain management programme. We have just started to use information leaflets for relatives to aid their understanding and co-operation with the aims of the programme.

Such programmes seem successful. A recent study by Nicholas, Wilson and Goyen (1992) compared the efficacy of cognitive-behavioural group treatment plus physiotherapy with physiotherapy alone. Patients receiving a combination of group treatment and physiotherapy showed significantly greater improvement which was maintained at the 6 month follow-up, and reflected in greater use of active coping strategies and perceived control over pain. In common with most previous research, this study found that reported pain intensity did not reduce in spite of subjects' increased ability to manage pain and enhance their quality of life. It seems that a realistic goal for such programmes is reduction of medication and increased ability to cope with pain, albeit at the same level of perceived pain.

(j) Rest and exercise

The commonly perceived relationship between pain, underlying tissue damage and rest is shown diagrammatically below:

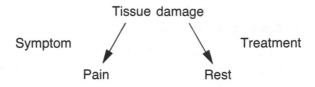

This relationship holds good for a number of common acute conditions such as bone fractures, the pain of which is directly related to tissue damage and relieved by a period of immobilization in a plaster cast while healing occurs. Unfortunately the applicability of this model even to acute back pain is much less certain and the notion that rest allows pain relief and healing is not proven. Traditional teaching that acute sciatica should be initially treated by several weeks of enforced bed rest is backed up by scanty evidence (Waddell, 1987) and doctors with back pain seldom follow it (Workmen's Compensation Board Symposium, 1986). By contrast the deleterious effects of bed rest are well documented; they include loss of muscle mass, osteoporosis, general malaise and depression. On a social level prolonged bed rest leads to loss of work, inability to function normally within the community and the family, and adoption of the sick role. Furthermore chronic back pain is characterized by the lack of relationship between symptoms and detectable underlying tissue damage. Teaching chronic back pain sufferers the inapplicability of this commonly perceived relationship to their condition is an important element of rehabilitation.

(k) Transcutaneous electrical nerve stimulation (TENS)

The use of TENS is based on the gate control theory of Melzack and Wall (1965) which suggests that stimulating large nerve fibres which carry touch sensation will inhibit transmission of pain signals in the spinal cord. The TENS machine is a box attached to pads which are placed close to the painful part to produce a buzzing sensation which can be adjusted in amplitude and frequency. It is often stated that one in three patients benefit for prolonged periods, however the recent study of Deyo *et al.* (1990) was unable to demonstrate any benefit from 'true' as opposed to 'sham' TENS.

9.6 OUTCOME

Who shall decide when doctors disagree?

Moral Essays – Alexander Pope

Perhaps the most intriguing question about outcome is how we should assess it. We have argued that the goal should be rehabilitation and useful outcome measures would therefore include return to work (a fairly rare phenomenon), reduced medication, and reduced reliance on 'healers' of whatever persuasion.

We have proposed that the provision of periods of analgesia should be seen as an aid to rehabilitation rather than an end in itself; this idea can be turned on its head. It is equally reasonable to argue that providing brief periods of pain relief hinders rehabilitation by reinforcing the sufferer's belief in the efficacy of medical therapy to finally 'cure' his pain. The methods of pain relief discussed in this chapter need to be assessed for their ability to help or hinder rehabilitation.

Our own belief, which we are unable to back up with firm evidence, is that in most patients TENS and tricyclic antidepressants do little to hinder rehabilitation and may help. Each of the other methods of analgesia discussed will help a few people, but distract the majority from the goal of rehabilitation.

Rehabilitation and pain management programmes also lack universal applicability but, being directed towards realistic goals, offer the greatest hopes of success.

9.7 CONCLUSIONS AND SUMMARY

Life is the art of drawing sufficient conclusions from insufficient premises.

Samuel Butler

Most patients referred to pain clinics with low back pain have chronic low back disability with loss of physical and social function. Their requests for causal explanations and cures for their pain can seldom be satisfied. The major aim of treatment should be rehabilitation. A large variety of specific treatments exist any of which may provide pain relief for some patients for varying lengths of time; there is no reliable method of predicting which patients will respond to which treatment. All of these treatments require evaluation in terms of contribution to rehabilitation.

ACKNOWLEDGEMENTS

We would like to thank Mr Raymond Chadwick for his constructive criticism of the text and for his literary expertise. We are also grateful to Mrs Christine O'Connor for reviewing the text and for her uncanny ability to spot split infinitives.

REFERENCES

Alcoff, J., Jones, E., Rust, P. and Newman, R. (1982) Controlled trial of imipramine for chronic low back pain. *Journal of Family Practice*, **14**, 841–6.

Battié, M. C., Bigos, S. J., Fisher, L. D. *et al.* (1989), A prospective study of the role of cardiovascular risk factors and fitness in industrial back pain complaints. *Spine*, **14**, 141–7.

Benzon, H. T. (1986) Epidural steroid injections for low back pain and lumbosacral radiculopathy. *Pain*, **24**, 277–95.

Block, A. R., Kremer, E. F. and Gaylor, M. (1980) Behavioral treatment of chronic pain: the spouse as a discriminative cue for pain behavior. *Pain*, **9**, 243–52.

Blumberg, B. S. and Sokoloff, L. (1961) Coalescence of caudal vertebrae in the giant dinosaur *Diplodocus*. *Arthritis and Rheumatism*, **4**, 592–601.

Bogduk, N. and Long, D. M. (1979) The anatomy of the 'so-called articular nerves' and their relationship to facet denervation in the treatment of low back pain. *Journal of Neurosurgery*, **51**, 172–7.

Calin, A. and Fries, J. F. (1975) Striking prevalence of ankylosing spondylitis in 'healthy' W27 positive males and females. A controlled study. *New England Journal of Medicine*, **293**, 835–9.

Calin, A., Porta, J., Fries, J. F. *et al.* (1977) Clinical history as a screening test for ankylosing spondylitis. *Journal of the American Medical Association*, **237**, 2613–14.

Deyo, R. A., Walsh, N. E., Martin, D. C., *et al.* (1990) A controlled trial of transcutaneous electrical nerve stimulation (TENS) and exercise for chronic low back pain. *New England Journal of Medicine*, **322**, 1627–34.

Dixon, A. St J. (1980) Introduction in *The Lumbar Spine and Back Pain*, 2nd edn, (ed. M. I. V. Jayson), Pitman Medical, Tunbridge Wells, pp. ix-xv.

Dunnell, K. and Cartwright, A. (1972) *Medicine Takers, Prescribers and Hoarders*, Routledge and Kegan Paul, London.

Editorial (1989) Risk factors for back trouble. *Lancet* i, 1305–6.

Frymoyer, J. W., Pope, M. H., Costanza, M. C., *et al.* (1980) Epidemiologic studies of low back pain. *Spine*, **5**, 419–23.

Grahame, R., Calin, A., Tudor, M., *et al.* (1974) HL-A 27 as a diagnostic aid, in *Proceedings of the 7th International Congress of Internal Medicine*, Tel Aviv.

Greenhalgh, T. (1992) A tutorial in alternative medicine. *British Medical Journal*, **305**, 655.

Hameroff, S. R., Cork, R. C., Scherer, K. *et al.* (1982) Doxepin effects on chronic pain, depression and plasma opioids. *Journal of Clinical Psychiatry*, **43**, 22–7.

Harper, A. C., Harper, D. A., Lambert, L. J. *et al.* (1992) Symptoms of impairment, disability and handicap in low back pain: a taxonomy. *Pain*, **50**, 189–95.

Humphrey, M. (1980) The problem of low back pain, in *Contributions to Medical Psychology*, (ed S. R. Rachman), Pergamon, Oxford.

Humphrey, M. (1989) *Back Pain*, Routledge, London.

Jajić, I. (1979) The role of HLA-B27 in the diagnosis of low back pain. *Acta Orthopaedica Scandinavica*, **50**, 411–13.

Jayson, M. I. V. (1986) A limited role for manipulation. *British Medical Journal*, **293**, 1454–5.

Jinkins, J. R., Whittemore, A. R. and Bradley, W. G. (1989) The anatomic basis of vertebrogenic pain and the autonomic syndrome associated with lumbar disk extrusion. *American Journal of Roentgenology*, **152**, 1277–89.

Kepes, E. R. and Duncalf, D. (1985) Treatment of backache with spinal injections of local anesthetics, spinal and systemic steroids. A review. *Pain*, **22**, 33–47.

Kirkaldy-Willis, W. H. (1983) *Managing Low Back Pain*, Churchill Livingstone, New York.

Kirwan, E. O'G. (1989) Back pain, in *Textbook of Pain*, 2nd edn, (eds P. D. Wall and R. Melzack), Churchill Livingstone, Edinburgh, pp. 335–40.

McCaffrey, M. (1983) *Nursing the Patient in Pain*, Harper and Row, London.

McQuay, H. J., Carroll, D. and Glynn, C. J. (1992) Low dose amitryptiline in the treatment of chronic pain. *Anaesthesia*, **47**, 646–52.

Macnab, I. (1977) *Backache*, Williams and Wilkins, Baltimore.

Meade, T. W., Dyer, S., Browne, W. *et al.* (1990) Low back pain of mechanical origin: randomised comparison of chiropractic and hospital outpatient treatment. *British Medical Journal*, **300**, 1431–7.

Melzack, R. and Wall, P. D. (1965) Pain mechanisms: a new theory. *Science*, **150**, 971–9.

Meyerding, H. W. (1941) Low backache and sciatica pain associated with spondylolisthesis and protruded intervertebral disc: incidence, significance and treatment. *Journal of Bone and Joint Surgery*, **23**, 461–70.

Mixter, W. J. and Barr, J. S. (1934) Rupture of the intervertebral disc with involvement of the spinal canal. *New England Journal of Medicine*, **211**, 210–15.

Mooney, V. and Robertson, J. (1976) The facet syndrome. *Clinical Orthopaedics and Related Research*, **115**, 149–56.

Nelson, M. A. (1973) Lumbar spinal stenosis. *Journal of Bone and Joint Surgery*, **55B**, 506–11.

Nicholas, M. K., Wilson, P. H. and Goyen, J. (1992) Comparison of cognitive-behavioral group treatment and an alternative non-psychological treatment for chronic low back pain. *Pain*, **48**, 339–47.

O'Brien, J. P. (1984) Mechanisms of spinal pain, in *Textbook of Pain*, (eds P. D. Wall and R. Melzack), Churchill Livingstone, Edinburgh, pp. 240–51.

O'Connor, M. and Glynn, C. J. (1991) Prevalence of HLA-B27 in patients with back pain attending a pain clinic. *Pain*, **44**, 147–9.

Ogsbury, J. S., Simon, R. H. and Lehman, R. W. (1977) Facet denervation in the treatment of low back pain syndrome. *Pain*, **3**, 257–63.

Papageorgiou, A. C. and Rigby, A. S. (1991) Review of UK data on the rheumatic diseases – 7. Low back pain. *British Journal of Rheumatology*, **30**, 208–10.

Richardson, P. H. and Vincent, C. A. (1986) Acupuncture for the treatment of pain: a review of evaluative research. *Pain*, **24**, 15–40.

Sandström, J., Andersson, G. B. J. and Rydberg, L. (1984) HLA-B27 as a diagnostic screening tool in chronic low back pain. *Scandinavian Journal of Rehabilitation Medicine*, **16**, 27–8.

Scoville, W. B. and Corkhill, G. (1974) Lumbar spondylolisthesis with ruptured disc. *Journal of Neurosurgery*, **40**, 529–34.

Shaw, M. D. M., Russell, J. A. and Grossart, K. W. (1978) The changing pattern of spinal arachnoiditis. *Journal of Neurology, Neurosurgery and Psychiatry*, **41**, 97–107.

Sullivan, M. J. L., Reesor, K., Mikail, S. and Fisher, R. (1992) The treatment of depression in chronic low back pain: review and recommendations. *Pain*, **50**, 5–13.

Waddell, G. (1980) Nonorganic physical signs in low back pain. *Spine*, **5**, 117–25.

Waddell, G. (1982) An approach to backache. *British Journal of Hospital Medicine*, **28**, 187–219.

Waddell, G. (1984) Chronic low back pain, psychologic distress, and illness behavior. *Spine*, **9**, 209–13.

Waddell, G. (1987) A new clinical model for the treatment of low back pain. *Spine*, **12**, 632–44.

Walsh, K., Varnes, V., Osmond, C. *et al.* (1989) Occupational causes of low back pain. *Scandinavian Journal of Work and Environmental Health*, **15**, 54–9.

Walsh, K., Cruddas, M. and Coggon, D. (1991) Interaction of height and mechanical loading of the spine in the development of low back pain. *Scandinavian Journal of Work and Environmental Health*, **17**, 420–4.

Walsh, K., Cruddas, M. and Coggon, D. (1992a) Low back pain in eight areas in Britain *Journal of Epidemiology and Community Health*, **46**, 227–30.

Walsh, K., Cruddas, M. and Coggon, D. (1992b) Risk of low back pain in people admitted to hospital for traffic accidents and falls. *Journal of Epidemiology and Community Health*, **46**, 231–3.

Ward, N., Bokan, J. A., Phillips, M. *et al.* (1984) Antidepressants in concomitant back pain and depression: Doxepin and desipramine compared. *Journal of Clinical Psychiatry*, **45**, 54–7.

Ward, N. G. (1986) Tricyclic antidepressants for chronic low back pain. Mechanisms of action and predictors of response. *Spine*, **11**, 661–5.

West, H. F. (1949) The aetiology of ankylosing spondylitis. *Annals of the Rheumatic Diseases*, **8**, 143–8.

Working Group on Back Pain (1979) *Report to Secretary of State for Social Services and Secretary of State for Scotland*, Her Majesty's Stationery Office, London.

Workmen's Compensation Board Symposium (1986) *Low Back Pain: A Multidisciplinary Approach*. Vancouver.

Yunnus, M. B. (1989) Fibromyalgia syndrome: new research on an old malady. *British Medical Journal*, **298**, 474–5.

CHAPTER 10

Psychological factors in surgical recovery

Peter Salmon

10.1 INTRODUCTION

The recovery of surgical patients has long been seen as a problem to which psychological techniques could bring important benefits. It has even been envisaged that surgical patients should routinely be helped by a psychologist (Kendall and Watson, 1981). It is more realistic, however, that psychological procedures could be administered by the nurses or doctors who are already involved in caring for the patient, and it is becoming common for surgical wards to give patients some sort of psychological preparation in this way. We shall see, however, that the evidence is far from clear as to whether the strategies that are often chosen benefit patients. This is not to propose that psychological factors should be neglected. On the contrary, it will be argued that they are inherent in the treatment and care which surgical patients receive routinely.

Specific forms of surgery entail specific psychological challenges, particularly if the length or quality of life is at stake, or if body image is threatened. These factors are neglected in the discussion that follows. Instead, this is intended to draw out the psychological issues which apply to surgery in general.

10.2 HISTORICAL CONTEXT

Psychological aspects of surgery have been researched from two distinct points of view. Studies by anaesthetists and nursing researchers have tended to focus on practical and humanitarian benefits for patients' well-being. Studies by psychologists, by contrast, have often been motivated by an interest in surgery as a convenient form of stress against which to test theories concerning stress in general. We shall first consider the results of this more theoretical approach before examining its convergence with those of the smaller number of more clinically oriented studies.

Freud was the first to suggest the theoretical value of studying surgery. He described how, in using play to 'work through' an unpleasant surgical or medical procedure, children might cope with such experiences. It was 30 years before another theorist returned to develop this suggestion, again from a psychoanalytic perspective: in his book 'Psychological Stress', Janis (1958) elaborated the theory that, if people prepared psychologically for an impending stressor, its emotional impact would be reduced. He, like Freud, described this preparation as 'working through' the stressor, coining the phrase 'work of worry' to describe this process before surgery. His concern with the emotional impact of surgery focused psychologists' interest for the decades which followed. Nevertheless, it has since become clear that emotional responses to surgery are only poorly related to other indices which might be used to index recovery.

10.3   INDICES OF RECOVERY

10.3.1   Emotional state

A major concern has been with anxiety reflecting, in large part, Janis' (1958) view that, preoperatively, it indicated the 'work of worry' and postoperatively, the impact of surgical stress. If, as Janis thought, the operation itself is the principal threat, then anxiety might be expected to increase preoperatively as the time of surgery draws nearer, and to decline rapidly postoperatively. This has sometimes been the case (Auerbach, 1973; Spielberger *et al.*, 1973; Martinez-Urrutia, 1975; Salmon, Evans and Humphrey, 1986). In each study, anxious mood measured around 24 hours preoperatively exceeded that measured a few days postoperatively. When Johnston (1980) subsequently examined changes in anxiety in more detail a more complex pattern emerged. In orthopaedic patients anxiety reached its maximum on the first day postoperatively and fell only slightly by the fifth day. Similar patterns have been described in other studies (Chapman and Cox, 1977; Vogele and Steptoe, 1986) and a longer-term study of gynaecological surgery patients found that anxiety was high throughout the hospital stay, and for the days at home immediately before admission, by comparison with levels measured at home two or five weeks postoperatively. Clearly, there is no universal pattern of change in anxiety and it is important to assess the pattern, without preconceptions, in any patient group which is of interest. Nevertheless, the different results indicate that it is naive to regard the operation itself as the sole source of threat and it should be expected that anxiety may extend far beyond the immediate preoperative and postoperative period.

Despite this evidence there have been few systematic attempts to identify sources of patients' anxiety apart from the operation. It is to be expected that particular operations will entail particular concerns about postoperative health or longevity. Many of these concerns will be rational but many may not; for example, many women facing gynaecological surgery for non-malignant disease worry that cancer will be discovered (Steptoe, Horti and Stanton, 1988). Subjective bodily changes produced by surgery might also be a source of anxiety (Salmon, Evans and Humphrey, 1986), especially if misinterpreted by patients.

Much less is known about surgical patients' emotions other than anxiety. Where depression has been measured, it has changed in a similar way to anxiety (Chapman and Cox, 1977; Vogele and Steptoe, 1986). It would be valuable to know more about how patients describe their emotional state during recovery. Patients' own reports have only rarely been published (Kelly, 1987). Nevertheless one dimension of emotional feeling – fatigue – is quite distinct from the emotions more typically studied and has been identified by Rose and King (1978) as the primary subjective problem during the postoperative convalescent period. Its persistence for long periods has been borne out by investigations of abdominal surgery patients, in whom feelings of fatigue were shown to be elevated up to 30 days postoperatively by comparison with preoperative levels (Christensen *et al.*, 1982, 1986). It is not yet clear how general this phenomenon is. Vogele and Steptoe (1986) described a more rapid decline of fatigue to preoperative levels in their samples of orthopaedic patients, together with a corresponding recovery in vigour.

How good patients feel, as opposed to how bad they feel is also an important subjective component of recovery and is probably independent of the extent of negative emotional responses or the kinds of indices of recovery considered below (Johnston, 1984). It is therefore unfortunate that this has been so rarely measured.

10.3.2 Behavioural changes

A variety of aspects of patients' behaviour have been used to index recovery. The studies that we shall go on to examine have routinely recorded the duration of patients' hospital stay and the amount of analgesic medication which they requested and received. Such measures have, however, been roundly criticized (e.g. Johnston and Jones, 1979). They are open to so many extraneous influences that they can hardly be regarded as indices of patients' underlying state. They may even be misleading if a patient who requests fewer analgesics, for example, suffers needlessly as a result or if early discharge puts a patient at risk. An alternative approach is to describe a patient's recovery by charting the speed of return to activities which were previously routine. Such a scale for gynaecological patients, based on the return to domestic tasks, has been described by Williams *et al.* (1976). Differences between patients in their usual activities limit this approach, although it might be possible to tailor a scale to each patient. This approach clearly requires patients to be followed up into their convalescent period at home, which would be a welcome contrast to the current concentration of research on the recovery period in hospital. The hospital stay is a mere fraction of the convalescent period. Rose and King (1978) suggested that information on changes in psychomotor functioning would be valuable, but Folkard, Simpson and Glynn (1979) found that herniorrhaphy patients recovered to normal efficiency on a variety of simple psychomotor tasks within 2–3 days postoperatively. More demanding tasks might detect longer-term changes.

10.3.3 Physiological changes

It might be expected that the most direct measures of recovery would be physiological ones: the healing of a wound or the reversion or palliation of the original disorder. But surprisingly little is known about how to measure these or about the influence which these changes have on surgeons' intuitive judgements of recovery. A different set of indices has received more attention. This is the constellation of endocrine responses which occur after all but minor surgery, the extent of which is related to the severity of surgery (Chernow *et al.*, 1987). The rise in cortisol has been described in most detail. It begins upon incision, reaches its maximum during the hours after surgery and may persist for up to five days following major surgery (Plumpton, Besser and Cole, 1969). Changes in adrenaline and noradrenaline are less consistent but, as with cortisol, the greatest changes are seen after surgery (e.g. Nistrup-Madsen *et al.*, 1978; Udelsman *et al.*, 1987). Increases also occur in other hormones, including oxytocin, anti-diuretic hormone and prolactin (Kaufman, 1982).

The endocrine mobilization by surgery is often regarded within anaesthesiology as a manifestation of Selye's (1976) stress response (Wilmore *et al.*, 1976). This response, which can be observed after a variety of physical insults, has long been regarded as adaptive. In the case of surgery there may therefore be valuable effects, particularly in coping with the immediate surgical trauma. However, prolonged or intense responses might be harmful. The hormones are catabolic and so may contribute to loss of muscle mass and delayed healing or even predispose to pressure sores (Ellis and Humphrey, 1982; Anand, 1986). More controversially, it has also been suggested that elevated cortisol levels contribute to the immunosuppression and vulnerability to metastases or infections which follow surgery (Walton, 1978; Salo, 1982). For these reasons it has been argued that to reduce or block these responses would benefit the surgical patient (Kehlet, 1984) and much anaesthetic practice is geared to minimizing them. Nevertheless, the case that these responses are harmful has not been proved (Baron *et al.*, 1991; Zeiderman *et al.*, 1991). A further reason to be cautious about the significance of endocrine responses is that it it is now realized that many of the metabolic effects of surgery are mediated, not by the endocrine response, but by the cellular release of cytokines in response to tissue damage (Hall, 1985; Brown and Grosso, 1989). Cytokines can act locally or systemically. Although their exact effects are not clear, they appear to modulate immune function and mediate fever and inflammation (Kehlet, 1989).

Furthermore, the use of endocrine measures as an index of recovery is limited because they return to baseline levels within a few days postoperatively, although patients would regard themselves as continuing to recover for some weeks more. Nevertheless, endocrine responses are important in the present context because of the evidence that endocrine responses to other forms of stress are sensitive to psychological aspects of the stress (Frankenhaueser, 1980). Speculatively, a psychological involvement in the endocrine effects of surgery would be consistent with the finding that endocrine responses are greatest shortly postoperatively, once patients have recovered consciousness. Moreover, just as patients' anxiety reactions could not be attributed entirely to the surgical trauma, it is possible that the endocrine responses are stimulated by other sources of stress postoperatively, such as the novelty of surrounding conditions or feelings of helplessness.

10.3.4 Interrelationships between different measures of recovery

With such a variety of ways to assess recovery, and in the absence of any definitive indices of physiological or behavioural improvement, it is hard to decide which measures should receive the most weight in interpreting the results of published research. If the different indices are all manifestations of a single underlying recovery process, the choice of a particular index is unimportant. Unfortunately the evidence is more complex. Relationships between different types of measure – subjective, behavioural and physiological – are minimal. There is little evidence that postoperative anxiety is related to behavioural or somatic indices. Where correlations reach significance they are small and unreliable (Wolfer and Davis, 1970; Ray and Fitzgibbon, 1981). There may be a sex difference because Wolfer and Davis found that anxiety correlated more extensively with objective indices (medication use, duration of stay, nurses' ratings) in gynaecological than in male abdominal surgery patients. Also, measurements of anxiety which are specifically related to hospitalization may be more closely related to analgesic use and pain (Wells *et al.*, 1986). Although relationships between subjective and endocrine measurements are generally absent or small, there is some evidence that postoperative fatigue is related to concurrent cardiovascular measures (Christensen, Bendix and Kehlet, 1982; Vogele and Steptoe, 1986). Nevertheless, the view that recovery is multidimensional receives concrete support from Johnston (1984) who carried out a principal components analysis of a range of recovery measures. Feelings of well-being were separate from those of emotional distress, and pain was separate from both of these: that is, low levels of distress or pain would be no guarantee that a patient 'felt better'.

Even within the different classes of measure – subjective, behavioural and physiological – interrelationships are very small. When different indices of emotional distress, such as anxiety and depression, have been measured within a single study, the correlations between them have rarely been reported. Such results as are available are consistent with the view that anxiety and depression represent a single dimension of emotional distress (Chapman and Cox, 1977; Vogele and Steptoe, 1986). Other subjective measures are probably distinct from this, however. Although significant correlations can be detected postoperatively between anxiety and subjective physical state or pain they are small (Wolfer and Davis, 1970; Martinez-Urrutia, 1975; Ray and Fitzgibbon, 1981). Feelings of arousal and fatigue are also unrelated to anxiety (Ray and Fitzgibbon, 1981; Ho *et al.*, 1988; Christensen *et al.*, 1986).

Turning to the more objective behavioural and physiological indices we find no more evidence of a unitary recovery process. There is little evidence that the most frequently used behavioural measures – analgesic requests and duration of postoperative stay – intercorrelate. Neither do the endocrine responses intercorrelate highly (Salmon *et al.*, 1988).

10.4   PSYCHOLOGICAL INFLUENCES ON POSTOPERATIVE RECOVERY

10.4.1   Preoperative emotional state

Janis (1958) set the scene for much subsequent research with his claim that the 'work of worry' reduced the impact of surgery and so facilitated recovery. He went on to argue that the work of worry would be associated with moderate levels of anxiety. Too little (or too much) anxiety would therefore increase the impact of surgery. Janis (1958) provided some evidence to support this theory but his results would not be regarded as rigorous by modern standards and it is better to regard this theory as based on astute clinical observation than on empirical investigation. More intensive investigations of the theory followed the development of the state-trait anxiety inventory by Spielberger, Gorsuch and Lushene (1970). Contrary to the prediction, preoperative anxiety was consistently related to postoperative anxiety in a positive, linear way (Spielberger *et al.*, 1973; Auerbach, 1973; Johnson, Leventhal and Dabbs, 1971; Johnston and Carpenter, 1980; Wallace, 1986). There was no evidence of the kind of curvilinear relationship which would support the theory.

Moreover, the relevance of preoperative anxiety to postoperative state is very circumscribed. In Wallace's (1986) results, preoperative anxiety was unrelated to postoperative anxiety when this was measured following discharge. Indeed, preoperative anxiety is sometimes unrelated to postoperative anxiety even shortly postoperatively (Ho *et al.*, 1988). Furthermore, if we look beyond postoperative anxiety to other indices of outcome, including other mood states, pain or physical symptoms, there is usually little or no relationship at all with preoperative anxiety (Wolfer and Davis, 1970; Ray and Fitzgibbon, 1981; Wallace, 1986; Johnson, Leventhal and Dabbs, 1971; Johnston and Carpenter, 1980).

There are two opposing conclusions that may be drawn from this pattern of results. One is that Janis (1958) was wrong: preoperative worry has little to do with postoperative recovery and certainly nothing to do with improving it. Another, however, is that his hypothesis has not yet been adequately tested. There are three bases for this proposal. First, since Janis was concerned with surgery as a psychological threat, his ideas might apply to more severe surgery than psychologists have typically investigated. An investigation of breast cancer patients (Dean and Surtees, 1989) was consistent with Janis' theory (although the results were not interpreted in this way). Women who were clinically distressed before surgery were less likely to have a recurrence of cancer during a 6–8 year period postoperatively. Second, the measurement of anxiety may not provide a valid index of the process of active mental preparation which Janis termed the work of worry. Ray and Fitzgibbon (1981) suggested that feelings of 'arousal' would be more indicative of this state. They showed that greater arousal before cholecystectomy predicted better postoperative state, indexed by lower self-rated pain, fewer requests for analgesic and hypnotic medication and shorter postoperative stay. Similarly, Ho *et al.* (1988) found that higher preoperative arousal in patients awaiting wisdom-tooth removal predicted lower anxiety postoperatively.

A third reason why it would be premature to regard Janis' theory as adequately tested is that outcome measures should perhaps be used which more directly reflect the stressfulness of surgery. In particular, the endocrine responses might be appropriate indices since they are generally regarded in anaesthesiology and psychology as stress responses. Consistent with Janis' theory, there are indications that preoperative distress does predict smaller endocrine responses (Salmon and Kaufman, 1990). Bursten and Russ (1965) rated their patients' state of distress a day or more before herniorrhaphy. Higher ratings predicted a smaller increase in cortisol levels during the first 45 minutes of surgery. Salmon *et al.* (1988) have also reported that postoperative circulating levels of cortisol were less in patients who rated themselves as in pain preoperatively and those of adrenaline were less in patients who had reported pain or anxiety. These relationships were seen with endocrine levels measured on the first two postoperative days, and also immediately after surgery.

10.4.2 Accuracy of expectations

A more complex influence of preoperative on postoperative state is indicated by Johnson's (1973) theory. This, like Janis' supposes that the preoperative period is a preparatory one, such that the way in which the patient anticipates surgery influences its emotional impact. The patient's task, according to this theory, is to anticipate accurately the intensity of pain and discomfort; distress will result to the extent that there is a discrepancy between anticipation and experience. Much of the supporting evidence for this is from patients who have undergone minor procedures. By contrast, Johnston (1981) found no support for the theory in surgical patients. Instead, her findings suggested that most postoperative distress occurred when patients had preoperatively underestimated the pain that they would experience. A more recent study of laparoscopy patients found little support for either hypothesis (Wallace, 1985). It is hard to escape the conclusion that the relationship between preoperative and postoperative emotional state is an unreliable one, and that preoperative factors other than emotional state are more important determinants of postoperative state.

10.4.3 Anxious personality

Although preoperative anxious state (State Anxiety) has not been reliably associated with postoperative recovery, there is some evidence that anxious personality (Trait Anxiety) is more predictive. In their review of the influence of personality on recovery, Mathews and Ridgeway (1981) found relatively consistent evidence that anxious personalities show greater distress than non-anxious people postoperatively and recover more slowly when this is indexed by pain ratings, length of stay or medication requests.

For clinical purposes, however, a measure of generally anxious personality may not be the most useful indicator of patients who are at risk of intense anxiety postoperatively. Trait Anxiety has long been viewed as a predisposition to respond with a state of anxiety to a wide variety of threatening situations; consistent with this, highly Trait

Anxious surgical patients do show greater State Anxiety preoperatively and postoperatively in many studies (Spielberger *et al.*, 1973; Auerbach, 1973; Martinez-Urrutia, 1975). However, high Trait Anxiety did not predict a greater *response* to surgery in these cases, merely greater levels both before and after it. Even this is not invariably the case: Ho *et al.* (1988) found such an association before, but not after in-patient wisdom tooth removal. They explained this by the evidence that Trait Anxiety is a predisposition to become anxious specifically in situations which involve diffuse psychological threat rather than the threat of physical trauma or pain. Trait Anxiety may therefore not be the best way of identifying patients who are at risk of intense anxiety responses to surgery.

More successful has been the use of a dispositional measure tailored to the situation. Martinez-Urrutia (1975) showed that an anxiety questionnaire that measured the disposition to anxiety about surgery was more predictive than was general Trait Anxiety of anxiety responses to surgery. This and similar results concerning other sources of stress have led Kendall (1978) to the view that an anxiety disposition only predicts State Anxiety in any situation when it is 'congruent' with that situation. Of course, as 'dispositional' measures become more situation-specific they become of less theoretical interest. In the absurd limiting case, the best dispositional predictor of anxiety in a situation is the disposition to become anxious in that particular situation! Against this, however, is the clinical absurdity of using a general personality scale to identify patients who will become anxious when some more specific questions would be more useful.

Since State Anxiety is not itself reliably associated with recovery, the postoperative effects of dispositional anxiety cannot be attributed to its association with State Anxiety. Mathews and Ridgeway (1981) suggested that Trait Anxiety might impair recovery by increasing the endocrine responses to surgery. More recent evidence suggests that this is unlikely. Salmon *et al.* (1989) found that, although Trait Anxiety predicted higher circulating noradrenaline levels preoperatively and three days postoperatively, it predicted lower circulating adrenaline levels before, during and after surgery, and lower cortisol levels postoperatively. The association of an anxious disposition with a lower cortisol response is hard to reconcile with existing evidence and theory (Frankenhaueser, 1980), but it is perhaps compatible with Janis' (1958) hypothesis of the stress-reducing effects of preoperative worry. The mechanisms which underly these effects of Trait Anxiety remain obscure however. Since Trait Anxiety has been shown to predict noradrenaline levels while patients were unconscious during surgery (Salmon *et al.*, 1989), it is possible that a constitutional difference between high and low Trait Anxious people underlies some of the results. Alternatively, differences in personality might lead to differences in medical treatment or nursing management which, in turn, influence the response to surgery.

10.4.4 Locus of control

A second personality dimension which has been applied to surgical patients because of its theoretical interest to psychologists is locus of control. People with internal locus of control believe that they have influence over the outcome of events; those with external locus of control believe that events are out of their control. Despite a great deal of research, there is little clear evidence that this dimension influences recovery (Mathews and Ridgeway, 1981). More specific scales concerned with beliefs in control over health and health care have been devised (Wallston, Wallston and DeVellis, 1978) but this writer's attempts to use them with abdominal surgical patients have been unsuccessful; patients have baulked at their length and the obscurity of the questions, and correlations with emotional or endocrine indices have been absent. It remains to be seen whether scales more specific to surgery would be more useful.

10.4.5 Type A personality

Type A personality describes people of extreme competitive drive, impatience and hostility. It has been associated with accentuated cardiovascular and catecholamine responses to psychologically stressful tasks in the laboratory and it has been identified as a risk factor for coronary heart disease although its status has been questioned (e.g. Myrtek and Greenlee, 1984). Kahn *et al.* (1980) found that Type A personality correlated with elevations of blood pressure during coronary artery bypass surgery; they suggested that Type A was associated with a 'constitutional' predisposition to accentuated responses, rather than causing such responses by conscious emotional or motivational mechanisms. Similar results were reported, also from patients undergoing cardiac surgery, by Krantz *et al.* (1982), but these findings could not be replicated in a subsequent report of herniorrhaphy and cholecystectomy patients (Kornfeld *et al.*, 1985). Blood pressure during surgery is a complex, multi-determined measure. Salmon *et al.* (1989) examined the endocrine responses which are major influences on the blood pressure response. Type A score correlated positively with circulating adrenaline levels postoperatively, but negatively with noradrenaline during surgery and afterwards. Contrary to the implication of Kornfeld *et al.*'s (1985) findings, this suggests that the importance of Type A personality extends beyond cardiac patients. Furthemore it appears to have different relationships with sympathetic (noradrenaline) and adrenomedullary (adrenaline) activation. As with Trait Anxiety, therefore, simple statements cannot be made about the beneficial or harmful effects of Type A personality on recovery.

10.4.6 Optimism

It is possible that the influence of personality on recovery extends beyond the traits that have traditionally featured in such research. For example, one rarely investigated personality dimension, optimism, has been related to recovery from cardiac surgery. Scheier and Carver (1987) found that dispositionally optimistic patients who underwent coronary artery bypass surgery were rated by care staff as recovering more quickly than less optimistic patients. In addition, they showed fewer ECG or biochemical signs of cardiac muscle damage during surgery.

10.4.7 Coping

Janis' (1958) account of the 'work of worry' was formulated in terms of patients' ways of coping with the threat of surgery rather than as the anxious emotional state with which it subsequently came to be identified. Worry meant taking an active, positive attitude to thinking through what was about to happen and developing realistic expectations of it. Since Janis' work, a number of investigators have continued to study psychological influences on recovery from the point of view of the patients' way of coping.

One way of dichotomizing coping styles has underpinned most of the work on this topic. Studies have compared, on the one hand, patients who cope with a stressor by avoiding thinking about it (termed 'avoidant' coping, or 'repression' in different theoretical schemes) and, on the other, people who confront it by finding out what they can and by using that information in thinking through what will – or may – happen ('vigilant' coping or 'sensitization'). These different patterns are typically regarded as stable traits or dispositions. Mathews and Ridgeway (1981) concluded that, on balance, the evidence suggests that avoidant patients fare better postoperatively. Discrepant findings have been reported, however: for example, Andrew (1970) found that both sensitizers and avoiders had shorter postoperative stays and requested less analgesic medication, by comparison with patients who could not be classified as belonging to either group. One reason for inconsistencies in the evidence may be the use of very different measurement procedures, based within different theoretical frameworks, and sometimes of uncertain reliability and validity. Recently, Miller (1987) has validated a questionnaire for distinguishing between coping styles which appears to be similar to those outlined above and might usefully be applied to surgical patients in future. She identifies 'monitors' as people who habitually cope with sources of stress by finding out what they can; blunters cope, by contrast, by distracting themselves. Steptoe and O'Sullivan (1986) demonstrated some validity for this distinction as applied to gynaecological surgery patients. For instance, monitors had learned more factual gynaecological knowledge than had blunters, and engaged in more health-related information-seeking behaviours (cervical smears and breast self-examination).

There are obvious limitations to treating coping as a dispositional, or personality, variable. That is, it does not allow for the possibility that a particular individual will cope differently with surgery and other stressors. This clearly cannot accommodate the observation that the seriousness of illness in hospital patients influences their way of coping (Feifel, Strack and Nagy, 1987a). An early report of a varied group of surgical patients directly compared the value of such dispositional measurements and 'situation-specific' assessments of patients' ways of coping with surgery and hospitalization. Vigilant and avoidant dispositions failed to predict outcome measures (postoperative stay, analgesic use and complications), but patients who had been rated by an interviewer preoperatively as coping vigilantly with the stress of hospitalization for surgery were discharged latest and developed the most postoperative complications (Cohen and Lazarus, 1973). Other evidence, from minor outpatient procedures, also suggests that assessments of how patients actually cope are superior to trait measures of usual coping style in predicting outcome (Kaloupek, White and Wong, 1984; Wong and Kaloupek, 1986). Overall, despite inconsistencies between results, studies of situation-specific coping conform to Mathews and Ridgeway's (1981) conclusion based on dispositional measures: patients faring worst on conventional measures of recovery tend to be vigilant copers (George *et al.*, 1980), even to the extent of 'catastrophizing' about what might go wrong (Chaves and Brown, 1987).

Although most studies have focused on vigilance and related concepts, it may be that quite separate ways of coping also have implications for recovery. A number of investigators have assessed a broad range of situation-specific modes of coping although, typically, styles related to vigilance and its converse feature prominently. Ho *et al.* (1988) identified a way of coping that they termed 'acquiescence', which was associated with lower distress following in-patient wisdom tooth removal. In general, passive, helpless coping with a variety of stressors is known to impair motivational state (Rosenberg *et al.*, 1988) and enhance adrenocortical responses to stress in man and animals (Frankenhaeuser, 1980). Intuitively, it is likely that surgical patients are often led to cope in this way by virtue of being denied opportunities for active involvement in their care. However whether 'active' or 'passive' coping affect physiological and psychological responses has not been studied in relation to surgery.

Mathews and Ridgeway (1981) argued that the apparent influence of coping on recovery could be attributed to the relationship of vigilant coping with anxious personality. However, the superiority of situation-specific over dispositional measures of coping argues against this. Moreover, in direct tests of this suggestion, measurements of coping and anxiety have been distinct (Ho *et al.*, 1988; Manyande and Salmon, 1992).

It is unlikely that simple conclusions about which is the most effective method of coping will ever be possible. Other research suggests that this will depend on specific properties of the surgery and situation. For instance, denial and avoidance may be effective responses to relatively short-term stressors or minor illnesses, but may prevent adaptation to longer-term stressors or more severe illnesses (Mullen and Suls, 1982; Feifel, Strack and Nagy, 1987b). It has also been argued that attempts at active coping – which may be effective in normal life – are counter-productive in hospital where the patient has no opportunity for participation or action (see Kaloupek, White and Wong, 1984). It is therefore important to examine what little is known about the influence of psychological aspects of the surgical ward setting on patients' recovery from surgery.

10.5　PSYCHOLOGICAL EFFECTS OF THE SURGICAL WARD

10.5.1　Control

This concerns patients' role in the organization of the ward and of their management. This might seem an inappropriate issue to discuss, if it is argued that patients are to be looked after by the experts and are neither competent, nor in some cases well enough, to play an active role. To adopt this view would be, however, to take a position of great psychological significance since a large literature attests to the harmful effects of being and feeling out of control of events. These extend from reduced pain tolerance (Seligman, 1975; Thompson, 1981) to increases in physiological or immunosuppressive responses to stress (Frankenhaueser, 1980). Apart from anecdotal material (e.g. Eisendrath, 1987), evidence in hospital patients is limited; but that which does exist is disturbing. DeWolfe, Barrel and Cummings (1966) measured feelings of comfort and distress in a sample of over 500 medical and surgical patients. The happier patients were those who were older and preferred an authoritarian staff approach. Consistent with this, Lorber (1975) found that the hospital patients who were judged 'problem' patients tended to be younger and better educated than 'good' patients. Taylor (1979) suggested that this was because such patients would want to be more involved in decisions over their treatment, and that this would lead to conflict with the hospital staff. By contrast, the acquiescent reaction of 'good' patients was likened to a state of helplessness. The view that successful adaptation to hospitalization for surgery entails giving up a feeling of being in control has received some empirical support. Raps *et al*. (1982) showed that medical patients' tendency to respond in a helpless way to an experimental stressor – loud noise – increased over the course of their stay in hospital; depressive symptoms increased in parallel. Rosenberg *et al*. (1988) confirmed that depression was associated with an absence of active coping efforts in medical patients.

There is one further, and possibly beneficial, consequence of surgical patients' dependent role that has rarely been considered systematically. The importance of a passive and dependent attitude to the doctor has been implicated in the placebo effect. However, although Ho *et al*. (1988) found that a placebo procedure (ultrasound treatment of zero intensity administered shortly after wisdom tooth removal) reduced postoperative facial swelling, they failed to detect any evidence that this was caused by an influence on coping.

10.5.2 Support in the surgical ward

Two types of social support are typically distinguished. Instrumental support refers to tangible, material forms of help and practical advice and obviously represents the doctors' and nurses' primary role. Expressive, or emotional, support is of more concern in the present context because of the evidence that its provision can reduce harmful psychological and physiological effects of stress (Cohen and Wills, 1985; Bovard, 1985). There is already evidence that the level of support that surgical patients feel that they have is related to their immunocompetence (Linn, Linn and Klimar, 1988; Levy *et al*, 1990). Therefore it is important that sufficient support should be available in the surgical ward. The central component of emotional support is the presence of someone who can communicate recognition of an individual's concerns and an acceptance that those concerns are genuine. Recognition of patients' concerns is not straightforward for staff caring for surgical patients, because the sources of patients' anxiety are so varied. They may be concerned that other diseases will be uncovered (Steptoe, Horti and Stanton, 1988) or, indeed, about factors unrelated to the surgery such as life at home in their absence (Volicer and Bohannon, 1975; Johnston, 1976, 1982; French, 1979; Ray, 1982).

Because of their continuous contact with their patients, nurses are in the best position of all carers to support surgical patients. However, it is unlikely that they are effective because the evidence is that they are poor at identifying the concerns that individual patients have. This conclusion emerged initially from Johnston's (1976) studies of the relationship between patients' own ratings of bodily and psychological state after gynaecological operations and their nurses' ratings of how they thought their patients felt. Nurses overestimated their patients' psychological distress and underestimated their physical complaints. Even apart from these systematic biases, the correlations between patients' ratings and nurses' estimates were very low. The nurses could not even accurately estimate the number of worries that individual patients identified on their questionnaires. Their only success was in recognizing worries which patients in general identified. That is, they apparently knew what an 'average' patient worried about, but they could not identify which patients worried and what they worried about. In a later study, using the same protocol, Johnston (1982) reported similar results. It might be hoped that a more encouraging picture would emerge should the study be repeated now but this is unlikely. Surgical nurses have also been found to assess their patients' level of pain inaccurately (Cohen, 1980; Teske, Daut and Cleeland, 1983) and these observations fit a general pattern of failure to perceive individual patients' concerns which characterizes nursing in different clinical areas (Davies and Peters, 1983; Bradley, Brewin and Duncan, 1983; Eddington *et al.*, 1990).

In her second study, however, Johnston (1982) showed that other patients, identified by the target patients in the same way as were the nurses – that is, as those with whom they had the most contact – identified the individual target patients' worries more accurately than did the nurses. The implication of these findings is that fellow patients may be particularly well placed to provide support (Kulik and Mahler, 1987).

Another source of support for patients is from outside the hospital. Frequent visits from spouses predicted faster recovery from cardiac surgery (measured by analgesic medication and postoperative stay, Kulik and Mahler, 1989), although it is likely that, in many cases, relatives are too distressed to provide support and the patient may feel obliged to support them. The emotional rapport which patients feel that they have with their doctor is also likely to be important; medical in-patients' perceptions of their physician's supportiveness were negatively related to their levels of depression in a study by Rosenberg *et al.* (1988).

10.6 PSYCHOLOGICAL PREPARATION TO FACILITATE RECOVERY FROM SURGERY

There are clearly two directions in which we can look for variables to manipulate in order to help surgical patients by psychological means. One approach is to try to change factors within the patients, in particular their ways of coping or their preoperative state, which are thought to influence recovery. Alternatively, we could remedy psychological deficits of the surgical ward setting, for example by allowing patients more feeling of control over their care, reducing sources of distress or arranging for better emotional support. It is striking that so much more effort has been targeted on to the patient variables than on to the situational factors. Fortunately, the effects of preoperative interventions have been reviewed repeatedly over recent years and a degree of consensus has developed about the relative efficacy of different types of approach (Kendall and Watson, 1981; Mathews and Ridgeway, 1984; Schultheis, Peterson and Selby, 1987; Weinman and Johnston, 1988; Kincey and Saltmore, 1990; Salmon, 1992).

10.6.1   Manipulating patients' preoperative emotional state

Interest in this derives from Janis' (1958) own suggestion as to how to facilitate mental preparation for surgery. He thought that, if patients had preoperatively been provided with information about what would happen to them, the 'work of worry' would be fostered and, as a result, their recovery facilitated. A second, and related theory, had proposed that postoperative distress would be reduced if patients accurately anticipated the pain and discomfort of surgery (Johnson and Leventhal, 1974). A large number of studies have therefore examined the effect of providing patients preoperatively with information about forthcoming events (see Suls and Wan, 1989).

It is clear that 'procedural' information – that is information which describes the events and procedures in an objective way from the observer's standpoint – is relatively ineffective. There is a little more support for the value of 'sensory' information – that is information about how the patient will feel, but this is largely from studies of patients undergoing minor investigative procedures such as endoscopy (Johnson and Leventhal, 1974) or barium enema (Wilson-Barnett, 1978). In the case of surgery, such information has less often been shown to be of value and has even been found to impede recovery (Langer, Janis and Wolfer, 1975). One problem may be that the information is intrinsically more distressing than for minor procedures. When patients undergoing major and minor surgery have been compared, information reduced distress only in the minor group (Lindeman and Stetzer, 1973). In a recent report, preoperative information facilitated patients' recovery from coronary artery bypass graft surgery (Anderson, 1987). In this case, however, the information went beyond what is normally entailed, by including filmed interviews with recovered patients. The equivocal status of information provision was foreseen by Janis himself (1971). He envisaged this as only one component of a package in which procedures to facilitate coping should also be included. In one report, doing so did indeed protect against harmful effects of information (Langer, Janis and Wolfer, 1975).

It is possible to be more specific about the type of patient who should benefit from information and those that may be harmed. First, information may counter the harmful effects of particularly high anxiety (Sime, 1976). Furthermore, it is likely that 'vigilant' patients benefit from being provided with information, whereas it may harm 'avoidant' ones; that is, the patients who normally cope with stress by gathering information may be helped while those who cope by ignoring information may be harmed (Mathews and Ridgeway, 1984). There are questionnaires which distinguish these two groups of patient. In practice, however, a rapid way of choosing the vigilant patients who should benefit from information could be simply to ask who would like it (Auerbach, Martelli and Mercuri, 1983).

It is possible that preparatory information works, when it does, according to the theoretical mechanisms outlined earlier: that is by fostering the work of worry or by improving the accuracy of patients' expectations of pain and discomfort. However, the evidence that we have seen for each of these theories is still very weak. Moreover, there is no evidence that the amount of information successfully communicated to the patient influences the effects of giving the information. In Andrew's (1970) study of hernia patients, in which hearing information about forthcoming surgery facilitated recovery in certain patients, there was, apparently, no correlation between this effect and the amount of the information which could be remembered. Information provision may therefore be merely a vehicle whereby some other process is facilitated.

One possible effect of giving information is to increase patients' feelings of being in control but, apart from one report that information can have this effect (Anderson, 1987), little evidence bears on the possibility. There is more evidence for an alternative explanation: that the provision of information conveys a degree of emotional support for the patient. Presenting information face-to-face as a social encounter has been shown to reduce postoperative anxiety more than by simply handing it over in a booklet (Leigh, Walker and Janaganathan, 1977) and there is evidence from minor, dental surgery that the effectiveness of information depended on the recipient's perception of the information-giver's warmth (Auerbach, Martelli and Mercuri, 1983). From studies of dental surgery it is also known that patients' postoperative adjustment is related to their perception of their surgeons' friendliness (Auerbach *et al.*, 1984). Giving information might therefore be seen by patients as a 'friendly' act and thereby increase their feeling of being supported. In most studies, it is unlikely that the general or irrelevant information received by control groups is able to control for this effect.

There are therefore a number of distinct ways in which receiving information preoperatively might help patients. At least in those who normally seek information to cope with stress, it may directly help to alleviate distress and facilitate other aspects of recovery. For other patients it might provide a way of communicating emotional support, provided that the information is not so distressing that it increases anxiety in patients who prefer not to find out about forthcoming stressors. Moreover, patients still value information as 'useful', even where no other effect can be detected (Ridgeway and Mathews, 1982).

10.6.2 Manipulating patients' way of coping with surgery

Providing information is a procedure which accepts, and may even reinforce, the passive role of patients as inactive recipients of expertise. An alternative procedure, which challenges this view, is a much more powerful facilitator of recovery. Postoperative pain and distress have been reduced in patients undergoing various types of surgery who have been trained preoperatively in cognitive coping techniques which are intended to help them to restrain, reinterpret or distract themselves from their distressing thoughts (Langer, Janis and Wolfer, 1975; Pickett and Clum, 1982; Ridgeway and Mathews, 1982; Wallace, 1984, Wells *et al.*, 1986; Anderson, 1987). In three of these studies, coping training was shown to be more effective than information-provision (Langer, Janis and Wolfer, 1975; Wilson, 1981 and Ridgeway and Mathews, 1982); in a fourth (Anderson, 1987), it was non-significantly more effective.

It is also possible to attribute the postoperative benefits (reduced infection rate and urinary cortisol excretion) of Boore's (1978) preoperative preparation of abdominal surgery patients to her having taught active (although not cognitive) coping techniques. The main ingredients of this were simple breathing and muscular exercises. Although it is not clear whether their effects might have been mediated physiologically, other evidence indicates that the cortisol response to a stressor should be reduced by giving people a feeling that they have some control (Frankenhaueser, 1980). In this context, it is interesting that an opposite difference in urinary cortisol excretion between prepared and non-prepared ear surgery patients was seen in an uncontrolled study by Salmon, Evans and Humphrey (1986). The prepared patients, although tending to be less anxious preoperatively, showed greater cortisol levels postoperatively than did patients experiencing more traditional nursing care in a different ward. The authors speculated that this might have resulted from encouragement of passivity by the emphasis in the nurses' preparation on the patients' compliance with nursing and medical requests.

Mathews and Ridgeway (1984) suggested that one potential advantage of cognitive coping procedures might be that, by contrast with the provision of information, they benefit vigilant and avoidant people equally. Little evidence in surgical in-patients bears on this. However, a study of dental out-patients suggests that this might not prove to be the case (Martelli *et al.*, 1987); it was the patients who preferred to have information who benefited most from a preoperative training designed to facilitate the patients' active attempts to cope. Further evidence that people differ in the value they gain from attempts to induce active cognitive coping emerged from Pickett and Clum's (1982) demonstration that cognitive coping skills training reduced postoperative anxiety in cholecystectomy patients: the effect was greatest in those with internal locus of control. Nevertheless, despite differing effectiveness in different sorts of patient, there remains no evidence that any type of patient can be harmed by coping training. Clinically, this is an important advantage over information provision.

There is too little evidence to suggest the mechanism through which cognitive coping training has its postoperative benefits. The most obvious possibility is that these result from an enhancement of feelings of being able to cope or of being in control. The interaction with locus of control, described above, is consistent with this. However, it is not clear that patients have to learn the specific coping techniques that are taught. It might well be enough that they *feel* that they have learned a coping strategy. Indeed, it is hard to imagine that much coping is learned during the brief periods of preparation that characterize this approach. A different mechanism that could be at work is the provision of support: it might be suspected that being taught an active skill by another person involves more two-way interaction even than does the provision of information and may therefore be seen by the patient as intensely supportive. Clearly, evidence is needed as to whether the sort of help that patients feel they have received resembles what the researchers think that they have given.

10.6.3   Relaxation

Training in simple relaxation skills is often envisaged as a form of training in coping, and is sometimes a component of coping skills training procedures. Even alone, it has been effective. It has reduced postoperative pain and medication use in a sample of cholecystectomy, herniorrhaphy and haemorrhoidectomy patients (Flaherty and Fitzpatrick, 1978). A report that it apparently shortened the duration of open heart surgery and reduced the volume of blood transfused (Aiken and Henrichs, 1971) should be treated with caution as the intervention was poorly controlled. In Wilson's (1981) study of abdominal surgery, postoperative analgesia was reduced, and self-reported postoperative mental and physical state were improved. However, urinary adrenaline levels were increased, indicating a greater stress response. Wilson attributed this to relaxation acting as an active coping task and there is other evidence that active coping tasks which people find difficult can increase sympatho-adrenal stress responses (Steptoe, 1983). Nevertheless, it is not clear that relaxation represents an active coping procedure. In a trial of minor abdominal surgery, Manyande *et al.* (1992) found that relaxation senstitized the plasma adrenaline and cortisol responses to surgery, despite reducing anxiety and analgesic use postoperatively. They speculated that relaxation training encouraged a passive, dependent attitude, perhaps antagonistic to the 'work of worry' described by Janis (1958), and thereby increased the stressfulness of surgery. Regardless of the explanation, these results confirm an association between better subjective state and greater adrenaline or cortisol responses (Salmon, Evans and Humphrey, 1986; Salmon *et al.*, 1988, 1989). Until the effects on clinical outcome of manipulating the stress response are clearly established, the use of relaxation or, indeed, of any other procedure intended to reduce patients' preoperative anxiety, should therefore be regarded as experimental.

10.6.4 Suggestion

A few patients can apparently be satisfactorily anaesthetized by hypnotic suggestion alone (Gibson and Heap, 1991). For the majority of surgical patients, however, suggestion should be regarded as a possible adjunct to more conventional procedures. There is some evidence that, given preoperatively, suggestions of improved recovery are followed by lower anxiety or less demand for analgesia. Where suggestion departs from other psychological techniques is in its potential for use during surgery when the patient is unconscious. However, despite some positive results (Evans and Richardson, 1988), this technique has not generally been shown to be effective (Block *et al.*, 1991; Liu, Standen and Aitkenhead, 1992).

It is important for future research to ascertain the extent to which suggestion merely changes patients' self-presentation or modifies underlying state. McClintock *et al.* (1990) found that hysterectomy patients receiving positive intraoperative suggestion apparently required somewhat less analgesia postoperatively, but did not experience less pain than controls according to visual-analogue self-ratings. There is a great deal of evidence that patients receive less analgesia postoperatively than is available, and therefore experience more pain than is necessary (Royal College of Surgeons of England, 1990). It is likely that, in part, this reflects their response to informal suggestion from various sources within and outside the surgical ward that they can and should bear the pain with the minimum of assistance.

10.6.5 Support

To date, the only preparatory procedure which directly reflects our analysis of the psychological deficits of surgical ward routine is the provision of additional social support for patients. Indeed, the first report that a psychological technique could facilitate recovery was, essentially, an account of the provision of emotional support. Egbert *et al.* (1963, 1964) demonstrated a number of benefits of a preoperative visit from an anaesthetist in two separate studies. Visited patients were judged to be calmer on the day of surgery than those who received a barbiturate premedication (Egbert, 1963), and required less morphine analgesia and had shorter postoperative stays than a routine control group (Egbert, 1964). The importance of the anaesthetist's visit as a social encounter was confirmed by Leigh, Walker and Janaganathan (1977), who found it to be more effective at reducing postoperative anxiety than simply presenting a booklet with the same information.

Around the time that researchers were approaching the issue of support from an anaesthetist's point of view, nursing researchers were making similar suggestions. Dumas and Leonard (1963) reported on having a nurse accompany gynaecology patients for an hour or so before surgery, during which time she assessed and managed their sources of distress. The effect was to reduce the incidence of vomiting in the recovery room immediately after surgery. Nursing researchers have also been concerned with enlisting fellow patients to provide support. In a comparison of group with individual preparation (which included information provision and teaching of specific postoperative exercises), Lindeman (1972) found that the group-prepared patients were discharged sooner than the individually prepared controls. In a subsequent report of group preparation in which the nurse merely facilitated a discussion between the patients, these patients were discharged sooner than routinely managed controls, received less analgesia and experienced less urinary retention (Schmitt and Woolridge, 1973).

10.6.6 Choice and control

The final subject of this review, although arguably the most provocative, is the least well researched. By comparison with teaching patients strategies to control their distressing thoughts, allowing them influence over more tangible aspects of their care has more profound implications for clinical and nursing practice. The reports which are now available do, however, suggest that the potential benefits are great. Firstly, even decisions over relatively trivial aspects of care can be of value. In an extreme demonstration of this, Totman (1976) reported that the benefits of a placebo hypnotic in surgical patients were enhanced in patients who had been asked to choose one of two placebos. When more profound choices over type of treatment have been evaluated, benefits have also been reported. Morris and Royle (1988) compared women who were asked to choose between 'lumpectomy' and mastectomy for breast cancer to those whose operation was chosen by the surgeon. They found lower levels of depression and anxiety preoperatively and two months postoperatively in women who chose and in their husbands. The patients were not, however, randomly allocated: women were ascribed to the choice and no-choice conditions according to the precise location of their tumour. There is other support for the view that patients' control over treatment for breast cancer is beneficial for postoperative psychological morbidity (Leinster, personal communication), although controlled evidence is awaited.

10.7   CONCLUSION: HOW SHOULD PATIENTS BE PREPARED PSYCHOLOGICALLY?

One approach to summarizing the evidence has been to submit all available studies to meta-analysis (Mumford, Schlesinger and Glass, 1982; Devine and Cook, 1983), which expresses average effect sizes in terms of the variability between patients in outcome measures. Since it is apparent that many negative results exist which have never been published, the apparent precision of this approach may be spurious. It is more useful to identify the trends which have become clear in the evidence. First, the provision of information is an unreliable strategy. Certainly, patients have a right to receive information if they so desire, but general policies regarding information should be seen as an ethical rather than psychological matter. From a psychological point of view, individual differences are crucial in predicting the effects of information: some patients will be helped and others harmed. Nevertheless, although information generally has no net effect across samples of patients undergoing major surgery, it is more likely to benefit patients undergoing relatively minor procedures.

Much more effective have been attempts to inculcate in the patient an attitude that they can actively cope with the surgery. Although it is possible that the effects of this depend on individual differences, definitive information is not yet available. These procedures – information provision and coping skills training – have arisen from the application of psychological ideas. By contrast, supportive approaches, although less carefully specified in psychological terms, are extensions of nursing and anaesthetic practice and may therefore be more successfully incorporated into existing ward practice. It is possible, also, that patients' perception of psychological procedures as supportive underlies or contributes to their effects. It should be stressed that support does not entail reassurance. Indeed, by encouraging unrealistically optimistic expectations, or by communicating a lack of empathy with patients' worries, attempts at reassurance might well be counter-productive. A focus on support would remedy one of the principal psychological deficits of the surgical ward. To remedy the remaining deficit – the lack of opportunity for patients to exert influence over their own lives – is more challenging to the professionals' expert role and its effects remain to be fully tested.

There remains, however, a serious threat to the validity of these recommendations. This arises from the limited range of outcome measures. Studies in which a physiological outcome index has been chosen for its unambiguous importance to recovery are the exception. Some clearly beneficial effects have been reported: for example, postoperative vomiting has been reduced (Dumas and Leonard, 1963) and hypertension has been reduced after cardiac surgery (Anderson, 1987). It is, however, more typical to find effects on measures that are, as discussed above, of uncertain significance, such as postoperative stay or analgesic requests. There are two responses which future research could make to this. One is to measure recovery in ways that unambiguously reflect the patients' interests, such as quality of life or well-being. The second is to focus on the processes that are thought to mediate recovery from surgery – for example the endocrine and metabolic responses – and investigate how psychological factors interact with these.

REFERENCES

Aiken, L. H. and Henrichs, T. F. (1971) Systematic relaxation as a nursing intervention technique with open heart surgery patients. *Nursing Research,* **20**, 212–17.

Anand, K. J. S. (1986) The stress response to surgical trauma: from physiological basis to therapeutic implications. *Progress in Food and Nutrition Science,* **10**, 67–132.

Anderson, E. A. (1987) Preoperative preparation for cardiac surgery facilitates recovery, reduces psychological distress, and reduces the incidence of acute postoperative hypertension. *Journal of Consulting and Clinical Psychology,* **55**, 514–20.

Andrew, J. M. (1970) Recovery from surgery, with and without preparatory instruction, for three coping styles. *Journal of Personality and Social Psychology,* **15**, 223–6.

Auerbach, S. M. (1973) Trait-state anxiety and adjustment to surgery. *Journal of Consulting and Clinical Psychology,* **40**, 264–71.

Auerbach, S. M., Martelli, M. F. and Mercuri, L. G. (1983) Anxiety, information, interpersonal impacts, and adjustment to a stressful health care situation. *Journal of Personality and Social Psychology,* **44**, 1284–96.

Auerbach, S. M., Meredith, J., Alexander, J. M. *et al.* (1984) Psychological factors in adjustment to orthognathic surgery. *Journal of Oral Maxillofacial Surgery,* **42**, 435–40.

Baron, J-F, Bertrand, M., Barre, E. *et al.* (1991) Combined epidural and general anesthesia versus general anesthesia for abdominal aortic surgery. *Anesthesiology,* **75**, 611–18.

Block, R. I., Ghoneim, M. M., Sum Ping, S. T. *et al.* (1991) Efficacy of therapeutic suggestions for improved postoperative recovery presented during general anesthesia. *Anesthesiology,* **75**, 746–55.

Boore, J. R. P. (1978) *Prescription for Recovery: the Effects of Pre-operative Prep-*

arations of Surgical Patients on Post-operative Stress, Recovery and Infection, Royal College of Nursing, London.

Bovard, E. W. (1985) Brain mechanisms in effects of social support on viability, in *Perspectives on Behavioral Medicine*, Vol. 2, (ed R. B. Williams), Academic Press, New York, pp 103–29.

Bradley, C., Brewin, C. and Duncan, S. L. B. (1983) Perceptions of labour: discrepancies between midwives' and patients' ratings. *British Journal of Obstetrics and Gynaecology*, **90**, 1176–9.

Brown, J. M. and Grosso, M. A. (1989) Cytokines, sepsis and the surgeon. *Surgery, Gynecology and Obstetrics*, **169**, 568–75.

Bursten, B. and Russ, J. J. (1965) Preoperative psychological state and corticosteroid levels of surgical patients. *Psychosomatic Medicine*, **27**, 309–16.

Chapman, C. R. and Cox, G. B. (1977) Determinants of anxiety in elective surgery patients, in *Stress and Anxiety*, Vol. 4, (eds C. D. Spielberger and I. G. Sarason), Hemisphere, Washington, pp. 269–90.

Chaves, J. F. and Brown, J. M. (1987) Spontaneous cognitive strategies for the control of clinical pain and distress. *Journal of Behavioral Medicine*, **10**, 263–76.

Chernow, B., Alexander, R., Smallridge, R. C. *et al*. (1987) Hormonal response to graded stress. *Archives of Internal Medicine*, **147**, 1273–8.

Christensen, T., Bendix, T. and Kehlet, H. (1982) Fatigue and cardiorespiratory function following abdominal surgery. *British Journal of Surgery*, **69**, 417–19.

Christensen, T., Hjortso, E., Mortensen, E. *et al*. (1986) Fatigue and anxiety in surgical patients. *Acta Psychiatrica Scandinavica*, **73**, 76–9.

Cohen, F. and Lazarus, R. S. (1973). Active coping processes, coping dispositions, and recovery from surgery. *Psychosomatic Medicine*, **35**, 375–9.

Cohen, F. L. (1980) Post-surgical pain relief: patients' status and nurses' medication choices. *Pain*, **9**, 265–74.

Cohen, S. and Wills, T. A. (1985) Stress, social support, and the buffering hypothesis. *Psychological Bulletin*, **98**, 310–57.

Davies, A. D. M. and Peters, M. P. (1983) Stresses of hospitalization in the elderly: nurses' and patients' perceptions. *Journal of Advanced Nursing*, **8**, 99–105.

Dean, C. and Surtees, P. G. (1989) Do psychological factors predict survival in breast cancer? *Journal of Psychosomatic Research*, **33**, 561–9.

Devine, E. C. and Cook, T. D. (1983) A meta-analytic analysis of effects of psychoeducational interventions on length of postsurgical hospital stay. *Nursing Research*, **32**, 267–74.

DeWolfe, A. S., Barrel, R. P. and Cummings, J. W. (1966) Patient variables in emotional response to hospitalization for physical illness. *Journal of Consulting and Clinical Psychology*, **30**, 68–72.

Dumas, R. G. and Leonard, R. C. (1963) The effect of nursing on the incidence of postoperative vomiting. *Nursing Research*, **12**, 12–15.

Eddington, C., Piper, J., Tanna, B. *et al*. (1990) Relationships between happiness, behavioural status and dependency on others in elderly patients. *British Journal of Clinical Psychology*, **29**, 43–50.

Egbert, L. D., Battit, G. E., Turndorf, H. *et al*. (1963) The value of the preoperative visit by an anaesthetist. *Journal of the American Medical Association* **185**, 553–5.

Egbert, L. D., Battit, G. E., Welch, C. E. *et al*. (1964) Reduction of postoperative pain by encouragement and instruction of patients. *New England Journal of Medicine*, **270**, 825–7.

Eisendrath, S. J. (1987) Issues of control in the general hospital surgical setting. *International Journal of Psychosomatics*, **34**, 3–5.

Ellis, F. R. and Humphrey, D. E. (1982) Clinical aspects of endocrine and metabolic changes relating to anaesthesia and surgery, in *Trauma, Stress and Immunity in Anaesthesia and Surgery*, (eds J. Watkins and M. Salo), Butterworth: London, pp. 189–208.

Evans, C. and Richardson, P. H. (1988) Improved recovery and reduced post-operative stay after therapeutic suggestions during general anaesthesia. *Lancet*, **2**, 491–3.

Feifel, H., Strack, S. and Nagy, V. T. (1987a) Degree of life threat and differential use of coping modes. *Journal of Psychosomatic Research*, **31**, 91–9.

Feifel, H., Strack, S. and Nagy, V. T. (1987b) Coping strategies and associated features of medically ill patients. *Psychosomatic Medicine*, **49**, 616–15.

Flaherty, G. G. and Fitzpatrick, R. (1978) Relaxation technique to increase comfort level of postoperative patients: a preliminary study. *Nursing Research*, **27**, 352–5.

Folkard, S., Simpson, J. E. P. and Glynn, C. J. (1979) The short- and long-term recovery of mental abilities following minor surgery using different anaesthetic agents, in *Research in Psychology and Medicine, Vol 1. Physical Aspects: Pain, Stress, Diagnosis and Organic Damage*, (eds S. J. Oborne, M. M. Gruneberg and J. R. Eiser), Academic Press: London, pp. 426–33.

Frankenhaueser, M. (1980) Psychobiological aspects of life stress, in *Nato Conference on Coping and Health*, (eds S. Levine and H. Ursin), Academic Press, New York, pp. 203–23.

French, K. (1979) Some anxieties of elective surgery patients and the desire for reasurance and information, in *Research in Psychology and Medicine, Col. 2: Social Aspects: Attitudes, Communication, Care and Training*, (eds D. J. Oborne, M. M. Gruneberg and J. R. Eiser), Academic Press, London, pp. 336–43.

George, J. M., Scott, D. S., Turner, S. P. *et al.* (1980) The effects of psychological factors and physical trauma on recovery from oral surgery. *Journal of Behavioral Medicine*, **3**, 291–310.

Gibson, H. B. and Heap, M. (1991) *Hypnosis in Therapy*, Lawrence Erlbaum: Hillsdale, NJ.

Hall, G. M. (1985) The anaesthetic modification of the endocrine and metabolic response to surgery. *Annals of the Royal College of Surgeons of England*, **67**, 25–9.

Ho, K. H., Hashish, I., Salmon, P. *et al.* (1988) A placebo effect on post-operative swelling. *Journal of Psychosomatic Research*, **25**, 135–41.

Janis, I. L. (1958) *Psychological Stress*, Wiley, New York.

Janis, I. L. (1971) *Stress and Frustration*, Harcourt Brace Jovanovich, New York.

Johnson, J. E. (1973) The effects of accurate expectations on the sensory and distress components of pain. *Journal of Personality and Social Psychology*, **27**, 261–75.

Johnson, J. E. and Leventhal, H. (1974) Effects of accurate expectations and behavioral instructions on reactions during a noxious medical examination. *Journal of Personality and Social Psychology*, **29**, 710–18.

Johnson, J. E., Leventhal, H. and Dabbs, J. M. (1971) Contribution of emotional and instrumental response processes in adaptation to surgery. *Journal of Personality and Social Psychology*, **20**, 55–64.

Johnston, M. (1976) Communication of patients' feelings in hospital, in *Commmunication between Doctors and Patients*, (ed M. Bennett), OUP, Oxford, pp 31–43.

Johnston, M. (1980) Anxiety in surgical patients. *Psychological Medicine*, **10**, 145–52.

Johnston, M. (1981) Emotional distress immediately following surgery, in *Behavioural Medicine* (eds J. W. G. Tiller and P. R. Marhi), Geigy, Melbourne.

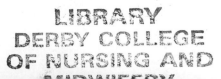

Johnston, M. (1982) Recognition of patients' worries by nurses and by other patients. *British Journal of Clinical Psychology*, **21**, 255–61.

Johnston, M. (1984) Dimensions of recovery from surgery. *International Review of Applied Psychology*, **33**, 505–20.

Johnston, M. and Carpenter, L. (1980) Relationship between pre-operative anxiety and post-operative state. *Psychological Medicine*, **10**, 361–7.

Johnston, M. and Jones, M. L. (1979) Evaluating the care of post-surgical patients in the community hospital, in *Research in Psychology and Medicine, Vol 2, Social Aspects: Attitudes, Communication, Care and Training*, (eds D. J. Oborne, M. M. Gruneberg and J. R. Eiser), Academic Press, London, pp. 353–60.

Kahn, J. P., Kornfeld, D. S., Frank, K. A. *et al.* (1980) Type A behavior and blood pressure during coronary artery bypass surgery. *Psychosomatic Medicine*, **42**, 407–14.

Kaloupek, D. G., White, H. and Wong, M. (1984) Multiple assessment of coping strategies used by volunteer blood donors: implications for preparatory training. *Journal of Behavioral Medicine*, **7**, 35–60.

Kaufman, L. (1982) The endocrine response to surgery and anaesthesia, in *Scientific Foundations of Anaesthesia*, (eds C. A. Scurr and S. Feldman), Heineman: London, pp. 290–307.

Kehlet, H. (1984) The stress response to anaesthesia and surgery: release mechanisms and modifying factors. *Clinics in Anaesthesiology*, **2**, 315–39.

Kehlet, H. (1989) Surgical stress: the role of pain and analgesia *British Journal of Anaesthesia*, **63**, 189–95.

Kelly, M. P. (1987) Managing radical surgery: notes from the patient's viewpoint. *Gut*, **28**, 81–7.

Kendall, P. C. (1978) Anxiety: states, traits-situations? *Journal of Consulting and Clinical Psychology*, **46**, 280–7.

Kendall, P. C. and Watson, D. W. (1981) Psychological preparation for stressful medical procedures. In *Medical Psychology: Contributions to Behavioural Medicine* (eds C. K. Prokop and L. A. Bradley), Academic Press: New York, pp. 197–221.

Kincey, J. and Saltmore, S. (1990) Surgical treatments, in *Stress and Medical Procedures*, (eds M. Johnston and L. Wallace), Oxford University Press, Oxford, pp. 120–37.

Kornfeld, D. S., Kahn, J. P., Frank, K. A. *et al.* (1985) Type A behavior and blood pressure during general surgery. *Psychosomatic Medicine*, **47**, 234–41.

Krantz, D. S., Arabian, J. M., Davin, J. E. *et al.* (1982) Type A behavior and coronary bypass surgery: intraoperative blood pressure and perioperative complications. *Psychosomatic Medicine*, **44**, 273–84.

Kulik, J. A. and Mahler, H. I. M. (1987) Effects of preoperative roommate assignment on preoperative anxiety and recovery from coronary-bypass surgery. *Health Psychology*, **6**, 525–43.

Kulik, J. A. and Mahler, H. I. (1989) Social support and recovery from surgery. *Health Psychology*, **8**, 221–38.

Lange, E. J., Janis, I. L. and Wolfer, J. A. (1975) Reduction of psychological stress in surgical patients. *Journal of Experimental Social Psychology*, 155–65.

Leigh, J. M., Walker, J. and Janaganathan, P. (1977) Effect of preoperative anaesthetic visit on anxiety. *British Medical Journal*, **2**, 987–9.

Levy, S. M., Herberman, R. B., Whiteside, T. *et al.* (1990) Perceived social support and tumor estrogen/progesterone receptor status as predictors of natural killer cell activity in breast cancer patients. *Psychosomatic Medicine*, **52**, 73–85.

Lindeman, C. A. (1972) Nursing intervention with the pre-surgical patient. *Nursing Research*, **21**, 196–209.

Lindeman, C. A. and Stetzer, S. L. (1973) Effects of preoperative visits by operating room nurses. *Nursing Research*, **22**, 4–15.

Linn, B. S., Linn, M. W. and Klimas, N. G. (1988) Effects of psychophysical stress on surgical outcome. *Psychosomatic Medicine*, **50**, 230–44.

Liu, W. H. D., Standen, P.J. and Aitkenhead, A. R. (1992) Therapeutic suggestions during general anaesthesia in patients undergoing hysterectomy. *British Journal of Anaesthesia*, **68**, 277–81.

Lorber, J. (1975) Good patients and problem patients: conformity and deviance in a general hospital. *Journal of Health and Social Behaviour*, **16**, 213–25.

Manyande, A. and Salmon, P. (1992) Recovery from minor abdominal surgery a preliminary attempt to separate anxiety and coping. *British Journal of Clinical Psychology*, **31**, 227–37.

Manyande, A., Chayen, S., Priyakumar, P. *et al.* (1992) Anxiety and endocrine responses to surgery: paradoxical effects of preoperative relaxation training. *Psychosomatic Medicine*, **54**, 275–87.

Martelli, M. F., Auerbach, M., Alexander, J. *et al.* (1987) Stress Management in the health care setting: matching interventions with patient coping styles. *Journal of Consulting and Clinical Psychology* **55**, 201–7.

Martinez-Urrutia, A. (1975) Anxiety and pain in surgical patients. *Journal of Consulting and Clinical Psychology*, **43**, 437–42.

Mathews, A. and Ridgeway, V. (1981) Personality and surgical recovery: a review. *British Journal of Clinical Psychology*, **20**, 243–60.

Mathews, A. and Ridgeway, V. (1984) Psychological preparation for surgery, in *Health Care and Human Behaviour*, (eds A. Steptoe and A. Mathews), Academic Press: London, pp. 231–59.

Mclintock, T. T. C., Aitken, H., Downie, C. F. A. *et al.* (1990) Postoperative analgesic requirements in patients exposed to positive intraoperative suggestions. *British Medical Journal*, **301**, 788–90.

Miller, S. M. (1987) Monitoring and blunting: validation of a questionnaire to assess styles of information seeking under threat. *Journal of Personality and Social Psychology*, **52**, 345–53.

Morris, J. and Royle, G. T. (1988) Offering patients a choice of surgery for early breast cancer: a reduction in anxiety and depression in patients and their husbands. *Social Science and Medicine*, **26**, 583–5.

Mulen, B. and Suls, J. (1982) The effectiveness of attention and rejection as coping styles: a meta-analysis of temporal differences. *Journal of Psychosomatic Research*, **26**, 43–9.

Mumford, E., Schlesinger, H. J. and Glass, G. V. (1982) The effects of psychological intervention on recovery from surgery and heart attacks. An analysis of the literature. *American Journal of Health*, **72**, 141–51.

Myrtek, M and Greenlee, M. W. (1984) Psychophysiology of Type A behavior pattern: a critical analysis. *Journal of Psychosomatic Research*, **28**, 455–66.

Nistrup-Madsen, S. Fog-Moller, F., Christiansen, C. *et al.* (1978) Cyclic AMP, adrenaline and noradrenaline in plasma during surgery. *British Journal of Surgery*, **65**, 191–3.

Pickett, C. and Clum, G. A. (1982) Comparative treatment strategies and their interaction with locus of control in the reduction of post-surgical pain and anxiety. *Journal of Consulting and Clinical Psychology*, **50**, 439–41.

Plumpton, F. S., Besser, G. M. and Cole, P. V. (1969) Corticosteroid treatment and surgery. 1 An investigation of the indications for steroid cover. *Anaesthesia*, **21**, 3–11.

Raps, C. S., Peterson, C., Jonas, M. *et al.* (1982) Patient behavior in hospitals:

helplessness, reactance, or both? *Journal of Personality and Social Psychology*, **42**, 1036–41.

Ray, C. (1982) The surgical patient: psychological stress and coping resources, in *Social Psychology and Behavioral Medicine* (ed. J. R. Eiser), Wiley, Chichester, pp. 483–507.

Ray, C. and Fitzgibbon, G. (1981) Stress arousal and coping with surgery. *Psychological Medicine*, **11**, 741–6.

Ridgeway, V. and Mathews, A. (1982) Psychological preparation for surgery: a comparison of methods. *British Journal of Clinical Psychology*, **21**, 271–80.

Rose, E. A. and King, T. C. (1978) Understanding post-operative fatigue. *Surgery, Gynecology and Obstetrics*, **147**, 97–101.

Rosenberg, S. J., Peterson, R. A., Hayes, J. R. *et al.* (1988) Depression in medical inpatients. *British Journal of Medical Psychology*, **61**, 245–54.

Royal College of Surgeons of England (1990) *Pain After Surgery: Report of Working Party*, Royal College of Surgeons, London.

Salmon, P. (1992) Psychological factors in surgical stress: implications for management. *Clinical Psychology Review*, **12**, 681–704.

Salmon, P., Evans, R. and Humphrey, D. (1986) Anxiety and endocrine changes in surgical patients. *British Journal of Clinical Psychology*, **25**, 135–41.

Salmon, P. and Kaufman, L. (1990) Preoperative anxiety and endocrine response to surgery. *Lancet*, **335**, 1340.

Salmon, P., Pearce, S., Smith, C. C. T. *et al.* (1988) The relationship of pre-operative distress to endocrine and subjective responses to surgery: support for Janis' theory. *Journal of Behavioural Medicine*, **11**, 599–613.

Salmon, P., Pearce, S., Smith, C. C. T. *et al.* (1989) Anxiety, Type A personality and endocrine responses to surgery. *British Journal of Clinical Psychology*, **28**, 279–80.

Salo, M. (1982) Effects of anaesthesia and surgery on the immune response, in *Trauma, Stress and Immunity in Anaesthesia and Surgery*, (eds J. Watkins and M. Salo), Butterworth, London, pp 211–53.

Scheier, M. F. and Carver, C. S. (1987) Dispositional optimism and physical well-being: the influence of generalized outcome expectancies on health. *Journal of Personality*, **55**, 169–210.

Schmitt, F. E. and Wooldridge, P. J. (1973) Psychological preparation of surgical patients. *Nursing Research*, **22**, 108–16.

Schultheis, K., Peterson, L. and Selby, V. (1987) Preparation for stressful medical procedures and person x treatment interactions. *Clinical Psychology Review*, **7**, 329–52,

Seligman, M. E. P. (1975) *Helplessness*, Freeman, San Francisco.

Selye, H. (1976) *The Stress of Life*, McGraw-Hill, New York.

Sime, A. M. (1976) Relationship of pre-operative fear, type of coping, and information received about surgery to recovery from surgery. *Journal of Personality and Social Psychology*, **34**, 716–24.

Spielberger, C. D., Auerbach, S., Wadsworth, M. *et al.* (1973) Emotional reactions to surgery. *Journal of Consulting and Clinical Psychology*, **40**, 33–8.

Spielberger, C. D., Gorsuch, R. K. L. and Lushene, R. E. (1970) *Manual for the State-Trait Anxiety Inventory*. Consulting Psychologists' Press, Palo Alto, CA.

Steptoe, A. (1983) Stress, helplessness and control: the implications of laboratory studies. *Journal of Psychosomatic Research*, **27**, 361–7.

Steptoe, A., Horti, J. and Stanton, S. (1988) Concern about cancer in women undergoing elective gynaecological surgery. *Social Science and Medicine*, **26**, 863–73.

Steptoe, A. and O'Sullivan, J. (1986) Monitoring and blunting coping styles in women prior to surgery. *British Journal of Clinical Psychology*, **25**, 143–4.

Suls, J. and Wan, C. K. (1989) Effects of sensory and procedural information on coping with stressful medical procedures and pain: a meta-analysis. *Journal of Consulting and Clinical Psychology*, **57**, 372–9.

Taylor, S. E. (1979) Hospital patient behavior; reactance, helplessness, or control? *Journal of Social Issues*, **35**, 156–84.

Teske, K., Daut, R. L. and Cleeland, C. S. (1983) Relationships between nurses' observations and patients' self-reports of pain. *Pain*, **16**, 289–96.

Thompson, S. C. (1981) Will it hurt less if I can control it? A complex answer to a simple question. *Psychological Bulletin*, **90**, 89–101.

Totman, R. (1976) Cognitive dissonance in the placebo treatment of insomnia – a pilot experiment. *British Journal of Medical Psychology*, **49**, 393–400.

Udelsman, R., Norton, J. A., Jelenich, S. E. *et al.* (1987) Responses of the hypothalamic-pituitary-adrenal and renin-angiotensin axes and the sympathetic system during controlled surgical and anaesthetic stress. *Journal of Clinical Endocrinology and Metabolism*, **64**, 986–94.

Vogele, C. and Steptoe, A. (1986) Physiological and subjective stress responses in surgical patients. *Journal of Psychosomatic Research*, **30**, 205–15.

Volicer, B. J. and Bohannon, M. W. (1975) A hospital stress rating scale. *Nursing Research*, **24**, 352–9.

Wallace, L. M. (1984) Psychological preparation as a method of reducing the stress of surgery. *Journal of Human Stress*, **10**, 62–77.

Wallace, L. M. (1985) Surgical patients' expectations of pain and discomfort: does accuracy of expectations minimise post-surgical pain and distress. *Pain*, **22**, 363–73.

Wallace, L. M. (1986) Pre-operative state anxiety as a mediator of psychological adjustment to and recovery from surgery. *British Journal of Medical Psychology*, **59**, 253–61.

Wallston, K. A., Wallston, B. S. and DeVellis, R. (1978) Development of the multidimensional health locus of control scales. *Health Education Monographs*, **6**, 161–70.

Walton, B. (1978) Anaesthesia, surgery and immunology. *Anaesthesia*, **33**, 322–48.

Weinman, J. and Johnston, M. (1988) Stressful medical procedures: an analysis of the effects of psychological interventions and of the stressfulness of procedures, in *Topics in Health Psychology*, (eds S. Maes, C. D. Spielberger, P. B. Defares *et al.*), Wiley: Chichester, pp. 205–18.

Wells, J. K., Howard, G. S., Nowlin, W. F. N. *et al.* (1986) Pre-surgical anxiety and post-surgical pain and adjustment: effects of a stress inoculation procedure. *Journal of Consulting and Clinical Psychology*, **54**, 831–5.

Williams, R. G. A., Johnston, M., Willis, L. S. *et al.* (1976) Disability: a model and measurement technique. *British Journal of Preventative Social Medicine*, **30**, 71–8.

Wilmore, D. W., Long, J. M., Mason, A.D. and Pruitt, B. A. (1976) Stress in surgical patients: a neurophysiologic reflex response. *Surgery, Gynecology and Obstetrics*, **142**, 257–69.

Wilson, H. F. (1981) Behavioral preparation for surgery: benefit or harm? *Journal of Behavioral Medicine*, **4**, 79–102.

Wilson-Barnett, J. (1978) Patients' emotional responses to barium X-rays. *Journal of Advanced Nursing*, **3**, 37–46.

Wolfer, J. A. and Davis, C. E. (1970) Assessment of surgical patients' pre-operative emotional condition and postoperative recovery. *Journal of Behavioral Medicine*, **19**, 407–14.

Wong, M. and Kaloupek, D. (1986) Coping with dental treatment: the potential impact of situational demands. *Journal of Behavioral Medicine*, **9**, 579–97.

Zeiderman, M. R., Welchew, E. A. and Clark, R. G. (1991) Influence of epidural analgesia upon postoperative fatigue. *British Journal of Surgery*, **78**, 1457–60.

CHAPTER 11

Anaesthesia for electroconvulsive therapy

Karen H. Simpson and A. G. Oswald

11.1 HISTORY

Although Oliver treated depression with camphor induced convulsions in 1785, interest in convulsive therapy did not grow until the 1930s, when von Meduna produced fits with intravenous metrazol. Cerletti first induced electrical convulsions in 1938, and in 1951 Slater showed that the widespread introduction of electroconvulsive therapy (ECT) was associated with a major reduction in mortality.

11.2 EFFICACY OF AND INDICATIONS FOR ECT

A number of random allocation trials compared ECT with anti-depressants for the treatment of depressive illness (Greenblatt, Grosser and Weschler; 1964; MRC, 1965). These showed that, although ECT acted faster, after some months patients treated with tricyclic anti-depressants tended to be equally well. Although the many randomized and double blind trials of the 1950s and 1960s led the Royal College of Psychiatrists, in 1977, to suggest that the evidence for the efficacy of ECT in severe depressive illness was 'substantial and incontrovertible', doubts have persisted into the 1990s. These have stimulated further research efforts and a number of double blind, random allocation trials have compared real and simulated ECT. Most of the studies using a biphasic sinusoidal stimulus have found real ECT to be superior (Freeman, Basson and Crichton, 1978; West, 1981). In one study the advantage was restricted to deluded patients and was lost at follow up after one month (Johnstone *et al.*, 1980). In another study, using a brief pulse stimulus, no difference was found between real and sham ECT (Lambourne and Gill, 1978). There are many possible explanations for the different findings, but there is fairly wide agreement between psychiatrists that these trials, taken together, do not strengthen or weaken the previous strong evidence for the efficacy of ECT in depressive illness.

A number of studies have found that the 'endogenous' symptoms of depression (sudden onset, sustained depression worse in the morning, early morning waking, retardation, loss of appetite, weight and libido) tend to predict good response to ECT, whilst the 'neurotic' symptoms of depression (fluctuating course from day to day, worse in the evening, hypochondriasis, hysterical features and emotional lability) tend to predict a poorer response. There is also some evidence that deluded depressives respond poorly to drugs and particularly well to ECT. Thus although ECT is mainly used where 'endogenous like' depressed patients have failed to respond to an adequate course of antidepressants, ECT is the preferred initial treatment when delusions or hallucinations form part of the depressive symptom cluster. As it works faster than antidepressant drugs, ECT may also be the preferred initial treatment when the patient is at risk, for example from dehydration or suicide. It has been suggested that ECT is often the best treatment for elderly patients as it may have fewer risks than drug treatment (Benbow, 1989). However this point of view has been challenged as there are few trials comparing the risks and benefits of ECT against more modern, less potentially toxic, antidepressants (Malcolm and Peet, 1989; Rifkin, 1988).

Although research has suggested that the benefits of ECT in the treatment of acute schizophrenia tend to be short lived, it may still be used where the acute illness has proved unresponsive to phenothiazines. It may also be the treatment of choice for schizophrenic stupor. There is no evidence that ECT is of any value in chronic schizophrenia. There has been little research into the efficacy of ECT for mania, but it is still used for severe manic illness not responsive to medication, and is probably an effective treatment. Puerperal psychoses often have a marked affective component and ECT is considered to be the treatment of choice by many.

11.3 ASSESSMENTS OF PATIENTS BEFORE ECT

The American Society of Anesthesiologists (ASA) have devised the most well known grading system for preoperative physical status (Saklad, 1949). The classification can be simplified as follows:

- normal healthy patient;
- mild systemic disease;
- severe systemic disease which limits activity but is not incapacitating;

- severe incapacitating systemic disease which is a constant threat to life;
- moribund patient who is not expected to survive for more than 24 hours with or without treatment.

Although the classification was designed to rank physical status, it is also a useful predictor of operative risk and correlates well with mortality (Keats, 1978). It is useful to apply this grading to patients having ECT so that morbidity and mortality can be compared in different centres. A detailed medical history should be taken and a full physical examination should be performed on patients requiring ECT (Abramczuk and Rose, 1979). A British study showed that patients were not examined prior to ECT in 7% of clinics (Pippard and Ellam, 1981).

The presence of cardiovascular problems is important as such profound haemodynamic changes accompany ECT (McKenna *et al.*, 1970). Respiratory function should be carefully assessed as anaesthesia can be hazardous in patients with severe chest disease. Bad or loose dentition should be noted as inhalation of dislodged teeth may occur during treatment or recovery. Gross obesity or a history of a hiatus hernia are important as they are associated with an increased risk of aspiration of gastric contents during anaesthesia. A full neurological examination is necessary as anaesthesia can be difficult in the presence of certain muscle or neurological problems. Any abnormality of the bones or joints must be noted as fractures or dislocations may occur during treatment. The anaesthetist should be aware of any arthritis in the jaws or neck as this may lead to airway problems. Patients with diabetes should have their illness stabilized prior to treatment. Any systemic problem such as anaemia, thyroid disease or adrenal problems should be dealt with prior to ECT. Specific enquiry should be made about current medication and drug allergies. Previous anaesthesia must be discussed; possible problems include: emesis, awareness, delayed recovery, suxamethonium apnoea, porphyria or susceptability to malignant hyperthermia. It is important not to add to the discomfort of patients awaiting ECT by performing unnecessary investigations, however all patients having anaesthesia should have a full blood count. Negroes and Eastern Mediterranean patients must be sickle cell tested. Serum urea and electrolytes should be measured in patients on diuretics or those suffering from dehydration, renal, cardiac or liver disease. All patients should have their urine tested for the presence of blood, glucose or protein. A chest X-ray is needed only if there are symptoms or signs of cardiorespiratory disease. An electrocardiogram (ECG) is required only if there is evidence of cardiovascular disease.

A study in 1981 reported that little information was supplied to anaesthetists about patients requiring ECT in 19% of British clinics (Pippard and Ellam, 1981). The most important part of assessment of patients prior to treatment is good communication between the psychiatrist, nurse and anaesthetist regarding the clinical status of the patient and the urgency of ECT. The psychiatrist should optimize the condition of the patient before requesting anaesthesia for ECT. The anaesthetist should bear in mind that treatment with antidepressants has a mortality risk (Avery and Winokur, 1976). Anaesthesia should be refused only after careful consideration and consultation.

11.4   CONTRAINDICATIONS TO ECT

There are few absolute contraindications to ECT and old age alone is insufficient reason to refuse treatment. As ECT may be the treatment of choice in some elderly depressed patients it is important to provide anaesthesia if at all possible. The risk from untreated depression is probably greater than that of brief careful anaesthesia.

It is suggested that ECT should be deferred in patients who have had a myocardial infarction within the preceding three months or those with untreated heart block or cardiac failure. The desirability of ECT in the presence of uncontrolled hypertension, severe myocardial ischaemia, stenotic valvular disease or aortic aneurism should be carefully considered. Patients with cardiac pacemakers can safely receive ECT as virtually no ECT current passes through the heart; the patient should be isolated from the ground and the ECG should be monitored during treatment and recovery. Thrombophlebitis was considered to be a contraindication to ECT because of the theoretical risk of embolization, but treatment may be given once the patient is anticoagulated.

ECT should be deferred in patients with acute upper respiratory tract infection. Most patients with chronic airways disease can be treated if their respiratory function is optimized, however those with bad chronic obstructive airways disease may not tolerate repeated anaesthesia. Upper airway obstruction due to arthritis, dental abscess, facial deformity, tumour or laryngeal disease usually precludes treatment.

Patients with myopathy, myasthenia gravis, muscular dystrophy and susceptibility to malignant hyperthermia should not be anaesthetized in a department remote from a main general hospital. Severe muscle spasm or muscle weakness may occur during anaesthesia or recovery, however there has been no report of malignant hyperthermia being triggered during ECT (Johnson and Santos, 1983).

A patient who has suffered a cerebrovascular accident within three months or who has an untreated intracranial aneurism should not receive ECT. It is possible to treat patients with cerebral tumours, however the mortality rate is reported as 28% within one month (Maltbie *et al.*, 1980). Acute closed angle glaucoma is a contraindication to ECT as intraocular pressure rises during treatment may damage the eye.

The desirability of ECT should be carefully considered if the patient is pregnant, however indications are that ECT can be given safely during pregnancy (Selvin, 1987). Patients with phaeochromocytoma should not receive ECT. Patients with a haemoglobin concentration of less than 10 g/dl should not usually receive elective anaesthesia until the anaemia is corrected. Patients with sickle cell trait can be treated safely, however those with sickle cell disease may develop an acute crisis and it is not appropriate to anaesthetize them in the ECT treatment unit. Patients with severe metabolic problems, for example hepatorenal disease, should not be treated in a department remote from the main hospital.

11.5 PREPARATION FOR ECT

A careful drug history should be taken as many drugs alter seizure threshold and may alter the efficacy of ECT. Patients are often taking tricyclic antidepressants which may increase the potential for cardiac arrhythmias, but may also protect against vagal stimulation. Benzodiazepines reduce the seizure intensity and duration during ECT (Standish-Barry, Deacon and Snaith, 1985). Patients on membrane stabilizing drugs such as anticonvulsants or beta blockers may have a modified response to ECT. Caffeine may augment seizure duration and alter the efficacy of treatment.

Medication for intercurrent medical conditions should usually be continued, as abrupt withdrawal of drugs may result in exacerbation of illness. Patients on long term steroids may need supplementary hydrocortisone prior to ECT. The only agents which should be withheld prior to ECT are oral hypoglycaemics because of the risk of hypoglycaemia and probably monoamine oxidase inhibitors (MAOIs) because of potential haemodynamic problems. A survey has shown that 42% of British psychiatrists stopped MAOIs for two weeks prior to ECT (Pippard and Ellam, 1981). The routine discontinuation of MAOIs prior to anaesthesia has been questioned (El Ganzouri *et al.*, 1985).

Every effort must be made to minimize the disruptive effect of ECT treatment on the daily life of the patient. Ideally ECT should be performed in a special unit close to the in-patient facilities. ECT should not usually be given in general operating theatres as this may be frightening for some patients and involves staff who are not appropriately trained in caring for psychiatric patients. The ECT treatment unit should have separate waiting, treatment and recovery areas. An audit of ECT practice in two regions in Britain showed that the physical surroundings in ECT treatment units had improved over the previous ten years (Pippard, 1992).

Morning treatments are preferable and patients should be dressed in their everyday clothes. Waiting must be kept to a minimum. An important part of preoperative preparation is reassurance of the patient by the ward and treatment unit staff. All patients should be starved for at least six hours prior to treatment. Heavy meals late in the evening prior to ECT should be avoided especially in patients taking antidepressant medication which slows gastric emptying. Obese patients or those with oesophageal reflux should receive antacid therapy prior to anaesthesia. Diabetic patients should have their blood glucose measured prior to treatment and normal diabetic management should be resumed as soon after ECT as possible.

Sedative premedication is undesirable as it may decrease seizure duration and prolong recovery. It has been suggested that deaths due to ECT were related to vagal bradycardia and could be prevented by routine atropinization (Bankhead, Torrens and Harris, 1950). Deaths were probably more related to hypoxaemia than vagal over-activity, and the routine use of atropine has been questioned (French, 1974). Atropine does not contribute to cardiac stability or produce consistent drying of secretions (Wyant and Macdonald, 1980). Injections producing a dry mouth and blurred vision are unnecessary, and the use of subcutaneous or intramuscular atropine prior to ECT has decreased in Britain (Pippard and Ellam, 1981).

11.6 ANAESTHESIA

11.6.1 General considerations

Anaesthesia must be given by an anaesthetist competent to deal with any of the complications of anaesthesia and ECT in a department which may be removed from the main hospital (Selvin, 1987). There is no place for the single-handed ECT machine operator-anaesthetist. In 1981, consultants gave anaesthesia for ECT in 28% of clinics and were involved in 43% of clinics in Britain (Pippard and Ellam, 1981). The involvement of consultants in anaesthesia for ECT should improve the quality of care for patients, facilitate staff training and strengthen the relationship between the departments of anaesthesia and psychiatry. Unfortunately the same study showed that 50% of British clinics rely totally on anaesthetists in training to provide anaesthesia for ECT, and worse still some used the duty emergency anaesthetist. This state of affairs has not improved in the ten years since the initial survey (Pippard, 1992). This situation has adverse effects on patient safety, the quality of care, training and staff morale. Most of the anaesthesia should be performed by a regular anaesthetist who can become a member of the team. The anaesthetist should receive concise, written clinical information about each patient and should be helped to understand and comply with the Mental Health Act.

Modification of ECT by anaesthesia has reduced fear, awareness and severe trauma. The anaesthetic technique has a direct effect on the outcome of treatment by altering physiological and psychological variables. As patients commonly receive multiple treatments, it is possible to tailor anaesthesia individually. Careful recording of anaesthetic regimens and patients' responses to each treatment are needed, so that these can be optimized (Rich and Smith, 1981). Anaesthetic drugs, doses, the nature of ventilation, cardiorespiratory changes, seizure quality and duration, time to recovery and postoperative problems should be clearly noted.

The ECT department must be adequately equipped with anaesthetic, monitoring and resuscitation equipment, which is regularly checked and maintained. A survey in 1991 suggested that only 70% of units had tipping trolleys (Pippard, 1992); this is unacceptable, as it is vital to be able to place a patient rapidly into a head-down position during any anaesthetic. The responsibility for keeping equipment in good working order must be clearly defined. The anaesthetist should have adequately trained assistance during ECT sessions.

11.6.2 Anticholinergic drugs

Although the benefit of vagolysis is not proven, 95% of clinics in Britain were still using atropine in 1981 (Pippard and Ellam). Six thousand uneventful administrations of ECT without atropine have been reported (Verheeke and Troch, 1982). As well as causing discomfort, atropine predisposes patients to cardiac arrhythmias. If an antisialogogue is needed, glycopyrrolate produces comparable antisialogogue activity to atropine but has a smaller effect on heart rate (Greenan, Dewar and Jones, 1983). All anticholinergic drugs reduce lower oesophageal sphincter tone and may predispose to regurgitation. As atropine can produce central nervous system effects, including confusion, the American Psychiatrists Association recommends methylscopolamine, which does not produce central effects (Frankel, 1978). There is no evidence that atropine causes confusion after ECT, as similar cognitive deficits were seen after the use of 0.6 mg atropine, 0.2 mg glycopyrrolate (which does not cross the blood-brain barrier) and placebo during ECT (Kelway *et al.*, 1986).

11.6.3 Anaesthetic induction agents

Gaseous induction of anaesthesia is best avoided in most patients requiring ECT as it is slow and may be frightening. Many patients have unpleasant childhood memories of anaesthetic masks. Anaesthesia is usually induced using intravenous drugs, and as patients need multiple anaesthetics, great care must be taken to preserve the veins. It has to be accepted that the use of an anaesthetic drug will reduce seizure duration compared with unmodified ECT (Ayd, 1961). The ideal agent should be safe with repeated use and produce smooth anaesthesia, good cardiovascular stability, rapid complete recovery and few post-treatment problems.

Methohexitone is the agent of choice, in a dose of 0.75–1.0 mg/kg. Higher doses decrease seizure duration and increase postictal amnesia (Miller *et al.*, 1985). It has been suggested that lower doses are needed during unilateral ECT (d'Elia and Raotma, 1975). Thiopentone increases cardiac arrhythmias 2–4 fold compared with methohexitone (Woodruff, Pitts and McClure, 1968). Seizure duration and the number of ECT treatments required are similar after the two drugs (Stromgren *et al.*, 1980). Thiopentone was reported to prolong recovery compared with methohexitone (Pitts *et al.*, 1968), however a later study showed that the time to return of spontaneous breathing and protective reflexes was similar following the two drugs (McCleave and Blakemore, 1975). Methohexitone is a painful injection and 10 mg of lignocaine can be added to reduce discomfort; the addition of this small dose of lignocaine does not reduce seizure activity (Simpson *et al.*, 1989). Ketamine was claimed to be an ideal drug for ECT anaesthesia (Brewer, Davidson and Hereward, 1972), however it causes sympathomimetic effects, emesis and prolonged recovery. The usual unpleasant emergence phenomena seen after ketamine do not seem to be a problem after ECT (McInnes and James, 1972). Diazepam has been recommended for ECT (Gomez and Dally, 1975), however as it does not produce sleep in one arm-brain circulation time it is not an anaesthetic induction agent. Diazepam is associated with more cardiac arrhythmias than methohexitone (Allen, Pitts and Summers, 1980) and produces a slow and variable onset of sleep with a prolonged hangover effect. Etomidate has been used for ECT as it has good cardiovascular stability and produces rapid recovery. It has similar characteristics to methohexitone (Gran, Bergholm and Bleie, 1984), but its effects on adrenocortical function call into question its use for repeated anaesthesia. Propofol produces smooth induction of anaesthesia followed by rapid and complete recovery. Propofol attenuates the tachycardia and hypertension seen during ECT better than methohexitone, but it does not alter the incidence of cardiac arrhythmias (Rampton, *et al.*, 1989). Propofol reduces seizure activity by about 40% and this may contraindicate its use for ECT (Simpson *et al.*, 1988; Rampton *et al.*, 1989).

11.6.4 Muscle relaxants

Relaxant drugs are used to prevent forceful and potentially damaging convulsions, without totally ablating signs of muscle activity. It is still important to remove dentures, insert a 'bite block' and protect the patient's limbs during a seizure. Curare was the first muscle relaxant used during ECT and virtually abolished the traumatic complications of treatment. As it has a prolonged duration of action a shorter acting drug is preferable. Suxamethonium remains the agent of first choice in a dose of 0.5 mg/kg (Pitts *et al.*, 1968; Konarzewski *et al.*, 1988). Its action is terminated by the patient's plasma cholinesterase enzyme. The dose of suxamethonium used and the seizure quality and duration must be recorded so that dosage can be optimized during the course of ECT. The seizure duration is inversely proportional to the dose of suxamethonium given (Miller *et al.*, 1985). The duration of action of suxamethonium is shortened by ECT (Bali, 1975) and is prolonged by lithium therapy (Martin and Kramer, 1982), although the latter effect is not clinically important. The 2% incidence of muscle pains following suxamethonium and ECT is less than the 70% expected, despite rapid ambulation (McCleave and Blakemore, 1975). The incidence of muscle pains is not related to the dose of suxamethonium used (Konarzewski *et al.*, 1988). Suxamethonium is contraindicated in patients with certain muscle diseases, susceptibility to malignant hyperthermia, high plasma potassium concentration, upper airway obstruction and genetically determined or acquired lack of plasma cholinesterase. If suxamethonium cannot be used for ECT then a small dose of 0.2 mg/kg atracurium is probably the next best option. This dose should be allowed adequate time to work and reversed after treatment.

11.6.5 Ventilation

The most important aspect of anaesthesia for ECT is the provision of oxygen; hypoxaemia does not augment treatment. In 1950 it was noted that '(cardiac) ectopic phenomena occurred almost uniformly during deepest cyanosis following a convulsion', and these could be corrected by administration of oxygen (Bankhead, Torrens and Harris, 1950). It has been suggested that oxygenation prior to ECT is unnecessary in healthy patients, as long as they are ventilated with room air following the convulsion (Woodruff, Pitts and McClure, 1968). It has since been proposed that inadequate ventilation, leading to cardiac arrhythmias, is an important cause of death during ECT (French, 1974). Despite this, as recently as 1979, Joshi stated that the use of oxygen during ECT was not essential. Hypoxemia is a frequent problem during ECT if preoxygenation is not adequate (Swindells and Simpson, 1987). It is vital to administer oxygen to all patients prior to applying an ECT stimulus, and most clinics in Britain use oxygen routinely (Pippard and Ellam, 1981).

Seizure duration is prolonged by 25% with the use of oxygen , 45%

with oxygen and partial paralysis and over 100% with oxygenation and total paralysis (Holmberg, Hard and Ramqvist, 1956). Hypoxaemia may play a role in the termination of seizures. It has now been shown that increasing oxygenation alone does not prolong convulsions (Bergholm, Gran and Bleie, 1984). Seizure duration is probably increased by ventilation and paralysis acting to reduce carbon dioxide concentration in the brain. Seizure duration was increased by 68% when the alveolar carbon dioxide concentration was reduced from 5 kPa to 2 kPa by hyperventilation of intubated patients (Bergholm, Gran and Bleie, 1984). Seizure duration can also be increased by passive hyperventilation using a face mask (Chater and Simpson, 1988). Therefore adequate ventilation during ECT ensures oxygenation and can increase seizure duration.

11.6.6   Anaesthetic and monitoring equipment

There is probably no need to have a complete anaesthetic machine in the ECT treatment unit as the main requirements are a source of oxygen and suction. Nitrous oxide and volatile agents are not usually necessary, however if these are supplied to the unit then adequate scavenging must be installed. There is no need to supply a mechanical ventilator to the treatment unit as it is an inappropriate site for a patient to be ventilated. It may occasionally be necessary to keep a patient anaesthetized after ECT, for example in the case of suxamethonium apnoea, however this can be achieved using total intravenous techniques via a syringe pump. Any patient needing prolonged ventilation must be immediately transferred to an intensive care unit.

As oxygenation during ECT is of paramount importance, the best monitor is probably a pulse oximeter; this is also the least disturbing for the patient as it only requires the use of a small ear or finger clip. A capnograph must be available as it is important to be able to detect end tidal carbon dioxide if faced with a difficult intubation. Routine ECG monitoring is not practical, especially as patients are often dressed in everyday clothes, however an ECG machine must be immediately accessible. Means of measuring the patient's blood pressure and temperature must be available in the ECT treatment unit. Adequate resuscitation equipment including a defibrillator must be kept in the department.

11.7   ADMINISTRATION OF ECT

11.7.1   General considerations

Many patients are fearful of ECT and know little about what is involved. A full explanation must be provided with the possible benefits weighed against the potential side-effects. Many patients are surprised to learn that they will receive an anaesthetic for the procedure which will last only for a few minutes. Written information for the patient to keep is very useful.

Mentally ill patients who are in hospital on a voluntary basis cannot be given ECT without their written consent. Severely depressed people may withhold their consent. They may be so withdrawn and mute that communication is impossible or they may believe that they are so 'bad' that they do not deserve treatment. They may be too paranoid to accept treatment or may be so indecisive that they cannot make up their mind. Where ECT is considered essential for such patients they can be detained under the Mental Health Act and the Mental Welfare Commission can be asked to appoint a doctor to provide a second opinion as to whether or not ECT should be given. If a detained patient gives informed consent to ECT and this is certified by a responsible medical officer, then the treatment can be given without a second opinion. The anaesthetist, treatment unit staff and psychiatrist must be aware to which category each patient belongs prior to treatment.

Almost all studies comparing bilateral ECT with unilateral ECT to the nondominant side for language have found that unilateral ECT causes less short term memory impairment and postictal confusion. However, several studies have also suggested that patients receiving unilateral ECT require one or two more treatments before full recovery is achieved. Nearly all right-handed people are left hemisphere dominant for language, and psychiatrists are increasingly using right unilateral ECT for such people. Only 40% of left-handed people are right hemisphere dominant, and there is no reliable way to firmly establish dominance. Thus, in left-handed people, bilateral treatment may be preferred, as unilateral treatment given to the dominant hemisphere in error may have more adverse effects.

In bilateral ECT the electrodes are placed on both sides of the head at a point 4 cm along a perpendicular line up from the midpoint of a line from the external auditory meatus to the lateral angle of the eye (frontotemporal position). In unilateral ECT one electrode is applied at this point, but many other positions have been suggested for the second electrode. Probably 12 cm along a line from the frontotemporal position to the vertex is satisfactory.

The padded electrodes should be moist and firmly applied to the head at points which have been degreased. The patient should be observed for at least 30 seconds after the stimulus for evidence of bilateral fitting. If no seizure is seen, the electrodes may be too close together or the hair between the electrodes may be too damp allowing too little current to penetrate the skull. The ECT machine may be set wrongly or the patient's seizure threshold may have risen for some reason. The patient must be given a maximum of two further stimuli before treatment is abandoned. The junior psychiatrist must have a clear understanding of the procedure to be followed if a patient fails to have a seizure. A survey has suggested that teaching of ECT practice to junior doctors by consultant psychiatrists could be improved (Pippard, 1992).

It seems likely that, for ECT to be effective, some maturing of cerebral processes between seizures is necessary, and treatment should be given two to three times each week. At least 48 hours should elapse between treatments. The number of ECT treatments is usually between 4 and 8, but may be as high as 12.

11.7.2   ECT machines

Many of the adverse cognitive effects of ECT are related to the amount of electrical energy used to produce a seizure. The minimum effective stimulus should be employed. ECT machines can be classified as sine wave or brief pulse stimulus generators depending on the electrical waveform they produce. In 1938 Cerletti and Bini defined the basic requirements for induction of a convulsion using a 50 Hz alternating supply, as 80–100 volts for 0.5–0.7 seconds, which gave 0.3–0.6 amps. The current was later reduced and rectified to decrease the amount of energy applied to about 40 milliamps for 1–2 seconds. Many ECT machines were designed to produce a variable unidirectional sine wave current with constant voltage. Instruments have since been designed to allow more precise control of electrical parameters by producing rectangular pulses of a defined number, voltage, spacing and direction (Blachly, 1976). Brief stimulus therapy used widely spaced square waves of short duration and decreased the energy delivered to approximately one-third that of a sine wave stimulus. As the skull has a high and variable resistance, of 200–500 ohms, only a small proportion of the energy generated during an ECT stimulus reaches the brain.

It is important to use a machine which will accurately deliver a measured amount of energy in Joules over a pre-set time. Most machines deliver 30–45 Joules over 0.5–1.5 seconds. Some machines incorporate electroencephalographic (EEG) monitoring. Regular servicing and updating of ECT machines is needed. In 1977 in 14 treatment units in Britain, there were 50 faults in 18 ECT machines, 30 faults in 16 reserve machines and a poor general standard of maintenance (Lambourne and Murrills, 1978). In 1981 Pippard and Ellam reported that 40% of units did not regularly maintain ECT machines, 28% were using obsolete machines and 48% had obsolete reserve machines. A survey of practice ten years later did not show much improvement in the state of ECT machines (Pippard, 1992). ECT machines must conform to British standards.

11.7.3 Monitoring seizures

A generalized convulsion must be produced for ECT to be beneficial, therefore it is important to monitor seizures. The minimum effective single clonic seizure duration is suggested to be 25 seconds (Fink and Johnson, 1982). A prolonged seizure of more than 120 seconds increases neurological problems without augmenting the therapeutic effect of treatment (Weiner *et al.*, 1980). Many factors influence seizure duration including: age, concomitant drug treatment, number of ECT treatments, doses of induction agent and relaxant, ventilation and blood pressure. Caffeine has been used to increase seizure activity (Coffey *et al.*, 1990). The electrode placement, current waveform and energy supplied have little effect on seizure duration as long as a supramaximal stimulus is received (d'Elia and Raotma, 1975; Daniel *et al.*, 1982; Robin and de Tissera, 1982). There is an intrinsic individual propensity for long or short seizure duration (Maletzky, 1978). It is sometimes difficult to detect seizures when ECT is modified by anaesthesia, especially when unilateral electrode placement is used.

Seizures may be monitored by EEG, cuff and electromyographic (EMG) methods. The EEG clearly records the onset, duration and nature of the seizure. The cuff method involves inflating a blood pressure cuff on the arm prior to administration of the muscle relaxant to show the unmodified convulsion. If unilateral electrode placement is to be used the cuff must be placed on the ipsilateral arm to check that a generalized seizure has occurred. The cuff method is highly correlated with EEG recording, but underestimates seizure duration by 10% (Fink and Johnson, 1982). The cuff method is inferior for the detection of prolonged seizures which occur in 4% of patients (Greenberg, 1985). The EMG method records motor discharge via electrodes on the calf or masseter muscles, and can be used in the presence of muscle relaxant. The duration of ECT induced tachycardia correlates well with both the isolated arm and the EEG methods of monitoring seizure duration (Larson, Schwartz and Abrams, 1984).

As powerful muscle contractions must be avoided, the quality of seizures should be graded. The response to therapy has been classified by Davies and Lewis (1949) and Ferguson (1952). The shock was graded as good (facial muscle contraction only), moderate (facial muscles, shoulders and other parts) and poor (severe contraction of all muscles including the back).

Patients should not be subjected to the risks of anaesthesia and the psychological and physical discomforts of treatment if seizure occurrence is not carefully monitored. A survey in Britain showed that 'in some hospitals fewer than 50% of the patients in a session received fits, usually because of incorrect criteria for a fit or because the staff did not look at the patient to see' (Pippard and Ellam, 1981). It is not sufficient to rely on physical signs such as 'gooseflesh', pallor or dilated pupils to indicate a successful treatment (McCleave and Blakemore, 1975). In the absence of EEG equipment, the simplicity and economy of the cuff method is recommended to monitor seizures. However the use of single-channel EEG monitoring offers greater control of treatment and reduces the incidence of missed seizures (Scott, Sherring and Trykes, 1989).

11.8   RECOVERY FROM ANAESTHESIA

Patients usually resume spontaneous breathing and regain protective reflexes within a few minutes of the end of the seizure. Possible problems during the recovery period include airway obstruction, ventilatory depression, cardiac arrhythmias, hypertension, hypotension, emesis, aspiration of gastric contents, delayed return of consciousness, agitation, confusion and headache. In patients who are slow to recover a cerebral event, prolonged seizure activity, lack of plasma cholinesterase and hypoglycaemia should be suspected.

The recovery area must be of sufficient size, well staffed and equipped with adequate monitoring and resuscitation equipment. One nurse was found to be responsible for five recovering patients in 21% of units in Britain (Pippard and Ellam, 1981). In view of the potential for mortality, this level of staffing is not acceptable. There should be one nurse or other trained member of staff for each patient who is not in control of their protective reflexes. Patients must be nursed in the lateral position and their colour, ventilation, heart rate and blood pressure must be monitored until stable. The anaesthetists and psychiatrist must remain within easy reach of the recovery area. Patients may become agitated in the recovery area and should be reassured by appropriately trained staff. Once patients have fully recovered they should be given something to eat and drink and returned to the ward, preferably accompanied by a nurse with whom they are familiar.

11.9   PHYSIOLOGICAL EFFECTS OF ECT

Bilateral and unilateral ECT have different effects on neuropsychological, EEG, endocrine and cardiovascular function, with bilateral ECT having the most profound effect (Lane *et al.*, 1989).

11.9.1   Central nervous effects

During unmodified ECT, unconsciousness and amnesia rapidly follow the shock. There is a brief period of muscular contraction concurrent with passage of the stimulus. The tonic phase follows 1–15 seconds later and lasts 5–20 seconds; this is gradually replaced by generalized clonic contractions lasting from a few seconds to a few minutes. The EEG is isoelectric for 1–5 seconds after the ECT stimulus. A rapid build-up of diffuse spike activity then occurs, accompanying the tonic muscle contraction. During the clonic phase, high voltage slow waves are usually present. ECT reduces total sleep time and increases rapid eye movement (REM) sleep. After initial cerebral vasoconstriction, cerebral blood flow increases by approximately 100–400%. There are regional differences in cerebral blood flow with the frontal area and basal ganglia having a higher flow than the occipital area and thalamus (Bajc *et al.*, 1989). Intracranial pressure is elevated. Cerebrospinal fluid pressure increases secondary to an increase in venous pressure. Cerebral hyper-perfusion is mainly related to increased blood pressure, however it still occurs if hypertension is blocked. The increase in cerebral blood flow provides for the elevated metabolic demands of the brain during the seizure. ECT stimulates brain glycolysis and lactic acid accumulates even if acidosis is prevented (Miller *et al.*, 1982). Raised cerebral per-fusion pressure results in increased permeability of the blood-brain barrier to macromolecules (Bolwig *et al.*, 1977).

11.9.2 Cardiovascular effects

The cardiovascular effects of ECT are due to activation of the autonomic nervous system and the Valsalva effect of forced expiration against a closed glottis. The latter is largely attenuated by the use of muscle relaxants. There is a parasympathetic-sympathetic sequence during the shock, followed by a similar but less marked sequence during the clonic phase which persists into the recovery period (Perrin, 1961). The heart rate rarely falls below 60 beats per minute during the bradycardia phase and almost always increases spontaneously. The transient early brady-cardia can be blocked by a large dose of atropine, but the need for this is questionable as a tachycardia of 130–160 beats per minute often fol-lows the bradycardia phase. The changes in blood pressure parallel those of heart rate, although the hypertensive response is somewhat attenuated by anaesthesia. Systolic blood pressure reaches 200–250 mm Hg during the hypertensive phase, due to catecholamine release (Jones and Knight, 1981). As the heart rate and blood pressure increase simul-taneously, the rate-pressure product often exceeds 35 000, with poten-tial deleterious effects on myocardial perfusion, especially in those patients with ischaemic heart disease. Beta blockade reduces the peak rate-pressure product to 16 000 (Jones and Knight, 1981). Patients with untreated essential hypertension do not show a greater hypertensive response to ECT than normal subjects (Stoker, Spencer and Hamilton, 1981). Severe hypertension should be controlled using beta blockers such as propranolol or esmolol (Jones, 1983; Weigner *et al.*, 1991) or nitrates. Esmolol may have less effect on seizure duration than propranolol (Weigner *et al.*, 1991). Venous return is impeded by raised intrathoracic and intra-abdominal pressure due to convulsive muscular activity and positive pressure ventilation.

11.9.3   Respiratory effects

If ECT is not modified by anaesthesia there is apnoea, forced expiration lasting 15–20 seconds after the end of the seizure, irregular breathing and finally hyperventilation. These changes are abolished by muscle paralysis. Oxygen saturation is reduced by apnoea and muscle activity during ECT. If no oxygen is administered, oxygen saturation falls below 90% (Fink, 1979). Care must be taken to ventilate adequately prior to the seizure, as a few breaths of oxygen are not always sufficient to prevent significant hypoxaemia occurring during the seizure (Swindells and Simpson, 1987). The extent of respiratory and metabolic acidosis which occur during ECT depends upon the adequacy of ventilation, the period of apnoea and the extent of muscle activity. Prolonged seizures produced by multiple monitored ECT result in adverse metabolic effects, even with good oxygenation (Weiner *et al.*, 1980).

11.9.4   Endocrine and metabolic effects

There is a release of catecholamines, adrenocorticotrophic hormone and corticosteroids during ECT, which leads to an increase in blood glucose (Gravenstein *et al.*, 1965; Jones and Knight, 1981). An insignificant increase of potassium has been reported after suxamethonium and muscle activity during ECT (McCleave and Blakemore, 1975). A diuresis with loss of sodium and a positive calcium balance occur after treatment, however these may be related to an improvement in mental state (Ottosson, 1974).

11.10   MODE OF ACTION

Ottosson (1960) showed that lignocaine, which reduces seizure activity, reduced the efficacy of ECT. He also showed that when an electrical stimulus greater than needed was used to produce a convulsion, no additional therapeutic effect was gained, but greater memory loss was induced. He concluded that the therapeutic effect of ECT varied with the duration of brain convulsive activity, but that memory disturbance varied with the amount of energy passed through the brain. Although this conclusion is still generally accepted, some doubt was cast on its validity when Robin and de Tissera (1982) found that fewer treatments were necessary with a high energy stimulus than with a low energy stimulus, even though fits of a similar duration were produced. This may explain the finding of Lambourne and Gill (1978) that real ECT using a brief pulse stimulus of low energy was no more effective than simulated ECT.

11.11 COMPLICATIONS OF ECT

ECT is a safe procedure with or without general anaesthesia. Computed tomography of the brain has not demonstrated any deleterious effect of ECT (Bergholm *et al.*, 1989). Any risks have to be weighed against the known benefits of treatment. Serious potential adverse effects include: myocardial infarction, cardiac arrhythmias, heart failure, chest infection, aspiration pneumonia, prolonged apnoea, pulmonary or fat embolus, cerebral haemorrhage and prolonged seizures. When unmodified ECT is used there is a 30–40% incidence of crush vertebral fractures which are rare when muscle relaxants are used.

There is a risk of skin burns if the ECT electrodes are not applied correctly. Headache and confusion can occur after ECT (Greenblatt, Grosser and Weschler, 1964). A study by Gomez (1975) showed a low incidence of minor side-effects in the 24 hours after ECT, with 8% muscle pains, 3% headaches, 2% sore throat or stuffy nose, 1% nausea, less than 1% confusion and 3% subjective memory impairment. Another study showed a higher incidence of side-effects when the patient's nursing and medical records were examined, with 16% headache, 9% confusion and 7% memory disturbance (Freeman and Kendell, 1988). When these patients were questioned one year later, 40% reported headaches, 27% confusion, 64% memory loss and 20% did not remember any adverse effects. Forty-nine per cent of these patients interviewed felt that there had been inadequate explanation given regarding the nature of ECT treatment.

The effect of ECT on memory has been extensively studied for many years. There is good evidence that a transient memory impairment occurs and lasts for 4–6 weeks after the final treatment. It consists of poor recall for recent events and impaired capacity to acquire new memories. Hamilton, Stocker and Spencer (1979) suggested that this memory deficit resulted from a rise in blood pressure during the fit with a temporary breakdown of the blood-brain barrier. Unilateral ECT causes less memory deficit than bilateral treatment. There is no evidence that ECT causes any long-term impairment of past memory or the capacity to acquire new memories.

11.12   MORTALITY AFTER ECT

A death rate of 0.04–0.1% was reported following ECT in the early days of treatment. Impastato and Almansi reviewed the literature in 1942 and suggested a mortality rate of 0.5% for patients aged more than 60 years and 0.02% for patients aged 20–30 years. Sixty-two deaths were reported in Britain between 1947 and 1952; there was an increase in deaths during the period studied, peaking with 19 deaths in 1951 (Maclay, 1953). Mortality was commoner in patients over 55 years old and may have been related to the use of curare with inadequate ventilation. In 1959 Barker and Baker reported 9 deaths in 259 000 treatments in Britain. In 1961 Perrin estimated the death rate in the United States of America to be one treatment in 12 500 and one patient in 950. Thirty six per cent of deaths occurred within one hour of treatment and were probably due to cardiac problems. Thirty to fifty per cent of deaths occurred after a successful first treatment, therefore surviving one ECT is no guarantee of safety.

The death rate following ECT has decreased more recently, as resuscitation methods are much better than previously. There were 3.6 deaths per year associated with ECT in England and Wales between 1957 and 1966 (Granville-Grossman, 1971). A study in Denmark reported only one death in 22 210 treatments in 3438 patients (Hesche and Roeder, 1976). In 1978 the American Psychiatrists Association survey revealed a death rate of 0.05%; 67% deaths were due to cardiac causes and commonly occurred during the recovery period (Frankel, 1978). In 1981 Pippard and Ellam reported one death during ECT and three deaths within 72 hours of treatment, a mortality rate of 0.03–0.006% of treatments. There is still a small risk of death during ECT which must be weighed against the risks with other forms of treatment (Avery and Winokur, 1976; Kendall, 1981).

11.13   CONCLUSION

ECT is a safe and effective treatment for many psychiatric problems. Regular review and updating of the service provided is essential and demands co-operation and communication between anaesthetists, nurses and psychiatrists.

REFERENCES

Abramczuk, J. A. and Rose, N. M. (1979) Preanaesthetic assessment and prevention of post-ECT morbidity. *British Journal Psychiatry*, **134**, 582–7.

Allen, R. E., Pitts, F. N. and Summers, W. K. (1980) Drug modification of ECT: Methohexital and diazepam. *Biological Psychiatry*, **15**, 257–64.

Avery, D. and Winokur, G. (1976) Mortality in depressed patients treated with electroconvulsive therapy and antidepressants. *Archives of General Psychiatry*, **33**, 1029–37.

Ayd, F. J. (1961) Methohexital: a new anaesthetic for electroconvulsive therapy. *Diseases of the Nervous System*, **22**, 388–90.

Bajc, M., Medred, V., Basic, M. *et al.* (1989) Acute effect of electroconvulsive therapy on brain perfusion assessed by Tc99 and single photon emission computed tomography. *Acta Psychiatrica Scandanavica*, **80**, 421–6.

Bali, I. M. (1975) The effect of modified electroconvulsive therapy on plasma potassium concentration. *British Journal of Anaesthesia*, **47**, 398–401.

Bankhead, A. J., Torrens, J. K. and Harris, T. H. (1950) The anticipation and prevention of cardiac ectopic complications in electroconvulsive therapy. A clinical and electrocardiographic study. *American Journal of Psychiatry*, **106**, 911–17.

Barker, J. C. and Baker, A. A. (1959) Deaths associated with electropexy. *Journal of Mental Science*, **105**, 339–48.

Benbow, S. M. (1989) The role of ECT in the treatment of depressive illness in old age. *British Journal of Psychiatry*, **155**, 147–52.

Bergholm, P., Gran, L. and Bleie, H. (1984) Seizure duration in unilateral electroconvulsive therapy. The effect of hypocapnia induced by hyperventilation and the effect of ventilation with oxygen. *Acta Psychiatrica Scandanavica*, **69**, 121–8.

Bergholm, P., Larson, J. L., Rosendahl, R. and Holsten F. (1989) Electroconvulsive therapy and cerebral computed tomography. *Acta Psychiatrica Scandanavica*, **80**, 566–72.

Blachly, P. H. (1976) New developments in electroconvulsive therapy. *Diseases of the Nervous System*, **37**, 356–8.

Bolwig, T. G., Hertz, M. M., Paulson, O. B. *et al.* (1977) The permeability of the blood-brain barrier during electrically induced seizures in man. *European Journal of Clinical Investigation*, **7**, 87–93.

Brewer, C. L., Davidson, J. R. T. and Hereward, S. (1972) Ketamine – a safer anaesthetic for ECT. *British Journal of Psychiatry*, **120**, 679–80.

British Standards Institution (1979) *Specifications for the Safety of Medical Equipment*. BS, 5742, Part 1.

Cerletti, U. and Bini, L. (1938) Un neuvo metodo di shockterapie 'L'elettroshock'. *Bollogna Academie Medicine Roma*, **64**, 136–8.

Chater, S. N. and Simpson, K. H. (1988) Effect of hyperventilation on seizure duration in patients having electroconvulsive therapy. *British Journal of Anaesthesia*, **60**, 70–3.

Coffey, C. E., Figiel, G. S., Weiner, K. D. and Sandey, W. B. (1990) Caffeine augmentation of electroconvulsive therapy. *American Journal of Psychiatry*, **147**, 579–85.

Daniel, W. F., Crovitz, H. F., Weiner, R. D. and Rodgers, H. J. (1982) The effects of ECT modifications on autobiographical and verbal memory. *Biological Psychiatry*, **17**, 919–24.

Davies, D. L. and Lewis, A. (1949) Effects of decamethonium iodide on respiration and on convulsions in man. *Lancet*, i, 775.

d'Elia, A. and Raotma, H. (1975) Is unilateral ECT less effective than bilateral ECT. *British Journal of Psychiatry*, **126**, 83–9.

El Ganzouri, A. R., Ivankovitch, A. D., Braverman, B. *et al.* (1985) MAOIs, should they be discontinued preoperatively. *Anesthesia and Analgesia*, **64**, 592–6.

Ferguson, A. L. (1952) Discussion on new muscle relaxants in electroconvulsive therapy. *Proceedings of the Royal Society of Medicine*, **45**, 875–9.

Fink, M. (1979) *Convulsive Therapy, Theory and Practice*, 1st Edn, Raven Press, New York.

Fink, M. and Johnson, L. (1982) Monitoring the duration of electroconvulsive therapy seizures. Cuff and EEG methods compared. *Archives of General Psychiatry*, **39**, 1189–91.

Frankel, F. H. (1978) *Report No. 14 of the American Psychiatrists Task Force on Convulsive Therapy*, American Association of Psychiatrists, Washington DC, pp. 200.

Freeman, C. P. L., Basson, J. V. and Crichton, A. (1978) Double blind controlled trial of electroconvulsive therapy (ECT) and simulated ECT in depressive illness. *Lancet*, **i**, 738–40.

Freeman, C. P. L. and Kendell, R. W. (1988) ECT, patients' experiences and attitudes. *British Journal of Psychiatry*, **137**, 8–16.

French, O. (1974) Electroshock therapy and inadequate ventilation. *Chest*, **66**, 468.

Gomez, J. (1975) Subjective side effects of ECT. *British Journal of Psychiatry*, **127**, 604–8.

Gomez, J. and Dally, P. (1975) Intravenous tranquillization with ECT. *British Journal of Psychiatry*, **127**, 609–11.

Gran, L., Bergholm, P. and Bleie, H. (1984) Seizure duration in unilateral electroconvulsive therapy. A comparison of the anaesthetic agents etomidate, Althesin and methohexitone. *Acta Psychiatrica Scandanavica*, **69** 472–83.

Granville-Grossman, K. (1971) *Recent Advances in Clinical Psychiatry*, J and A Churchill, London, pp. 13.

Gravenstein, J. S., Anton, A. H., Weiner, S. M. and Tetlow A. G. (1965) Catecholamine and cardiovascular response to electroconvulsive therapy in man. *British Journal of Anaesthesia*, **37**, 833–9.

Greenan, J., Dewar, M. and Jones, C. J. (1983) Intravenous glycopyrrolate and atropine at induction of anaesthesia, a comparison. *Journal of the Royal Society of Medicine*, **76**, 369–71.

Greenberg, L. B. (1985) Detection of prolonged seizures during electroconvulsive therapy, a comparison of electroencephalogram and cuff monitoring. *Convulsive Therapy*, **1**, 32–7.

Greenblatt, M., Grosser, G. H. and Weschler, H. (1964) Differential response of hospitalized depressed patients to somatic therapy. *American Journal of Psychiatry*, **120**, 935–43.

Hamilton, M., Stocker, M. J. and Spencer, C. M. (1979) Post ECT cognitive defect and elevation of blood pressure. *British Journal of Psychiatry*, **135**, 77–8.

Hesche, J. and Roeder, E. (1976) Electroconvulsive therapy in Denmark. *British Journal of Psychiatry*, **128**, 241–5.

Holberg, G., Hard, G. and Ramqvist, N. (1956) Experiments in the prolongation of convulsions induced by electric shock treatment. *Acta Psychiatrica and Neuroligica Scandanavica*, **31**, 61–70.

Impastato, D. J. and Almansi, R. (1942) The electrofit in the treatment of mental disease. *Journal of Nervous and Mental Diseases*, **96**, 375–409.

Jones, R. M. (1983) ECT for patients with hypertensive heart disease. *American Journal of Psychiatry*, **140**, 139–40.

Jones, R. M. and Knight, P. R. (1981) Cardiovascular and hormonal responses to electroconvulsive therapy. *Anaesthesia*, **36**, 795–9.

Johnson, G. C. and Santos, A. B. (1983) More on ECT and malignant hyperpyrexia. *American Journal of Psychiatry*, **140**, 266.

Johnstone, E. C., Deakin, J. G. W., Lawler, P. *et al*. (1980) The Northwick Park ECT trial. *Lancet*, **ii**, 1317–20.

Joshi, V. G. (1979) Modifying ECT with a safe, simple and economic technique. *British Journal of Psychiatry*, **134**, 128.

Keats, A. S. (1978) The ASA classification of physical status – recapitulation. *Anesthesiology*, **49**, 233–6.

Kelway, B., Simpson, K. H., Smith, R. J. and Halsall, P. J. (1986) Effects of atropine and glycopyrrolate on cognitive function following anaesthesia and electroconvulsive therapy (ECT). *International Journal of Clinical Psychopharmacology*, **1**, 296–302.

Kendell, R. E. (1981) The present status of electroconvulsive therapy. *British Journal of Psychiatry*, **139**, 265–83.

Konarzewski, W. H., Milosavljevic, D., Robinson, M. *et al*. (1988) Suxamethonium dosage in electroconvulsive therapy. *Anaesthesia*, **65**, 474–6.

Lambourne, J. and Gill, D. (1978) A controlled comparison of simulated and real ECT. *British Journal of Psychiatry*, **133**, 514–19.

Lambourne, J. and Murrills, A. J. (1978) Actual practice of ECT in a health region of Britain. *British Journal of Psychiatry*, **133**, 520–3.

Lane, R. D., Zeitlin, S. B., Abrams, R. and Swartz, C. M. (1989) Differential effects of right unilateral and bilateral ECT on heart rate. *American Journal of Psychiatry*, **146**, 1041–3.

Larson, G., Swartz, C. and Abrams, R. (1984) Duration of ECT induced tachycardia as a measure of seizure length. *American Journal of Psychiatry*, **141**, 1269–70.

Maclay, W. S. (1953) Death due to treatment. *Proceedings of the Royal Society of Medicine*, **46**, 13–20.

Malcolm, K. and Peet, M. (1989) ECT and old age. *British Journal of Psychiatry*, **155**, 713–14.

Maletzky, B. (1978) Seizure duration and clinical effect in electroconvulsive therapy. *Comprehensive Psychiatry*, **19**, 541–50.

Maltbie, A. A., Wingfield, R. S., Volow, M. R. *et al*. (1980) Electroconvulsive therapy in the presence of a brain tumour. *Journal of Nervous and Mental Diseases*, **168**, 400–5.

Martin, B. A. and Kramer, P. M. (1982) Clinical significance of the interaction between lithium and a neuromuscular blocker. *American Journal of Psychiatry*, **139**, 1326–8.

McCleave, D. J. and Blakemore, W. B. (1975) Anaesthesia for electroconvulsive therapy. *Anaesthesia and Intensive Care*, **3**, 250–6.

McInnes, E. C. and James, N. McI. (1972) A comparison of ketamine and methohexital in electroconvulsive therapy. *Medical Journal of Australia*, **1**, 1031–2.

McKenna, G., Engle, R. P., Brooks, H. and Dalen, J. (1970) Cardiac arrhythmias during electroshock therapy, significance, prevention and treatment. *American Journal of Psychiatry*, **127**, 530–3.

Medical Research Council Clinical Psychiatry Committee (1965) Clinical trial of the treatment of depressive illness. *British Medical Journal*, **i**, 881–6.

Miller, A. L., Faber, R. A., Hatch, J. P. and Alexander H. D. (1985) Factors affecting amnesia, seizure duration and efficacy of ECT. *American Journal of Psychiatry*, **142**, 692–6.

Miller, A. L., Shamban, A. T., Corddry, D. H. and Kiney, C. A. (1982) Cerebral metabolic responses to electroconvulsive shock and their modification by hypercapnia. *Journal of Neurochemistry*, **38**, 916–24.

Ottosson, J. O. (1960) Experimental studies of the mode of action of ECT. *Acta Psychiatrica Scandanavica*, Suppl 1, 145.

Ottosson, J. O. (1974) Systemic biochemical effects of electroconvulsive therapy, in *Psychobiology of Convulsive Therapy*, (eds M. Fink, S. Kety, J. McGaugh and T. Williams), V. H. Winston and Sons, Washington DC, pp. 209–20.

Perrin, G. M. (1961) Cardiovascular and other psychologic changes accompanying ECT. *Acta Psychiatrica et Neurolologica Scandanavica*, **36S**, 10–24.

Pippard, G. M. (1992) Audit of ECT in two NHS regions. *British Journal of Psychiatry*, **160**, 621–38.

Pippard, J. and Ellam, L. (1981) Electroconvulsive treatment in Great Britain. *British Journal of Psychiatry*, **139**, 563–8.

Pitts, F. N., Woodruff, R. A., Craig. A. G. and Rich, C. L. (1968) The drug modification of ECT II. Succinyl choline dosage. *Archives of General Psychiatry*, **19**, 595–9.

Rampton, A. J., Griffin, R. M., Stuart, C. S. *et al.* (1989) Comparison of methohexitone and propofol for ECT. *Anesthesiology*, **70**, 412–17.

Rich, C. L. and Smith, N. T. (1981) Anaesthesia for electroconvulsive therapy, a psychiatric viewpoint. *Canadian Anaesthetists Society Journal*, **28**, 153–7.

Rifkin, A. (1988) ECT versus antidepressants, a review of the evidence. *British Journal of Clinical Psychiatry*, **49**, 3–7.

Robin, A. and de Tissera, A. (1982) A double blind controlled comparison of the therapeutic effects of low and high energy electroconvulsive therapies. *British Journal of Psychiatry*, **141**, 357–66.

Royal College of Psychiatrists (1977) Memorandum on the use of electroconvulsive therapy. *British Journal of Psychiatry*, **131**, 261–72.

Saklad, M. (1949) Grading of patients for surgical procedures. *Anesthesiology*, **2**, 281–4.

Scott, A. I. F., Sherring, P. A. and Trykes, S. (1989) Would monitoring by EEG improve the practice of ECT? *British Journal of Psychiatry*, **154**, 853–7.

Selvin, B. L. (1987) Electroconvulsive therapy – 1987. *Anesthesiology*, **67**, 367–85.

Simpson, K. H., Halsall, P. J., Carr, C. M. E. and Stewart, K. G. (1988) Propofol reduces seizure duration in patients having anaesthesia for ECT. *British Journal of Anaesthesia*, **1**, 343–4.

Simpson, K. H., Halsall, P. J., Sides, C. and Keeler, J. (1989) The use of lignocaine to reduce pain on injection of methohexitone during anaesthesia for ECT. *Anaesthesia*, **44**, 688–9.

Slater, E. T. O. (1951) Evaluation of electric convulsion therapy as compared with conservative methods of treatment of depressive states. *Journal of Mental Sciences*, **97**, 567–9.

Standish-Barry, H. M. A. S., Deacon, V. and Snaith, R. P. (1985) The relationship of concurrent benzodiazepine administration to seizure duration in ECT. *Acta Psychiatrica Scandanavica*, **71**, 269–71.

Stoker, M. J., Spencer, C. M. and Hamiliton, M. (1981) Blood pressure elevation during electroconvulsive therapy and associated cognitive deficit. *Electroconvulsive Therapy – and Appraisal*, (ed. R. L. Palmer), Oxford University Press, pp. 106–24.

Stromgren, L. S., Dahl, J., Fjeldborg, N. and Thomsen, A. (1980) Factors influencing seizure duration and number of seizures applied in unilateral electroconvulsive therapy. Anaesthetics and benzodiazepines. *Acta Psychiatrica Scandanavica*, **62**, 158–65.

Swindells, S. R. and Simpson, K. H. (1987) Oxygen saturation during electroconvulsive therapy. *British Journal of Psychiatry*, **150**, 685–7.

Verheeke, G. and Troch, E. (1982) Atropine in electroconvulsive therapy. *Anaesthesia and Intensive Care*, **10**, 166.

Weigner, M. B., Partridge, B. L., Haugher, R., and Mirow, A. (1991) The prevention of the cardiovascular and neuroendocrine response to ECT. *Anesthesia and Analgesia*, **73**, 556–62.

Weiner, R. D., Volow, M. R., Gianturco, D. T. and Cavenar, J. O. (1980) Seizures terminable and interminable with ECT. *American Journal of Psychiatry*, **137**, 1416–18.

West, E. (1981) Electric convulsion therapy in depression. *British Medical Journal*, **282**, 355–7.

Woodruff, R. A., Pitts, F. N. and McClure, J. N. (1968) The drug modification of ECT I. Methohexital, thiopental and preoxygenation. *Archives of General Psychiatry*, **8**, 605–11.

Wyant, G. M. and Macdonald, W. N. (1980) The role of atropine in electroconvulsive therapy. *Anaesthesia and Intensive Care*, **8**, 445–51.

CHAPTER 12

Anxiety and pain: terrible twins or supportive siblings?

Frank J. Vingoe

12.1 INTRODUCTION

It has been noted (Vingoe, 1981) that the 'subjective characteristics of pain' involve more than the physiology of the organism, but also 'the sum total of past experience and the totality of the present situation in which the individual finds himself' (p. 130). Beecher (1959) emphasized that the affective, psychological or **reaction component** of pain is quite significant. He stressed the importance of central nervous system processing of any original pain stimulus, noting 'that it can determine the presence or absence of suffering; it is an intimate part of the pain experience.'

The personality and cultural background of a person may be important in pain perception and behaviour. Thus, it would be highly likely that various emotional states, including anger, anxiety, depression, euphoria, intense pleasant sensations, etc. would all influence a person's perception of pain. It would be expedient to conclude that negative emotions increased pain perception while positive emotions decreased it. Unfortunately, as the literature shows, pain perception is far from simple. Clearly, variables in addition to the above, such as Locus of Control, expectation of experiencing pain, suggestibility, etc. may be important in pain perception. However, limitations of space dictate that the balance of the chapter will be devoted to the evidence concerning the influence of anxiety on pain.

Bond and Pearson (1969) found that advanced cancer patients experiencing pain were more neurotic than those not experiencing pain. However, there was no indication of whether the neuroticism was present prior to the pain or developed after the experience of pain. Klusman (1975) in studying fear and anxiety in a sample of women pre- and post-childbirth and child care classes, noted that 'Anxiety level was found to exert a significant effect on self-ratings of pain during the transition stage of labour.' Klusman concluded that anxiety enhances the perception of pain. Whether or not anxiety exacerbates pain perception is not as simple as it might seem. Bond and Pearson (1969) found that while extroverted neurotic women experiencing pain received analgesics, the introverted neurotic women experiencing pain did not. This could be explained on the basis that the extroverts would have more of a tendency to report their feelings of pain. However, these results also suggest that neuroticism/anxiety may act in interaction with other variables in its influence on pain perception.

12.2   ANXIETY

Almost thirty years ago, Coleman (1964) indicated that the twentieth century has been called the 'Age of Anxiety', perhaps suggesting that anxiety had increased over the years, although there is no firm evidence for this suggestion. Indeed, much of the following statement from Coleman probably applies as easily to the nineteenth century as it applies in the 1990s:

> Periodic breakdowns and runaways of the economic machinery –
> as well as automation and other technological innovations – have
> taken their toll in the millions of victims of unemployment and
> dislocation. The human population explosion is creating difficult
> political and social problems and tensions. Racial discrimination,
> with it unreasoned feelings of superiority, hatred, and resentment,
> hurts both the individual and the community. Homes broken by
> divorce leave emotional scars upon parents and children alike.
> Excessive competition, conflicting pressure groups, interpersonal
> bureaucracy, rapid social change, and the ever present threat of
> global atomic war further aggravates modern man's anxieties.
> (p. 2)

It is difficult to deny the importance of the concept of anxiety, particularly since many factor analytic studies of personality measures result in the preponderance of accountable variance being attributed to Anxiety/Neuroticism and Extraversion. Many studies show that scales of anxiety and neuroticism are moderately to highly correlated. Nietzel and Bernstein (1981) note that 'Anxiety is one of psychology's central concepts' which has been used in every major theory of personality and psychopathology.

There seem to be many synonyms for anxiety, such as, 'distress', 'fear', or 'stress', so that some may feel that there is no clear definition of anxiety.

12.2.1 Psychoanalytic view of anxiety

The definition, meaning, or interpretation of anxiety varies according to the theoretical point of view of the person who describes the concept. For example, the psychoanalytic view would be that various repressed feelings or impulses of which the individual is unaware (i.e., are unconscious) may serve to threaten the person. These feelings and impulses are felt as anxiety, and act as a warning of dangers and unacceptable impulses which are threatening to become conscious. The person is not aware of the source of the anxiety, since the source is from the unconscious (Freud, 1936). Freud named the above type of anxiety as 'neurotic anxiety' in contrast to 'fear' or 'realistic anxiety' which has a definite object, and 'moralistic anxiety', which involves a conflict between one's basic 'instincts' and one's conscience or superego.

12.2.2 Behavioural-cognitive view of anxiety

Nietzal and Bernstein (1981) saw no particular advantage in distinguishing the terms anxiety and fear. Considering anxiety from a learning point of view, there are specific eliciting stimuli which lead to anxiety, and reinforcing stimuli which maintain it. While the concept of prepared fears and the evidence for the genetic basis of neurosis may be considered (Rachman, 1990), the Behavioural-Cognitive or Learning View of anxiety is that the principles of learning, including stimulus generalization and one's reinforcement history are crucial for an understanding of the development and maintenance of anxiety.

12.2.3 Information-processing view

Following on an earlier, more behavioural, approach to anxiety is the Information-Processing paradigm, much concerned with the concept of Attention and Multiple-Channel processing (Williams *et al.*, 1988; MacLeod and Rutherford, 1992). In this paradigm, the controversy regarding the specifics of the interaction between affect (emotion) and cognition is important and must be based on empirical research. Differential processing is postulated for information of which one is unaware, as compared to information of which one is aware. Williams *et al.* (1988) demonstrate the definite effect of non-conscious processing in discussing many well-designed experimental projects.

12.2.4 Some unitary measures of anxiety

Most people would probably agree that they know when they are anxious by feelings of uneasiness, worry, or in being afraid (i.e. evidence from subjective self-report – a cognitive view).

Perhaps at the simplest level a visual analogue scale may be used which consists of a 100 millimetre line from zero to 100, in which the individual has to mark off a place indicating the degree of his or her anxiety, where 100 is the highest degree of anxiety one could expect to feel, and zero indicates being perfectly calm. This measure has been referred to as the Subjective Units of Distress/Disturbance Scale (SUDS), which can use 100 points (Wolpe, 1982), but can also be restricted to a zero to 10 scale. This SUDS is frequently used in behavioural therapy.

More objectively, a person may be said to be anxious when certain types of behaviour, such as tremor, excessive sweating, or a tendency to withdraw, can be objectively observed (i.e., evidence based on objective behavioural observation, see Nietzal and Bernstein, 1981). The Hamilton Anxiety Scale (Hamilton, 1959) is based on behavioural observation.

The Behavioural Avoidance Test (BAT), is an *in-vivo* test which measures the degree of approach – avoidance behaviour – of a patient towards a feared object or situation. For example, if the individual is snake phobic, how close is that individual willing to move towards a non-poisonous snake. The distance from the snake is then a measure of avoidance.

Further, when certain physiological changes, such as increased heart rate, increased skin conductance, and increased or irregular respiration rate occur, it may be concluded that a condition of anxiety is present (Lang, 1968, 1971).

Some or all of these suggestive indicants may, however, be related to factors other than anxiety, for example, another emotion, exercise, medication, or changes in environmental temperature. Therefore, different factors may result in similar indicants/symptoms being experienced or observed. Many people may wish to use the term fear or stress rather than anxiety to refer to their condition. Thus, the same or a similar condition in different people, or in the same person at different times, may be labelled differently.

12.2.5 The three response systems

In reference to theories of emotion, including anxiety, Lang (1985) has indicated the importance of considering the three components of emotion (i.e., physiological, behavioural, and cognitive). The Gate-Control theory of pain (Melzack and Dennis, 1983; Melzack and Wall, 1982), in emphasizing sensory, affective and evaluative aspects of pain experience, is analogous. Lacy's (1967) ideas regarding autonomic, behavioural and cortical arousal are also valuable with regard to understanding anxiety and pain. Hugdahl (1981) should be read for its critique of the Three Systems Model of fear. Hugdahl recommends that treatment should be selected on the basis of the individual's response profile (i.e., his/her relative standing in behavioural, cognitive and physiological indicants) of anxiety.

12.2.6 Response desynchrony

It has frequently been noted that the objective BAT measure, cognitive measure, and psychophysiological measures of anxiety are not necessarily consistent in indicating the presence of anxiety, i.e., they frequently have a low correlation with each other. This has been referred to as Response Desynchrony (Rachman and Hodgson, 1974). For example, a significant minority of people may not be aware they are anxious yet show many of the clinical or behavioural indicants of anxiety. The following case study illustrates the point.

Case study 12.1

One of the patients treated by the author complained of a lift phobia and, when asked about this and asked to rate herself on the 10-point SUDS scale, she marked an 8, indicating that she had relatively high distress or anxiety associated with taking a lift and, indeed, in coming for her appointment she would tend to walk up four flights of stairs to the author's consulting room. She was asked if she would be willing to go down to one of the less busy lifts and see how she would feel going into the lift with her therapist. She agreed to this with some trepidation.

She was asked to step inside the lift with the therapist. We remained in the lift for a minute or two keeping the lift door open. She was observed during this time and there were no indications of physiological anxiety, although instrumentation was not used and, when asked how she felt then, she said she felt fine. We then proceeded to travel one floor above, a few floors below, and so forth, and this particular patient remained free of any indication of anxiety. This case demonstrates that, in fact, one should not rely upon measures of anxiety alone, since one could be misled into thinking that a problem is much more difficult to solve than, in fact, is the case. Rachman (1990, pp. 255–66) provides an interesting and informative discussion on the over-prediction of fear.

12.2.7 Trait and state anxiety

Spielberger, Gorsuch and Lushene (1970), who developed the State Trait Anxiety Inventory (STAI), indicate that Trait Anxiety (A Trait) 'refers to relatively stable individual differences in anxiety proneness, that is, the difference between people in the tendency to respond to situations perceived as threatening with elevation of A-State intensity. These authors refer to State Anxiety 'as a transitory emotional state or condition of the human organism that is characterized by subjective, consciously perceived feelings of tension and apprehension, and heightened autonomic nervous system activity' (p.3). They note that anxiety states 'may vary in intensity and fluctuate over time' (p.3).

If one is not feeling particularly anxious and things are going along reasonably well, with a relative absence of perceived stressors in one's environment, then the anxiety measured at that time would be referred to as Trait Anxiety following Spielberger, Gorsuch and Lushene, 1970. However, if one is expecting an operation in the very near future or has a feeling that one is going to be hurt or suffer pain in the near future, then this hypothesized increase in anxiety, based upon a particular perceived stressor, whether at the present time or anticipated for the near future, would be referred to as State Anxiety. Trait Anxiety then is a generalized predisposition to respond to stressors as perceived idiosyncratically by the particular individual. Research (Chapman and Cox, 1977) has found that pre-surgical levels of State Anxiety tend to vary as a function of Trait Anxiety.

12.2.8 Anxiety questionnaires

The Cognitive and Somatic Anxiety Questionnaire (CSAQ) (Schwartz, Davidson and Coleman, 1978) is concerned with differentially measuring cognitive as well as somatic anxiety. Evidence that this scale effectively differentiates these factors is supported by Delmonte and Ryan (1983). Steptoe and Kearsley (1990) compared the CSAQ to the somatic and cognitive scales of the Lehrer and Woolford (1982) Anxiety Symptom Questionnaire (LWASQ) (i.e., omitting the behavioural scale) and the Worry-Emotionality Scale (WES) (Morris, Davies and Hutchens, 1981), and concluded by recommending the CSAQ for the measurement of somatic and cognitive anxiety.

However, the full LWASQ (including somatic, behavioural and cognitive anxiety) was compared to other scales by Scholing and Emmelkamp (1992), who reported on the psychometric characteristics and validity of this questionnaire and supported its use to measure treatment effectiveness. Scholing and Emmelkamp (1992) compared the LWASQ with the CSAQ and the WES, both of which measure only two aspects of anxiety. The LWASQ was recommended for both research and clinical practice in that:

- It is the only scale that measures the main three aspects to anxiety;
- The factorial structure is clear for both analogue and clinical groups;

- It is the best of the three scales in assessing unique variance;
- It possesses good internal consistency (reliability);
- the scale possesses adequate ability to discriminate between several normal and clinical groups, and to detect treatment progress.

12.2.9 Anticipatory anxiety

In analogue research, i.e. research carried out in the laboratory, and in real life situations, anticipatory anxiety can occur. In a laboratory setting, in which the subject expects to be stimulated by an objective stressor, such as an electric shock, there is more likely to be general agreement that, on average, the person would experience anticipatory anxiety or stress prior to experiencing the shock which then, of course, may result in a feeling of pain.

In a clinical situation a person may report feeling quite anxious about something that might happen in the future, but the patient may be unable to specify to what the anxiety refers, although indeed in some cases questioning might reveal a great deal of anxiety about death or the development of some terminal disease. Others, including some health professionals, may feel that the patient is malingering or is imagining things, in cases in which there is no objective stimulus or situation which could conceivably elicit anxiety. The anxious person may be convinced that something dire is about to happen and is anxious for that particular reason, but basically the person may be unable to specify the object of this anticipatory anxiety. In short, anticipatory anxiety may have a known object or not.

12.3 ANXIETY AND PAIN

A question that can be raised is: Is pain, like anxiety, an actual emotion? If it is an emotion, then one would suppose that one would respond to the pain stimulus in many ways as one responds to some other stressor, which evokes anxiety. Indeed, both the feeling of pain and anxiety are usually considered as stressful responses.

12.3.1 Confounding of pain and other emotions

A question that could be raised then with reference to anticipatory anxiety in a case where the anticipated stressor is expected to cause pain is as follows: Is the measurement of anxiety at that time compounded with one's attitude towards pain, as compared to the situation where the anticipatory anxiety is related to a stressor that does not involve expected pain? One might anticipate, for example, that pain perception would be magnified by high state anxiety if the expected stressor normally involves pain. There are obviously other anticipated situations which may have a varying probability of actually occurring (from 0.0 where a threat is made but not carried out, to 1.0, a case in which the probability of the threat occurring is 100%). One's attitudes, beliefs, and other cognitions relating to the threat value of some hypothetical or actual future event, are surely of the greatest importance whether or not the stressor involves pain.

Sternbach (1968) takes a whole chapter to define pain, and he notes that 'pain is a hurt that we feel'. We frequently equate a feeling with an emotion. Sternbach stresses that pain 'is the essential personal and individual quality of the phenomena.' He further points out that while we can observe pain behaviour, we cannot actually observe a person's feeling of pain. Sternbach notes that each person's perception of pain is unique or idiosyncratic. On the basis of his discussion, pain can be considered from a cognitive point of view, in that we interpret or attach meaning to our pain. Sternbach also refers to the behavioural aspect of pain, noting that this could be at the cellular level in the nervous system, or overt measurable behaviour. The psychophysiological aspects of pain are also important for Sternbach. Consistent with the ideas of the Gate-Control theory of pain (Melzack and Wall, 1982), Sternbach would agree that there is a definite emotional or affective aspect to pain as is characteristic of anxiety.

In their excellent book on pain, Turk, Meichenbaum and Genest (1983) note that pain is 'An unpleasant sensory **and emotional experience** associated with actual or **potential** tissue damage, or described in terms of such damage.' (IASP, Subcommittee on Taxonomy, 1979, p. 250, emphasis added) (Cited by Turk, Meichenbaum and Genest, 1983, p. 82).

On the basis of Sternbach's (1968) work, noted above, and the definition provided by Turk, Michenbaum and Genest (1983), pain can certainly be considered to have an emotional component or factor. Further, it seems plausible to consider any emotional or mood state to be such as to influence one's perception of pain. For example, heightened anxiety, depression, being in a state of anger, all may influence pain, although the specific interaction would depend upon the total situation, as well as the type and degree of emotion. Wade *et al.* (1990) point out that the experience of pain is multi-dimensional, and they refer to the work of Melzack and Wall on the Gate Control Theory of pain, indicating that pain consists not only of a sensory dimension, but also of a cognitive-evaluative and an affective-motivational dimension. Wade *et al.* (1990) note that: 'The experience of pain is not necessarily associated with one particular emotion, such as, depression, but also may be accompanied by anxiety, frustration, anger or fear, depending upon a variety of circumstances' (p. 304).

12.3.2 Prediction of pain and pain behaviour

It would seem reasonable that most people would like to have some control over their pain. Unfortunately, there can be uncontrollable aspects to pain (Arntz and Schmidt, 1989) and many who suffer from chronic pain may perceive much or all of their pain as uncontrollable. Further, perceived uncontrollability may very well lead to depression and even feelings of helplessness (Seligman, 1975).

Wade *et al.* (1990) developed a number of Visual Analogue Scales (VAS) in order to measure the various emotions. While controlling for pain sensation intensity, they determined the specific 'contribution of anger, frustration, anxiety, fear, and depression to pain-related unpleasantness and clinical indices of depression' (p. 304). All subjects in their study were patients who were referred by anaesthesiologists for psychological evaluation. The psychological battery included the Beck Depression Inventory (BDI), the Minnesota Multiphasic Personality Inventory (MMPI), as well as the Pain Experienced, and VASs noted above. In addition to the VAS depression, anxiety, frustration, fear, and anger scales, another scale was developed and was referred to as Pain Unpleasantness. One end of this scale was labelled as 'not bad at all' and the other end was labelled as 'the most intense bad feeling imaginable'.

Wade *et al.* (1990) noted that the main purpose of their study was to determine the specific feelings which contrbuted to the unpleasantness and depression pain patients suffer. The authors found that pain patients' highest level of negative emotion was on the frustration scale. While Wade *et al.* were also interested in predicting clinical depression, the following comments will apply only to the Pain-Related Emotional Unpleasantness Scale. After statistically controlling the pain sensation intensity, it was found that anxiety and frustration were the most important predictors of pain unpleasantness. The authors, however, were quick to point out that the relationship between the VAS scales and the Pain Unpleasantness Scale did not specify a causal relationship. They indicate the possibility that 'prolonged or intense anger and anxiety [may] exacerbate the overall emotional unpleasantness associated with pain, making pain less tolerable (p. 309). Wade *et al.* indicate that each emotion VAS makes a unique contribution to the overall magnitude of pain-related emotional unpleasantness. They conclude that their 'findings suggest that anger and frustration make important contributions to the emotional unpleasantness associated with chronic pain' (p. 309).They suggest that the use of treatment approaches which target these particular symptoms may prove very useful.

Anderson *et al.* (1988) worked with patients suffering from rheumatoid arthritis (RA) and attempted to determine the degree to which depression, anxiety, and helplessness predicted pain behaviour, as well as the functional status of these patients. Pain behaviour was measured using a standardized observation method. Anderson *et al.* (1988) point out that previous work had suggested that both anxiety and depression contributed to rheumatoid arthritic pain and functional disability, independently of disease activity (p. 26). These authors were also interested in the concept of learned helplessness, which they defined as 'a behaviour pattern characterized by emotional, motivational, and cognitive deficits in coping with stressful situations' (p. 26). Anderson *et al.* were interested in determining 'whether helplessness can predict pain behaviour and disability after controlling for important medical status variables, such as, duration of disease and rheumatoid disease activity.' They were concerned with determining what percentage of the variance in pain behaviour and functional status of rheumatoid arthritic patients could be predicted on the basis of measures of depression, anxiety, and helplessness. All patients were diagnosed as having classic rheumatoid arthritis. Lubin's (1967) Depression Adjective Checklist (DAC) was used to measure depression. The Trait Form of the STAI was used to measure the tendency to experience anxiety, and the measure of helplessness used was the Arthritis Helplessness Index (AHI), which is a measure 'that assesses the extent to which patients believe they can control their arthritis symptoms.' Pain behaviour was based upon a 10-minute videotape session, in which the subject was required to perform a standardized sequence of movements. Mean scores all indicated moderate levels of depression, anxiety, and helplessness.

While total pain behaviour, guarding and rigidity were predicted by the duration of the disease, neither depression, anxiety, nor helplessness predicted a significant amount of the variance in these three dependent variables once demographic and medical status variables were controlled.

Referring to the fact that previous studies had found that depression was a good predictor of pain behaviour in low back pain (LBP) patients (Keefe *et al.*, 1986), the authors felt that depression might 'play a larger role in the pain behaviour of LBP patients compared to RA patients, due to differences in the aetiology of depression and the extent or severity of tissue or joint damage' (p. 30). In their discussion, Anderson *et al.* (1988) suggested that in RA patients physiological variables might play a greater role in chronic pain than either psychological variables or learning processes. Finally, while the authors found that helplessness was significantly related to the rheumatoid arthritis index and depression, it failed to predict pain behaviour or functional disability.

In comparing the contrasting results of the above two studies, it should be pointed out that Wade *et al.* (1990) were interested in a cognitive type of pain dependent variable, while Anderson *et al.* (1988) focused on behavioural dependent variables (pain behaviours). Further, the type of patients used were quite different. While Anderson *et al.*

used RA patients, Wade *et al.* included LBP, myofacial pain, and causal-gic patients primarily.

12.3.3.　Anticipation of pain

Patients who are awaiting an operation tend to anticipate a degree of pain and distress associated with the operation. This, however, has been referred to as pre-operational anxiety/stress (Janis, 1958). There are other situations which involve an anticipation of both pain and anxiety. Those individuals, for example, who suffer from needle phobia may anticipate a certain amount of pain, and are quite anxious about having injections. One questions whether the anticipation of a stress event expected to result in pain can be accurately assessed by using separate pain and anxiety measures?

A specific situation which is useful in terms of studying both pain and anxiety, of course, is the dental situation, since many people seem to be rather afraid of receiving dental treatment. Many of those with high anticipatory anxiety and a high expectation of feeling significant pain may actually over-predict the degree of pain they will experience and/or over-predict the degree of anxiety they will suffer. Kent (1986) compared the discrepancy between the discomfort dental patients expected in the dental situation and their actual experience to changes in dental anxiety which were reported three months after their dental appointment. Kent pointed out that anxious patients have a pessimistic outlook about the degree of pain they will experience. On the other hand, reasonably accurate expectations were found to be associated with those of low anxiety in a previous study carried out by Kent.

While waiting in the dentist's reception area, patients were asked to participate in a study on the anxiety people feel when they visit a dentist. The Corah Dental Anxiety Scale (DAS) (Corah, Gale and Illig, 1978) was used, and patients were asked to indicate their reason for attending. Further, they were required to indicate the degree of pain they expected to experience during that visit, on a 100 mm VAS. Following treatment, patients were required to complete another VAS indicating the amount of pain they had actually experienced while in the dental chair. Thus, a pain discrepancy score was obtained. They were also asked to indicate the degree of confidence regarding their prediction of the degree of pain they would experience on another visit to the dentist, and how confident they would be in experiencing the same amount of pain if the treatment was similar to that obtained during their initial visit. Anxiety was also assessed three months after the initial visit. The results indicated that when the discrepancy between expected and experienced pain decreased, the patients' confidence increased. When there was a large discrepancy between expected and experienced pain, there seemed to be a low rating on the confidence of the typicality of the appointment. Kent

(1986) recommended that it is important that the therapist encourage the patient to consider a discomfort-free exposure as typical.

12.3.4 Desired and perceived control of pain

The extent to which one feels one has control of a potential noxious stimulus is important in actually coping with that stimulus. Logan *et al.* (1991) carried out a study on desired and felt control with reference to stress in a dental setting. These authors felt that the desire for control was a very important variable to assess, as well as the degree of felt control. More than 150 patients were used, and were required to complete the Iowa Dental Control Index (IDCI) and the Dental Fear Survey (DFS). The DFS measured three factors: avoidance, fear of specific dental stimuli, and autonomic arousal. The authors pointed out that previous research had found that higher scores on the DFS were related to higher rates of dental appointment cancellation and greater waiting room activities. The IDCI was used to allocate patients to four sub-groups. The IDCI contains two items on the desire for dental control scale, and two items on the felt dental control scale. An analysis of the scales indicated that the 'high desire for control/low felt control subject sub-group had significantly higher fear scores than each of the remaining three groups'. Basically, it was concluded that 'patients who report having a high desire for dental control, coupled with low feelings of such control, appear to be at risk for dental fear'. Those subjects who reported a relative absence of a desire for control in a dental situation and reported low felt control, were not more fearful of dental treatment than patients who reported high levels of felt control.

On a basis of the three studies carried out by Logan *et al.* (1991) it was indicated that when patients both desire control and feel they have little control, they are most likely to experience negative emotions.

Relating their results to Lazarus' work on stress (Lazarus and Folkman, 1984), the authors note that 'desired control may reflect the level of threat subjects feel in dental settings, whereas felt control reflects patients' confidence in their individual coping strategies'. Logan *et al.* (1991) suggested that dental distress is causally related to the discrepancy between desired and felt control in the dental situation. They noted that if this interpretation is correct, then 'increasing patients' perception of control should have a particularly therapeutic impact upon patients in the high desire/low felt group because increasing control should reduce the key discrepancy' (p. 358).

12.3.5 Fear expectancy model of avoidance behaviour

Gross (1992) reported on three studies involving pain, anxiety, and dental avoidance. Reviewing previous work, he noted that the fear of pain may be worse than the actual experience of pain itself. In order to accomplish dental work, people with extreme dental phobias may have to be admitted to hospital and given general anaesthesia. Gross pointed out that it was not clear whether the fear of pain, anxiety or panic is primarily responsible for dental avoidance. Gross referred to the fear expectancy model of avoidance behaviour, which consists of three factors: danger expectancy, anxiety expectancy, and anxiety sensitivity. He defined anxiety sensitivity as 'the fear of anxiety' and, in the study reported, he referred to pain sensitivity as the fear of pain. An anxiety sensitivity scale had been constructed by previous workers, and could be distinguished from the construct of anxiety *per se*. However, a measure of pain sensitivity was not available, and Gross' major purpose was to develop a measure of pain sensitivity and determine if pain sensitivity could predict dental avoidance and dental pain. The Dental Phobias and Pain Sensitivity Inventory (DPPSI) was then developed for Gross' study. The DPPSI is made up of 33 items which relate to dental and medical treatment. All 33 items are rated on a zero to 7-point scale, and relate to fear, avoidance, and pain sensitivity. A factor analysis of the DPPSI revealed the following factors: dental phobia, health concerns, medical phobia, injections/venipuncture phobia and, finally, 'the fifth factor (which) was interpreted as a pain sensitivity factor, as fears related to painful dental procedures, injection into one's gums, and severe pain correlated highest and positively with this factor' (p. 9). It was pointed out 'that the fear of severe pain (was) loaded on several factors – which suggests that the fear of pain is a generalized and transsituational fear.'

The second study undertaken by Gross was the development of a Pain Sensitivity Index (PSI), which was 'based on the Anxiety-Sensitivity Scale (ASS) (Reiss and McNally, 1985, p. 9)' and contains 16 items which were subsequently factor analysed into five main factors, the first factor accounting for 32% of the variance. 'The first factor obtained was interpreted as a Pain Sensitivity factor (p. 9)'. The remaining four factors together accounted for only 31% of the variance. The interpretation of each of the remaining four factors is as follows: 'The second factor was characterized by feeling uncomfortable when other people discussed their painful experiences. The third factor was characterized by concerns about appearing in pain to other people. Whereas the fourth factor was characterized by cognitive interference due to pain, the fifth factor was characterized by painful memories' (Gross, 1992, p. 10).

The third study carried out by Gross included 40 undergraduate psychology students and their friends, and a group of 25 dental patients. In addition to administering the DPPSI and the PSI to subjects, the fear questionnaire, which is made up of four subscales involving:

agoraphobia,* 'blood injury phobia', social phobia, and anxiety/ depression was also administered. Finally, a 4-item Panic Scale was also administered. Intercorrelations between the results were determined. Basically, the results indicated that pain sensitivity correlated significantly with injection pain and drill pain. While pain sensitivity and injection pain did not correlate significantly with the view that the construct of pain sensitivity is different from that with avoidance, drill pain did. Gross concluded that evidence was found 'In support of anxiety sensitivity, the PSI but not the ASS was found to correlate significantly with blood-injury phobia* (many of the situations described by items on this subscale of the Fear Questionnaire, such as, having minor surgery, often involve pain).' (Gross, 1992, p. 11).

Gross suggests that 'pain intensity and pain sensitivity are important components of dental avoidance. In other words, perceived pain is different to reactions to pain; however, pain sensitivity is only one of the reactions that people may experience in relation to pain . . . cognitions may influence the relationship between pain and dental avoidance' (p. 12). It is further noted by Gross that 'Cognitions may interact with biological factors, for instance, pain sensitive persons may interpret physical arousal as pain cues. Finally, Gross argues 'As pain sensitivity is regarded as a stable personality component, it could contribute to an understanding of chronic and multiple pains which are accompanied by anxiety. It is argued that the expectancy model of fear could be expanded to include pain sensitivity and pain expectation . . .' (Gross, 1992, p. 12).

Milgrom, Vignehsa and Weinstein (1992) carried out a study concerning the frequency and aetiology of dental fear in more than 1500 children from six Singapore secondary schools. The schools were chosen as being representative of all State-supported schools. The Dental Fear Survey (DFS) a 20-item self report fear inventory, was administered, as was the Dental Beliefs Survey (DBS) where high scores are related to perceptions of vulnerability and lack of control. Subjects were also asked about their most recent dental visit. The results indicated that in the population studied the reported rate of high dental fear was 115 children per 1000 population. The authors note that the three variables of importance in the prediction of self-reported fears were found to be perceived control over aversive stimuli, recency of last dental visit, and painful treatment. They felt that those who stay away from dental treatment tend to develop the greatest fear.

---

* Rachman (1990, pp. 79–84) provides a very interesting discussion of 'blood-injury phobia', suggesting that perhaps it should not be called a phobia after all, since it does not satisfy some of the criteria for the typical phobias. Those who are adversely affected by the sight of blood show an avoidance response, but their physiological reactions are not like those exhibited in response to other feared stimuli. Finally, the sight of blood fails to evoke a phobic reaction in a person who is recumbent.

With reference to pain, they note 'While motivation and cognitive factors can enhance pain . . . , pain may reinforce fear and fear-related behaviours (Milgrom, Vignehsa and Weinstein 1992). With reference to the perception of control, Milgrom *et al.* note that this may moderate the aversiveness of treatment. They note 'The finding that high levels of fear are most likely when Ss report lack of control, and pain during the last visit points to the importance of control in mediating the fearfulness of a painful experience. Longer intervals between treatment were associated with greater fear. It may be that delay is related to an expectation of having dental problems that would require aversive painful, treatment' (p. 371). Milgrom, Vignesha and Weinstein (1992) further report that 'The probability of a stressful experience resulting in fear and avoidance is enhanced when perceptions of control are low.' (p. 371).

Berggren (1992) studied over 100 adult patients at a Dental Fear Research and Treatment Centre in Sweden. These patients were placed on a one-year waiting list and, after a short interview, were later sent a packet of questionnaires. These questionnaires included the Dental Anxiety Scale (DAS) (Corah, 1969) and the Dental Fear Survey (DFS) Kleinknecht, Klepac and Alexander (1973). In addition, the Fear Survey Schedule-II (Geer, 1965) was used, together with some additional items. Included was an item measuring fear of pain, which could be rated on a one to 7-point scale, one indicating no fear of pain, and seven indicating a totally terrifying reaction. Among the results was the finding with reference to feared objects and situations, that 'the separate item "pain" elicited the highest mean scores for both men and women' (p. 398). Among other quite common extreme fears were a fear of suffocating, death of a loved one, and fear of hypodermic needles. Berggren concluded 'However, there is still a question of whether dental fear and general fearfulness are both reactions among individuals prone to phobic reactions, and that the inter-relationship between these fears is a component of a personality, or if dental fear may have influenced the individual's appraisal of other situations or generalized to other situations' (p. 400). A more specific question is whether those individuals who are prone to high anxiety or to many phobic reactions would tend to have a greater fear of pain and, in fact, to report a greater degree of subjective pain and exhibit more pain behaviour than those individuals who are not particularly subject to high anxiety or many phobic reactions.

Part of the research noted by Lacroix and Barbaree (1992) concerned the use of affective or behavioural responses to predict future pain intensity, severity and duration. Mood state was assessed using the Profile of Mood States (POMS) (McNair, Lorr and Droppleman, 1971). Lacroix and Barbaree used a Group of 25 headache subjects, who had had two sequential headaches, and determined if the relationship between mood or behavioural disturbance during the first headache could explain the intensity, duration and overall severity of the second headache. Headache intensity was based on a 5-point scale. Pain duration was in hours, and the Headache Severity Index was derived from the headache intensity multiplied by headache duration. The Headache Severity Index was found to be independent of the other two measures. Partialling out the duration of the first headache, it was found that the Mood Factor score during the first headache was significantly correlated with the duration of the second headache. However, the mood during the first headache was not significantly correlated with the intensity of the second headache. Partialling out the pain severity of the first headache, it was found that the Mood Factor score during the first headache was significantly predictive of the pain severity during the second headache.

An important factor found by Lacroix and Barbaree (1992) was that mood and behavioural disruption continued 24 hours following the time when the actual headache pain had ended. The authors note that 'The affective response to one's first headache is related to the duration and overall severity of the subsequent headache' (p. 477). In contrast to the ability of mood to predict the duration and severity of the subsequent headache, behavioural disruptions during the first headache were not found predictive for the duration or severity of the second headache. It was suggested by the authors that treatment techniques which tend to reduce the affective response to pain might serve also to prevent or to diminish the degree of future pain. In referring to the range of responses to pain, the authors suggest that the term Pain Elicited Response would be useful in summarizing them, in that,

(1) it 'reflects the large number of quantifiable behavioural and psychological changes that co-occurs (*sic*) with the perception of pain sensations';
(2) it 'refers to the disturbances that are triggered by the perception of pain, and also those which may persist following pain termination . . .'; and
(3) 'The use of the term "Pain Elicited Responses" further encourages the study of a broad range of disturbances which accompany pain, while simultaneously avoiding terminology often used which either invoke abnormal personality constructs or psychiatric labels.' (p. 477–78).

Lacroix and Barbaree (1992) thus remind us that emotional responses may accompany pain but may continue some time after the pain. Obviously, these emotional responses are different from anticipatory anxiety or other anticipatory emotional feelings which are associated with some actual or assumed noxious stimulus which is expected to occur at some point in the relatively near future.

12.3.6 Analogue study of pain and fear

In an analogue study on pain and fear, McNeil and Brunetti (1992) used 48 beginning psychology student subjects assigned to one of three groups: (1) pain, (2) fear and (3) pain and fear. The pain scripts used referred to pain (i) in the mouth, or (2) in the lower leg, while the fear scripts referred to either the anticipation of (1) dental procedures, or (2) a dog attack. The combined script involved the former pain and fear or the latter pain and fear. McNeil and Brunetti (1992) found that physiological (heart rate) and (self-reported affective) response to pain imagery and fear imagery scripts were very similar, although they did differ in amplitude. For example, a greater heart rate response and more negative emotional ratings were made in reference to action or neutral scripts which were used as a control procedure.

McNeil and Brunetti (1992) indicated that 'Pain was rated as significantly more negative than either fear or pain plus fear. Additionally, pain scripts had the lowest dominance ratings, suggesting that the Pain Group felt less in control' (p. 518). The authors suggested that 'Response to pain is different than response to fear, with more intense verbalizations in the former and stronger cardiac acceleration in the latter' (p. 518). The authors note that 'From the perspective of Rachman and Lopatka's (1986) work, no *additivity* was demonstrated in the Pain plus Fear scripts' (p. 518). The authors suggest that future research might involve the use of personally relevant scenes, as they have been found to be highly vivid, and also it would be useful to measure self-reported imagery-ability, since this can be a significant individual difference variable. They also suggest that future work should determine the relationship between pain and fear by 'inducing pain and fear by using stimulation other than imagery scripts' (p. 519). McNeil and Brunetti conclude that 'To fully understand the relationship between pain and fear, . . . the effects of pain on fear must also be studied. By studying pain and fear in combination, much should be learned about each of these states as independent constructs' (p. 519).

12.3.7 Pain confronters and pain avoiders

In a very significant article, Rose *et al.* (1992) compared three chronic pain groups with three pain-free comparison groups by using the fear avoidance model of exaggerated pain perception. Rose *et al.*, using a work of Philips and colleagues (Philips, 1974; Philips and Hunter, 1981) who suggested that physiological, subjective and behavioural aspects of pain might be desynchronous under certain conditions, indicated that 'The central concept of the model is fear of pain and consequent pain avoidance or confrontation.' They further noted that both the fear of pain and consequent pain avoidance or confrontation has an affect upon the behavioural response of the patient to acute pain. The authors contrast a non-adaptive pain avoider with an adaptive pain confronter. They indicate that the person who confronts pain exhibits behaviours which increase the range of physical and social activities, enabling the individual to calibrate his/her pain experience as compared to the sensory-discriminative stimulus. They note that 'The adaptive pain confronter maintains synchrony between pain sensation and pain behaviour. By contrast, the non-adaptive pain avoider is considered to be motivated to avoid any fresh exposure to pain' (p. 316). Rose *et al.* note that 'The pain avoider will avoid pain experience and painful activities. Physicially, this may lead to loss of mobility, loss of muscular strength, and weight gain. Psychologically, the consequences of avoiding physical activity includes fewer opportunities for calibrating pain sensation against pain experience. This leads to desynchrony between sensation and pain behaviour, and may lead to invalid status' (p. 360). The foregoing is based on the work of Lethem *et al.* (1983) who 'Proposed a continuum between avoidance and confrontation of pain' and indicated that an individual's fear of pain enabled that individual to be placed on this continuum. Rose *et al.* (1992) indicate that both 'fear of, and the tendency to avoid pain is determined by the "psycho-social context" in which initial injury or disease takes place (p. 360). They indicate that the psycho-social context is influenced by four factors which are 'stressful life events, personal pain history, personal pain coping strategies, and personality characteristics' (p. 360). Following Lethem *et al.* (1983) Rose *et al.* (1992) indicate that 'The previous experience of severe pain may sensitize the individual to fear of pain and lead to an avoidance response whenever more pain is threatened.'

Basically, Rose *et al.* compared three groups who had recovered from shingles, acute low back pain or fractures, with the chronic pain groups of post-herpetic neuralgia (PHN), chronic low back pain (CLBP), and reflex sympathetic dystrophy (RSD) patients. The authors used the Modified Somatic Perception Questionnaire (MSPQ) which includes 13 questions related to the autonomic nervous system, such as, sweating or blurring of vision. A Weighted Life Events Questionnaire was also used, as well as ratings on externally produced pain such as joint sprains, internally produced pain such as headaches, and results of minor accidents, such as banging one's finger with a hammer. Subjects were asked about previous pain coping strategies they had used in reference to a particular type of pain. Two options referred to passive coping strategies, while two referred to acting coping strategies.

The results of a discriminant function analysis indicated that there was a correct prediction of recovery or chronicity; the exception was that the difference in mean Fear Avoidance Model scores between the fracture patients and the RSD patients was not significant. Rose *et al.* (1992) indicate that the results of their study supports the Fear Avoidance Model, in that, it 'provides a unified psychological theory which explains the development of chronic pain resulting from a benign, acute pain experience, across a range of pathologies' (p. 364). Further, the recovered patients and the chronic pain patients were differentiated in terms of stressful life events, personal pain history, and personality characteristics. However, the personal pain coping strategies were not significantly different for the two groups. In conclusion, Rose *et al.* note that 'the findings of this study reinforce the concept of psychological phenomena which influence the onset of chronic pain regardless of physical signs and symptoms associated with specifically "labelled" pathology' (p. 364). The authors note that further research may lead to the development of a scale which can be used with acute pain patients, enabling a prediction to be made regarding the course their condition will follow, i.e. recovery or chronicity.

12.4   ATTENTION, ANXIETY AND PAIN

Rachman (1990) in discussing Londoners' reaction to World War II air raids, drew on data from Dr. Henry Wilson (1942, p. 284) and found that a large number of people who suffered from mild fears unrelated to air raids were present in the 485 people who did not suffer from acute fear related to air raids. This suggested that these mild, unrelated, fears may have served as inoculations against developing air raid fears. Further support for this general idea is, as Rachman pointed out, that those employed in essential services, such as firemen and policemen, who were also repeatedly exposed to dangerous situations, did not, for the most part, develop adverse psychological reactions. Rachman further noted that Aubrey Lewis, a well-known British psychiatrist, suggested that being involved 'in a socially useful occupation might have provided a form of innoculation against stress.' (p.25).

Arntz, Dreesen and Merkelbach (1991) commented on the idea held by many that anxiety increases pain, and noted that the dual process theory of habituation could be interpreted as supporting that view. The authors also refer to research supporting the view that anxiety may reduce pain. They note that whether or not anxiety increases pain has not been established. They postulate that a third factor, such as attention, may modulate the relationship between anxiety and pain. They point to a significant number of studies which suggest that attention to the pain may increase it, while distraction may decrease it. Arntz *et al.* indicate that 'it seems evident that if the focus of fear/anxiety is directed away from the pain, the pain experience is reduced; and conversely, if the pain itself is focused upon because of pain-related fear/anxiety, the pain experience will be stronger'. They suggest that in previous studies concerning anxiety and pain, anxiety may very well have been confounded with attention.

Using 55 spider-phobic subjects in a 2 by 2 design (low vs. high anxiety) and (attention vs. distraction from pain), they tested whether anxiety increased or decreased pain, whether attention to the experimental pain increased it or, finally, whether the interaction hypothesis that only anxiety and attention to the pain increases pain. Ten cm VASs were used to measure S response to (1) anxiety during shock; (2) experienced pain, and (3) attention to pain during pain stimulation. Skin conductance and heart-rate measures were also obtained. Experimental pain was via electric shock. Anxiety was induced by suggestions that the shock apparatus might be at fault, disturbances in heart rate could be caused and skin might be burned due to the use of improper electrode paste.

The authors indicate that three unambiguous conclusions may be drawn from their data:

(1) 'attention to pain is clearly related to stronger pain responses';
(2) the hypothesis that anxiety is related to stronger pain responses is refuted; and
(3) there is little support for the idea that anxiety results in a lesser response to pain.

The authors, therefore, conclude that: attention appears to be the critical factor: subjective pain, skin conductance responses (SCRs) and (marginally significant) heart-rate responses (HRRs) were less when the S directed his/her attention away from the pain stimulation.

Arntz *et al.* (1991) suggest that further research which examines the effect of distraction on long-term habituation of pain responses might be both fruitful and clinically relevant. The authors are keen to note that: 'The lack of influence of anxiety does not mean that anxiety is never relevant with respect to clinical pain, he/she may pay a lot of attention to the pain thereby increasing the pain . . . Pain-related anxiety merely motivates the S to direct attention to the pain.' Arntz *et al.* note that anxiety reduction techniques are appropriate when anxiety is the motivating factor in the patient's attention to his/her pain.' Arntz *et al.* further indicate that, with reference to chronic pain, distraction techniques, because they decrease experienced pain and foster subjective habituation, may be a powerful factor in the psychological treatment of pain. Further, feelings of helplessness and a perceived decreased control over pain and life in general may be significantly diminished.

12.5 SUMMARY AND CONCLUSIONS

The introductory section stressed the importance of past and present experience, including experience of pain, in the perception of pain. It was also noted that emotional/psychological factors affect the central nervous system processing of any pain stimulus. While cultural and learning factors are important, the introductory section stressed emotional and psychological factors, including locus of control in pain perception and behaviour.

The second section of the chapter gave an indication of the psycho-analytic, behavioural-cognitive and information-processing views of anxiety. Various means of measuring unidimensional anxiety were discussed, stressing one of the three response systems: cognitive or self-report, behavioural or avoidance, and physiological. The reality of response desynchrony rather than response consistency and measurement was indicated. Further the State versus Trait concepts of anxiety were differentiated, and the concept of anticipatory anxiety was discussed. The importance of Trait Anxiety in response to various stressors, including pain, was indicated, and a short overview of some of the questionnaires measuring anxiety was provided. The final topic in the section discussed anticipatory anxiety, which may not have an object or, in cases in which an object is anticipated, there may be a greatly exaggerated degree of anxiety attached to it.

The third section considered anxiety and pain together, these concepts frequently being confounded, sometimes with other emotions also. There follows a discussion of some of the work on the prediction of pain and pain behaviour. As indicated by Rachman (1990) the literature supports the notion that many tend to over-estimate anticipated pain.

Wade *et al.* (1990) found that anxiety, frustration, and anger contributed to the unpleasantness of experiencing chronic pain. However, Kent (1986) found that anxiety, common depression, and helplessness were not useful in predicting pain behaviour. Differences in a type of pain patient used and specific dependent variables of interest may explain these apparently divergent results.

Working with dental patients Kent found that there tended to be an over-estimation of pain based on later pain experience, and he recommended that the therapist encouraged the dental patient to consider a discomfort-free exposure as typical of a visit to a dentist. Many of the studies reported in this chapter used dental patients as subjects. Logan *et al.* (1991) were quite interested in the desire-for-control over noxious stimulation, and also felt-control over noxious stimulation. They found that of four groups studied the group with the high desire-for-control, but low felt-control, had significantly higher fear scores than the remaining three groups. The recommendations, on the basis of this study, was that the stress of treatment should be on increased control.

Gross (1992) was interested in the fear and expectancy model of avoidance behaviour, consisting of three factors: danger expectancy, anxiety expectancy and anxiety sensitivity. Gross' major effort was directed to developing a measure of pain sensitivity, and determining if this could predict dental avoidance and dental pain. Gross concluded that the concept of pain sensitivity could be differentiated from that of anxiety sensitivity and suggested that pain intensity and pain sensitivity were important components of dental avoidance. Gross concluded that pain sensitive people may interpret physical arousal as cues for pain. He argued that pain sensitivity is a stable personality component and could contribute to an understanding of chronic and multiple pains which are accompanied by anxiety. Therefore, he further argued that the expectancy model of fear could be expanded to include pain sensitivity and pain expectation.

Milgrom, Vignehsa and Weinstein (1992), studying children in Singapore secondary schools, found that 11.5% of children exhibited high dental fear. It was concluded that perceived control over aversive stimuli, recency of last dental visit, and painful treatment, were all of importance in the prediction of self-reported fear. The authors also felt that pain can reinforce fear and fear-related behaviours. Milgrom *et al.* laid stress upon the importance of felt lack of control in mediating the fearfulness of a painful experience.

Berggren (1992), who studied Swedish dental patients, found that many of these patients had other common extreme fears, such as a fear of suffocating, fear of death of a loved one, and fear of hyperdermic needles. His study raised the question of whether individuals who are prone to high anxiety or to many phobic reactions, would tend to exhibit a greater degree of subjective pain and, possibly, exhibit more pain behaviour than those individuals who are not subject to high anxiety or many phobic reactions.

LaCroix and Barbaree (1992) studied headache patients and attempted to predict the characteristics of the second headache from information gained from an initial headache. It was found that the mood factor score during the initial headache was significantly predictive of pain severity during the second headache. The authors suggested that treatment technique should attempt to reduce the affective response to pain, in that this might also tend to prevent or diminish the degree of future pain. Finally, an important point made by LaCroix and Barbaree was that emotional responses may not only accompany head pain but may continue some time after the head pain.

In an analogue study on pain and fear, McNeil and Brunetti (1992) induced fear imagery, pain imagery, or a combination of fear and pain imagery, in beginning psychology students. They found that pain was rated as significantly more negative than either fear or pain plus fear. McNeil and Brunetti concluded that in order to understand clearly the relationship between pain and fear, the effects of pain on fear need to be studied, as well as the effect of fear on pain.

Rose *et al*. (1992) developed the concept of Pain Confronters and Pain Avoiders. They worked with three chronic pain groups, as compared to three pain-free comparison patient groups, and were interested in interpreting their data in terms of the Fear Avoidance Model of exaggerated pain perception. They pointed out that the central concept of the model is fear of pain, and consequent pain avoidance or confrontation. They concluded that the adaptive pain confronter maintained synchrony between pain sensation and pain behaviour, but the non-adaptive pain avoider is motivated to avoid any fresh exposure to pain. The authors argue that the tendency to avoid pain is determined by the psychosocial context, which is influenced by four factors, including: stressful life events, personal pain history, personal pain coping strategies and personality characteristics. The authors found that the recovered patients who were in the control groups, and the chronic pain patients, could be differentiated in terms of stressful life events, personal pain history, and personality characteristics and they interpreted the results as supporting the Fear of Avoidance Model. Rose *et al*. conclude by suggesting that further research could lead to the development of a scale which could be used with acute pain patients, enabling a prediction to be made regarding the course their pain condition will follow (i.e. by recovery or chronicity).

The final section of the chapter, on attention, anxiety and pain, points out that attention may modulate the relationship between anxiety and pain. Basically, the research of Arntz, Dreesen and Merckelbach (1991) has to do with whether or not the fear or anxiety that may be experienced by a person influences a pain experience. If the fear or anxiety is directed away from the pain, then they postulate that the pain experience is reduced. On the other hand, if there is pain-related fear or anxiety, the pain experience will be stronger. These authors used phobic subjects in a two-by-two design, i.e. low versus high anxiety and attention versus distraction from pain, and they found that the following unambiguous conclusions could be drawn from their data: First, that attention to pain was clearly related to stronger pain responses; second, that there was no evidence that anxiety is related to a stronger pain response and, third, that there was little support for the idea that anxiety results in a lesser response to pain. The authors concluded that attention appears to be the critical factor, and conclude that further research should examine the effect of distraction on long-term habituation of pain responses. With reference to treating anxiety, Arntz *et al*. indicate that anxiety reduction techniques would be appropriate when anxiety is the motivating factor in the patient's attention to his or her pain. However, distraction techniques would tend to foster subjective habituation, and may be a very powerful factor in the psychological treatment of pain, as well as counteracting a tendency towards feeling helpless or in perceiving decreased control over pain.

REFERENCES

Anderson, K.O., Keefe, F.J., Bradley, L.A. *et al.* (1988) Prediction of pain behaviour and functional status of rheumatoid arthritis patients using medical status and psychological variables. *Pain*, **33** (1), 25–32.

Arntz, A., Dreessen, L. and Merckelbach, H. (1991) Attention, not anxiety, influences pain. *Behaviour, Research and Therapy*, **29** (1), 41–50.

Arntz, A. and Schmidt, A.J.M. (1989) Perceived control and the experience of pain, in *Stress, Personal Control and Health*, (eds A. Steptoe and A. Appels), Wiley, Chichester, (pp. 131–62).

Beecher, H.K. (1959) *Measurement of Subjective Responses: Quantitative Effects of Drugs*. Oxford University Press: New York.

Berggren, U. (1992) General and specific fears in referred and self-referred adult patients with extreme dental anxiety. *Behaviour, Research and Therapy*, **30** (4), 394–401.

Bond, M.R. and Pearson, I.B. (1969) Psychological Aspects of Pain in Women with Advanced Cancer of the Cervix. *Journal of Psychosomatic Research*, **13**, 13–18.

Chapman, C.R. and Cox, G.B. (1977) Anxiety, Pain and Depression surrounding elective surgery: A multivariate comparison of abnormal surgery patients with kidney donors and recipients. *Journal of Psychosomatic Research*, **21**, 7–15.

Coleman, J.C. (1964) (Third Ed.) *Abnormal Psychology and Modern Life*, Scott, Foresman and Company, Chicago.

Corah, N.L. (1969) Development of a dental anxiety scale. *Journal of Dental Research*, **48**, 596.

Corah, N., Gale, E. and Ilig, S. (1978) Assessment of a dental anxiety scale. *Journal of American Dental Association*, **97**, 816–19.

Delmonte, M.M. and Ryan, G.M. (1983) The Cognitive-Somatic Anxiety Questionnaire (CSAQ) : A factor analysis. *British Journal of Clinical Psychology*, **22**, 209–12.

Freud, S. (1936) *The Problem of Anxiety*, Norton, New York.

Geer, J.H. (1965) The development of a scale to measure fear. *Behaviour, Research and Therapy*, **3**, 45–53.

Gross, P.R. (1992) Is pain sensitivity associated with dental avoidance? *Behaviour, Research and Therapy*, **30** (1), 7–13.

Hamilton, M. (1959) The assessment of anxiety states by rating. *British Journal of Medical Psychology*, **32**, 50–5.

Hugdahl, K. (1981) The Three-Systems-Model of Fear and Emotion – A Critical Examination. *Behaviour, Research and Therapy*, **19**, 75–85.

International Association for the Study of Pain, Subcommittee on Taxonomy (1979) Pain terms: A list with definitions and notes on usage. *Pain*, **6**, 249–52.

Janis, I. (1958) *Psychological Stress*, Academic Press, New York.

Keefe, F. J., Wilkins, R.H., Cook, Jr. W. A. *et al.* (1986) Depression, pain, and pain behavior. *Journal of Consulting and Clinical Psychology*, **54**, 665–9.

Kent, G. (1986) The typicality of therapeutic 'surprises'. *Behaviour, Research and Therapy*, **24** (6), 625–8.

306 *Anxiety and pain*

Kleinknecht, R.A., Klepac, R.K. and Alexander, L.D. (1973) Origins and Characteristics of fear in dentistry. *Journal of the American Dental Association*, **86**, 842–8.

Klusman, L.E. (1975) Reduction of Pain in Childbirth by the Alleviation of Anxiety During Pregnancy. *Journal of Consulting and Clinical Psychology*, **43**, 162–5.

Lacy, J.I. (1967) Somatic response patterning and stress: Some revisions of activation theory, in *Psychological Stress*, (eds M. H. Appleby and R. Turnbull), Appleton-Century-Crofts, New York.

Lacroix, R. and Barbaree, H.E. (1992) Pain-elicited responses and their role in predicting future pain duration and severity. *Behaviour, Research and Therapy*, **30**, (5) 471–8.

Lang, P.J. (1968) Fear reduction and fear behaviour: Problems in treating a construct, in *Research in Psychotherapy, (Vol. 3)*, (ed. J. M. Schein), American Psychological Association, Washington DC.

Lang, P.J. (1971) The application of psychophysiological methods to the study of psychotherapy and behaviour change, in *Handbook of Psychotherapy and Behaviour Change: An Empirical Analysis*, (eds A. E. Bergin and S. L. Garfield), Wiley, New York.

Lang, P.J. (1985) The cognitive psychophysiology of emotion: Fear and anxiety, in *Anxiety and the Anxiety Disorders*, (eds A. H. Tuma and J. D. Maser), (pp. 131–70), Erlbaum, Hillsdale, N.J.

Lazarus, R. and Folkman, S. (1984) Coping and Adaptation, in *The Handbook of Behavioral Medicine*, (ed. W. Gentry), Guilford, New York.

Lehrer, P.M. and Woolford, R.L. (1982) Self-report assessment of anxiety: Somatic, cognitive and behavioural modalities. *Behavioral Assessment*, **4** 167–77.

Lethem, J., Slade, P.D., Troup, J.D.G. and Bentley, G. (1983) Outline of a fear-avoidance model of exaggerated pain perception – 1. *Behaviour, Research and Therapy*, **21**, 401–8.

Logan, H.L., Baron, R.S., Keeley, K. *et al.* (1991) Desired control and felt control as medicators of stress in a dental setting. *Health Psychology*, **10** (5), 352–9.

Lubin, B. (1967) *Manual for the Depression Adjective Check List*, Educational and Industrial Testing Service. San Diego, California.

MacLeod, C. and Rutherford, E. (1992) Anxiety and the selective processing of emotional information: mediating roles of awareness, trait and state variables and personal relevance of stimulus materials. *Behaviour, Research and Therapy*, **30**, (5), 479–91.

McNair, D.M., Lorr, M. and Droppleman, L.F. (1971) *Manual for the profile of mood states*. Educational Industrial Testing Service, San Diego, California.

McNeil, D.W. and Brunetti, D.G. (1992) Pain and fear: A bioinformational perspective on responsivity to imagery. *Behaviour, Research and Therapy*, **30** (5) 513–20.

Melzack, R. and Dennis, S.G. (1983) Neurophysiological Foundations of Pain, in *The Psychology of Pain*, (ed. R. A. Sternbach), Raven Press, New York: pp. 1–26.

Melzack, R. and Wall, P.D. (1982) *The Challenge of Pain*, Basic Books, New York.

Milgrom, P., Vignehsa, H.V. and Weinstein, P.W. (1992) Adolescent dental fear and control: Prevalence and theoretical implications. *Behaviour, Research and Therapy*, **40** (4), 367–73.

Morris, L.W., Davies, M.A. and Hutchins, C.H. (1981) Cognitive and emotional components of anxiety: Literature review and a revised worry-emotionality scale. *Journal of Education Psychology*, **73**, 541–55.

Nietzel, M.T. and Bernstein, D.A. (1981) Assessment of anxiety and fear, in

Behavioural Assessment: A Practical Handbook, 2nd edn, (eds Hersen, M. and Bellack, A.S.) Pergamon Press, Oxford.

Philips, C. (1974) A psychological analysis of tension headache, in *Contributions of Medical Psychology*, (ed. S. Rachman) Vol. I, Pergamon, Oxford.

Philips, C. and Hunter, M. (1981) Pain behaviour in headache sufferers. *Behaviour Analysis and Medication*, **4**, 259–66.

Rachman, S. (1990) *Fear and Courage*, 2nd edn, Freeman, Reading.

Rachman, S. and Hodgson, R.I. (1974) Synchrony and desynchrony in fear and avoidance. *Behaviour, Research and Therapy*, **12**, 311–18.

Rachman, S. and Lopatka, C. (1986) Do fears summate? III. *Behaviour, Research and Therapy*, **24**, 653–60.

Reiss, S. and McNally, R.J. (1985) Expectancy model of fear, in *Theoretical Issues in Behaviour Therapy*, (eds Reiss, S. and Botzin, R. R.), Academic Press, Orlando.

Rose, M.J., Klenerman, L., Atkinson, L. and Slade, P.D. (1992) An application of the fear avoidance model to three chronic pain problems. *Behaviour, Research and Therapy*, **30** (4), 359–65.

Seligman, M.E.P. (1975) *Helplessness: On Depression Development and Death*, Freeman, San Francisco.

Scholing, A. and Emmelkamp, P.M.G. (1992) Self report assessment of anxiety: A cross validation of the Lehrer Woolfolk Anxiety Symptom Questionnaire in three populations. *Behaviour, Research and Therapy*, **30** (5), 521–31.

Schwartz, G.E., Davidson, R.J. and Golman, D.J. (1978) Patterning of cognitive and somatic processes in the self-regulation of anxiety: Effects of meditation versus exercise. *Psychosomatic Medicine*, **40**, 321–8.

Spielberger, C.D., Gorsuch, R.L. and Lushene, R.E. (1970) *Manual for the State-Trait Anxiety Inventory*, Consulting Psychologist Press, Palo Alto, California.

Steptoe, A. and Kearsley, N. (1990). Cognitive and somatic anxiety. *Behaviour, Research and Therapy*, **28** (1), 75–81.

Sternbach, R.A. (1968) *Pain: A Psychophysiological Analysis*, Academic Press, New York.

Turk, D.C., Meichenbaum, D. and Genest, M. (1983) *Pain and Behavioural Medicine: A Cognitive Behavioral Perspective*. Guilford Press, London.

Vingoe, F.J. (1981) *Clinical Psychology and Medicine: An Interdisciplinary Approach*, Oxford University Press, Oxford.

Wade, J.B., Price, D.D., Hamer, R.M., *et al.* (1990) An emotional component analysis of chronic pain. *Pain*, **40** (3), 303–10.

Williams, J.M.G., Watts, F.N., MacLeod, C. and Matthews, A. (1988) *Cognitive Psychology and Emotional Disorders*. Wiley, Chichester.

Wilson, H. (1942) Mental reactions to air raids. *The Lancet*, **1**, 284–7.

Wolpe, J. (1982) *The Practice of Behavior Therapy*, 3rd edn, Pergamon, Oxford.

Index

Figures given in italic represent tables, those given in bold represent figures